American College of Physicians

MKSAP® 15

Medical Knowledge Self-Assessment Program®

Hematology and Oncology

Hematology and Oncology

Hematology Contributors

Jack E. Ansell, MD, FACP, Book Editor[2]
Chairman, Department of Medicine
Lenox Hill Hospital
New York, New York

Marc J. Kahn, MD, FACP[1]
Professor of Medicine
Hematology/Medical Oncology
Senior Associate Dean for Admissions and Student Affairs
Tulane University School of Medicine
New Orleans, Louisiana

Randy L. Levine, MD, FACP[1]
Director of Research for Hematology and Oncology
  Fellowship
Director of Blood Bank and Transfusion Services
Lenox Hill Hospital
New York, New York

Karen Quillen, MD[2]
Associate Professor of Medicine
Director, Blood Bank
Boston University School of Medicine
Boston, Massachusetts

Vaishali Sanchorawala, MD[2]
Associate Professor of Medicine
Boston University School of Medicine
Director, Stem Cell Transplant Program
Boston Medical Center
Boston, Massachusetts

Oncology Contributors

Bernard A. Mason, MD, FACP, Book Editor[1]
University of Pennsylvania School of Medicine
Clinical Professor of Medicine
Pennsylvania Hospital
Philadelphia, Pennsylvania

Mary E. Cianfrocca, DO[2]
Assistant Professor
Division of Hematology/Oncology
Feinberg School of Medicine
Northwestern University
Chicago, Illinois

Nancy L. Lewis, MD[2]
Director, Phase I Clinical Trial Program
Cooper Cancer Institute
Voorhees, New Jersey

Jyoti D. Patel, MD[2]
Assistant Professor
Division of Hematology/Oncology
Feinberg School of Medicine
Northwestern University
Chicago, Illinois

Russell J. Schilder, MD[2]
Senior Member
Director, Graduate Medical Education
Fox Chase Cancer Center
Philadelphia, Pennsylvania

Associate Editor

Richard S. Eisenstaedt, MD, FACP[2]
Clinical Professor of Medicine
Temple University School of Medicine
Chair, Department of Medicine
Abington Memorial Hospital
Abington, Pennsylvania

Editor-in-Chief

Patrick C. Alguire, MD, FACP[1]
Director, Education and Career Development
American College of Physicians
Philadelphia, Pennsylvania

Hematology and Oncology Reviewers

John E. Bennett, MD, MACP[1]
Lee Berkowitz, MD, FACP[1]
Duane R. Hospenthal, MD, PhD, COL, MC, FACP[2]
Dan L. Longo, MD, FACP[1]
Robert T. Means, Jr., MD, FACP[2]
Richard H. Moseley, MD, FACP[1]
Steven Ricanati, MD[1]
Barbara L. Schuster, MD, MACP[2]

Hematology and Oncology Editorial Staff

Margaret Wells, Managing Editor
Sean McKinney, Director, Self-Assessment Programs
Charles Rossi, Senior Associate of Clinical Content
   Development
John Murray, Editorial Coordinator

ACP Principal Staff

Steven E. Weinberger, MD, FACP[2]
Deputy Executive Vice President
Senior Vice President, Medical Education and Publishing

D. Theresa Kanya, MBA[1]
Vice President, Medical Education and Publishing

Sean McKinney[1]
Director, Self-Assessment Programs

Margaret Wells[1]
Managing Editor

Charles Rossi[1]
Senior Associate of Clinical Content Development

Becky Krumm[1]
Senior Staff Editor

Ellen McDonald, PhD[1]
Senior Staff Editor

Amanda Neiley[1]
Staff Editor

Katie Idell[1]
Production Administrator/Editor

Valerie Dangovetsky[1]
Program Administrator

John Murray[1]
Editorial Coordinator

Shannon O'Sullivan[1]
Editorial Coordinator

Developed by the American College of Physicians

---

1. Has no relationships with any entity producing, marketing, re-selling, or distributing health care goods or services consumed by, or used on, patients.

2. Has disclosed relationships with entities producing, marketing, re-selling, or distributing health care goods or services consumed by, or used on, patients. See below.

Conflicts of Interest

The following contributors and ACP staff members have disclosed relationships with commercial companies:

Jack E. Ansell, MD, FACP
Consultantship
Bristol-Myers Squibb, Bayer/Scios, Sanofi-Aventis, St. Jude Medical, Roche Diagnostics, HemoSense, Aryx Pharma, Aton Pharma, Instrumentation Labs, Regado Biosciences, ITC, Inc.

Mary E. Cianfrocca, DO
Research Grants/Contracts
GlaxoSmithKline
Speakers Bureau
GlaxoSmithKline, Genentech, Genomic Health

Richard S. Eisenstaedt, MD, FACP
Speakers Bureau
Ortho Biotech

Duane R. Hospenthal, MD, PhD, COL, MC, FACP
Research Grants/Contracts
Schering-Plough, Merck
Speakers Bureau
Merck, Pfizer

Nancy L. Lewis, MD
Research Grants/Contracts
Pfizer, Raven, Boehringer-Ingelheim, Wyeth, Incyte, PharmaMar USA Inc., Merck, Novartis, Sonus, EMD Pharmaceuticals, AstraZeneca, PharmaMar, Amgen, Lilly, BiPar Sciences, Bristol-Myers Squibb

Robert T. Means, Jr., MD, FACP
Honoraria
Beckman Coulter

Jyoti D. Patel, MD
Speakers Bureau
Genentech
Research Grants/Contracts
Lilly Pharmaceuticals, Genentech

Karen Quillen, MD
Research Grants/Contracts
Novo Nordisk

Vaishali Sanchorawala, MD
Research Grants/Contracts
Celgene, Millenium Pharmaceuticals
Speakers Bureau
Ortho Biotech, LLP

Russell J. Schilder, MD
Research Grants/Contracts
Bristol-Myers Squibb
Consultantship
Biogen Idec
Speakers Bureau
Biogen Idec, Ortho Biotech, Lilly

Barbara L. Schuster, MD, MACP
Honoraria
American Journal of Medicine (Editorial Board)

Steven E. Weinberger, MD, FACP
Stock Options/Holdings
Abbott, GlaxoSmithKline

Acknowledgments

The American College of Physicians (ACP) gratefully acknowledges the special contributions to the development and production of the 15th edition of the Medical Knowledge Self-Assessment Program® (MKSAP 15) of Scott Thomas Hurd (Senior Systems Analyst/Developer), Ricki Jo Kauffman (Manager, Systems Development), Michael Ripca (Technical Administrator/Graphics Designer), and Lisa Torrieri (Graphic Designer). The Digital version (CD-ROM and Online components) was developed within the ACP's Interactive Product Development Department by Steven Spadt (Director), Christopher Forrest (Senior Software Developer), Ryan Hinkel (Senior Software Developer), John McKnight (Software Developer), Sean O'Donnell (Senior Software Developer), and Brian Sweigard (Senior Software Developer). Computer scoring and reporting are being performed by ACT, Inc., Iowa City, Iowa. The College also wishes to acknowledge that many other persons, too numerous to mention, have contributed to the production of this program. Without their dedicated efforts, this program would not have been possible.

Continuing Medical Education

The American College of Physicians is accredited by the Accreditation Council for Continuing Medical Education (ACCME) to provide continuing medical education for physicians.

The American College of Physicians designates this educational activity for a maximum of 166 *AMA PRA Category 1 Credits*™. Physicians should only claim credit commensurate with the extent of their participation in the activity.

AMA PRA Category 1 Credit™ is available from July 31, 2009, to July 31, 2012.

Learning Objectives

The learning objectives of MKSAP 15 are to:
• Close gaps between actual care in your practice and preferred standards of care, based on best evidence
• Diagnose disease states that are less common and sometimes overlooked and confusing
• Improve management of comorbidities that can complicate patient care
• Determine when to refer patients for surgery or care by subspecialists

• Pass the ABIM certification examination
• Pass the ABIM maintenance of certification examination

Target Audience

• General internists and primary care physicians
• Subspecialists who need to remain up-to-date in internal medicine
• Residents preparing for the certifying examination in internal medicine
• Physicians preparing for maintenance of certification in internal medicine (recertification)

How to Submit for CME Credits

To earn CME credits, complete a MKSAP 15 answer sheet. Use the enclosed, self-addressed envelope to mail your completed answer sheet(s) to the MKSAP Processing Center for scoring. Remember to provide your MKSAP 15 order and ACP ID numbers in the appropriate spaces on the answer sheet. The order and ACP ID numbers are printed on your mailing label. If you have not received these numbers with your MKSAP 15 purchase, you will need to acquire them to earn CME credits. E-mail ACP's customer service center at custserv@acponline.org. In the subject line, write "MKSAP 15 order/ACP ID numbers." In the body of the e-mail, make sure you include your e-mail address as well as your full name, address, city, state, ZIP code, country, and telephone number. Also identify where you have made your MKSAP 15 purchase. You will receive your MKSAP 15 order and ACP ID numbers by e-mail within 72 business hours.

Permission/Consent for Use of Figures Shown in MKSAP 15 Hematology and Oncology Multiple-Choice Questions

Figures shown in Self-Assessment Test Items 3, 36, and 44 are reprinted with permission from the ASH Image Bank. Copyright © American Society of Hematology; accessible at www.ashimagebank.org.

Figure shown in Self-Assessment Test Item 99 is reprinted with permission from Woo SB, Hellstein JW, Kalmar JR. Systematic Review: Bisphosphonates and Osteonecrosis of the Jaws. Ann Intern Med. 2006;144(10):753-761. [PMID: 16702591] Copyright © 2006, American College of Physicians.

Disclosure Policy

It is the policy of the American College of Physicians (ACP) to ensure balance, independence, objectivity, and scientific rigor in all its educational activities. To this end, and consistent with the policies of the ACP and the Accreditation

Council for Continuing Medical Education (ACCME), contributors to all ACP continuing medical education activities are required to disclose all relevant financial relationships with any entity producing, marketing, re-selling, or distributing health care goods or services consumed by, or used on, patients. Contributors are required to use generic names in the discussion of therapeutic options and are required to identify any unapproved, off-label, or investigative use of commercial products or devices. Where a trade name is used, all available trade names for the same product type are also included. If trade-name products manufactured by companies with whom contributors have relationships are discussed, contributors are asked to provide evidence-based citations in support of the discussion. The information is reviewed by the committee responsible for producing this text. If necessary, adjustments to topics or contributors' roles in content development are made to balance the discussion. Further, all readers of this text are asked to evaluate the content for evidence of commercial bias so that future decisions about content and contributors can be made in light of this information.

Resolution of Conflicts

To resolve all conflicts of interest and influences of vested interests, the ACP precluded members of the content-creation committee from deciding on any content issues that involved generic or trade-name products associated with proprietary entities with which these committee members had relationships. In addition, content was based on best evidence and updated clinical care guidelines, when such evidence and guidelines were available. Contributors' disclosure information can be found with the list of contributors' names and those of ACP principal staff listed in the beginning of this book.

Educational Disclaimer

The editors and publisher of MKSAP 15 recognize that the development of new material offers many opportunities for error. Despite our best efforts, some errors may persist in print. Drug dosage schedules are, we believe, accurate and in accordance with current standards. Readers are advised, however, to ensure that the recommended dosages in MKSAP 15 concur with the information provided in the product information material. This is especially important in cases of new, infrequently used, or highly toxic drugs. Application of the information in MKSAP 15 remains the professional responsibility of the practitioner.

The primary purpose of MKSAP 15 is educational. Information presented, as well as publications, technologies, products, and/or services discussed, is intended to inform subscribers about the knowledge, techniques, and experiences of the contributors. A diversity of professional opinion exists, and the views of the contributors are their own and not those of the ACP. Inclusion of any material in the program does not constitute endorsement or recommendation by the ACP. The ACP does not warrant the safety, reliability, accuracy, completeness, or usefulness of and disclaims any and all liability for damages and claims that may result from the use of information, publications, technologies, products, and/or services discussed in this program.

Publisher's Information

Unauthorized Use of This Book Is Against the Law

MKSAP 15 ISBN: 978-1-934465-25-7
Hematology and Oncology ISBN: 978-1-934465-32-5

Printed in the United States of America.

For order information in the U.S. or Canada call 800-523-1546, extension 2600. All other countries call 215-351-2600. Fax inquiries to 215-351-2799 or e-mail to custserv@acponline.org.

Errata and Norm Tables

Errata for MKSAP 15 will be posted at http://mksap.acponline.org/errata as new information becomes known to the editors.

MKSAP 15 Performance Interpretation Guidelines with Norm Tables, available December 31, 2010, will reflect the knowledge of physicians who have completed the self-assessment tests before the program was published. These physicians took the tests without being able to refer to the syllabus, answers, and critiques. For your convenience, the tables are available in a printable PDF file at http://mksap.acponline.org/normtables.

Table of Contents

Hematology

Hematopoietic Stem Cells and Their Disorders

Blood Cell Production

Hematopoiesis is the generation, development, and differentiation of the cellular elements of blood. Hematopoietic pluripotent stem cells, characterized by surface expression of the CD34 molecule, are self-renewing cells that reside in the bone marrow and either proliferate or differentiate in response to hematopoietic stressors (such as infections or bleeding) or growth factors. Proliferative abnormalities or perturbations in differentiation of stem cells result in bone marrow failure or abnormal maturation, as occurs in the myelodysplastic syndromes, myeloproliferative disorders, and acute leukemias.

Bone Marrow Failure

Neutropenia

Neutropenia is an abnormally low neutrophil count, defined as an absolute neutrophil count (ANC) less than 1500/μL (1.5×10^9/L) (ANC is calculated by adding neutrophils plus band forms). Neutropenia is further classified as mild (ANC 1000-1500/μL [1.0-1.5×10^9/L]), moderate (ANC 500-1000/μL [0.5-1.0×10^9/L]), severe (ANC 200-500/μL [0.2-0.5×10^9/L]), and profound (ANC <200/μL [0.2×10^9/L]). Ethnic variants of neutrophil counts occur in certain populations, such as blacks, Yemenite Jews, and Arabs, and mild neutropenia is not abnormal in these populations. Patients with mild neutropenia rarely develop complications, but the risk of infection increases as the neutrophil count falls below 1000/μL (1.0×10^9/L). Infections are usually due to invasion of colonizing bacteria from the oropharynx and gastrointestinal tract, and patients may present with high fevers without localizing findings.

Neutropenia is usually an acquired, self-limited disorder that is due to a medication or postinfectious state (**Table 1**). Bone marrow aspirate findings may vary in both drug-induced and postinfectious neutropenia. Hypocellular bone marrow may indicate the disorder known as large granular lymphocytic syndrome (confirmed by finding large circulating lymphocytes with abundant cytoplasm and azurophilic granules) or the early onset of aplastic anemia. The bone marrow may also appear hypercellular with a "left shift" (increased numbers of metamyelocytes, myelocytes, and promyelocytes) or may show late maturation arrest of the myeloid cells or agranulocytosis. Hypercellular bone marrow may indicate peripheral

TABLE 1 Common Drugs Associated with Neutropenia and Agranulocytosis
Angiotensin-converting enzyme inhibitors
Antibiotics
Amoxicillin
Cefazolin
Cephalexin
Cefotaxime
Cefuroxime
Chloramphenicol
Clindamycin
Norfloxacin
Metronidazole
Trimethoprim-sulfamethoxazole
Antiarrhythmic agents
Amiodarone
Procainamide
Antiepileptic agents
Carbamazepine
Phenytoin
Sodium valproate
H_2-receptor blockers
Cimetidine
Ranitidine
Hydrochlorothiazide
NSAIDs
Diclofenac
Indomethacin
Naproxen
Phenylbutazone
Propylthiouracil
Sulfasalazine

Reprinted with permission from Hoffman R, Benz E, Shattil S, Furie B, Cohen H. Hematology: Basic Principles and Practice. 4th ed. Philadelphia, PA: Churchill Livingstone; 2004:Table 46-15. Copyright 2004, Elsevier.

destruction due to hypersplenism or autoimmune disease. However, hypercellular bone marrow with dysplastic morphologic findings suggests myelodysplasia. Associated megaloblastic anemia and thrombocytopenia suggest the presence of vitamin B_{12} or folate deficiency.

Cyclic neutropenia, a disorder in the regulation of stem cells, should be considered in neutropenic patients with recurrent infections and fluctuating leukocyte counts. Patients have predictable periodic fluctuations of granulocyte, lymphocyte, monocyte, and reticulocyte counts, and the counts return to normal without treatment. Most patients experience cycles every 21 days, but cycles may range from every 2 weeks to every 4 weeks.

Treatment of neutropenia depends on the severity, chronicity, and cause of the disorder. Therapy is not needed if the neutropenia is mild and due to a causative agent that can be withdrawn or an infection that is resolving. However, complete cultures and empiric antibiotics that cover staphylococci and enteric pathogens are required when the ANC falls below $1000/\mu L$ $(1.0 \times 10^9/L)$ in a febrile patient. If the neutropenia persists and there is no response to antibiotics after 5 days, empiric antifungal agents are added. If there is still no response to antimicrobial therapy and the patient remains neutropenic and critically ill, granulocyte colony-stimulating factor is added to the treatment regimen. Colony-stimulating agents have been shown to decrease the duration of neutropenia, but they have not been shown to influence mortality, and they add only a minimal benefit. Therefore, the use of these agents should be limited to those patients in whom the neutropenia is expected to be prolonged.

Aplastic Anemia

Aplastic anemia occurs when the hematopoietic stem cells do not repopulate the bone marrow, resulting in severely diminished or absent committed progenitor cells. The disorder can be either acquired or congenital. Patients present with transfusion-dependent anemia, thrombocytopenia, and severe neutropenia with markedly reduced bone marrow cellularity (<25% cellularity). Aplastic anemia is classified by the severity of the neutropenia. Moderate aplastic anemia is diagnosed when the ANC is 500 to $1000/\mu L$ $(0.5-1.0 \times 10^9/L)$. Severe aplastic anemia occurs when two or more of the following are present: ANC 200 to $500/\mu L$ $(0.2-0.5 \times 10^9/L)$, platelet count less than $20,000/\mu L$ $(20 \times 10^9/L)$, and reticulocyte count less than $40,000/\mu L$ $(40 \times 10^9/L)$. Very severe aplastic anemia is diagnosed when the ANC is less than $200/\mu L$.

No cause is identified in approximately 50% of patients with acquired aplastic anemia. Causes in the remaining patients include toxins, ionizing radiation, drugs, nutritional deficiencies, and infections. Some patients have an associated thymoma or autoimmune disorder such as systemic lupus erythematosus. An abnormal expression of suppressor T cells has been found in 30% to 80% of patients with idiopathic aplastic anemia, and many of these patients respond to immunosuppressive therapy.

A small percentage of patients have paroxysmal nocturnal hemoglobinuria (PNH), which can occur de novo and transform into aplastic anemia or can develop as a complication of aplastic anemia. Patients with PNH have an abnormal anchor protein (glycosylphosphatidylinositol) that causes lack of expression of the surface markers CD55 and CD59 (complement inhibitors) and increased sensitivity to

complement activation. The end result is chronic hemolysis and a hypercoagulable state, pancytopenia, and a bone marrow that can appear aplastic, megaloblastic, or consistent with the diagnosis of a myelodysplastic syndrome. The most sensitive test for diagnosing PNH is flow cytometry of erythrocytes, granulocytes, lymphocytes, and monocytes, which will demonstrate the lack of expression of CD55 and CD59.

Initial treatment of aplastic anemia involves withdrawal of any potentially causative agents and a CT scan of the chest to rule out an associated thymoma. If a thymoma is found, surgical excision can be curative. Hematopoietic stem cell transplantation (HSCT) is first-line therapy for very young patients (<20 years of age) with severe or very severe acquired aplastic anemia. Because of the high mortality rate associated with this procedure, HSCT is generally not recommended as initial therapy for older patients. However, some transplant centers report satisfactory results in patients up to 45 years of age when HLA-identical siblings are used as donors.

For patients who are not transplant candidates, immunosuppressive therapy with intravenous antithymocyte globulin plus corticosteroids and cyclosporine can result in both partial and complete responses in 60% to 80% of patients. Many of these patients become transfusion independent, although response is often delayed for 3 to 6 months, and relapses occur when the cyclosporine is tapered. Growth factors such as granulocyte colony-stimulating factor should not be given as primary therapy, and the use of growth factors as concomitant therapy is controversial. These agents are expensive, and some reports suggest a lower response rate to immunosuppressive therapy and a higher relapse rate when granulocyte colony-stimulating factor is used. Finally, it is important to identify which patients with aplastic anemia also have PNH, since eculizumab, an antibody that inhibits the activation of terminal complement components, may decrease intravascular hemolysis and transfusion dependence in these patients.

Congenital aplastic anemia is an inherited hematopoietic stem cell disorder that usually presents in childhood but may not become manifest until the third decade of life. The most common form of congenital aplastic anemia is Fanconi anemia, an autosomal recessive or X-linked disorder (multiple different genes appear to be responsible) characterized by pancytopenia, hypocellular bone marrow, short stature, café-au-lait spots, and abnormalities of the thumb. Not all patients have congenital anomalies or short stature. Diagnostic studies show excessive chromosomal breakage in cultured peripheral cell lymphocytes or dermal fibroblasts. HSCT is the only curative treatment.

Pure Red Cell Aplasia

Pure red cell aplasia (PRCA) is an acquired disorder characterized by profound anemia and absence of reticulocytes and erythroid precursors in the bone marrow. Most cases are idiopathic, although PRCA may occur in association with thymomas, systemic lupus erythematosus, or as a precursor to a myelodysplastic syndrome. The peripheral blood smear may show large granular lymphocytes, suggesting a direct autoimmune toxicity. Parvovirus B19 infection is associated with PRCA in susceptible individuals, including patients who have a chronic hemolytic disorder such as sickle cell disease or who are unable to produce neutralizing antibodies, such as patients with HIV infection. Patients with parvovirus B19 infection have a characteristic bone marrow showing giant proerythroblasts with a maturation arrest. Certain medications have also been implicated in causing PRCA (**Table 2**). One unusual cause is exposure to exogenous recombinant erythropoietin, which can lead to development of cross-reacting antibodies that attack the erythroid precursors, resulting in PRCA.

Initial management of PRCA involves removal of any potentially causative agents and determination of the presence of a thymoma, which, when excised, can result in improvement or cure in a small number of patients. If parvovirus B19 is implicated, intravenous immune globulin is effective. Immunosuppressive therapy with corticosteroids, cyclophosphamide, or cyclosporine is indicated when the cause is unknown. Supportive care with transfusions may be needed until patients respond to more definitive treatment.

TABLE 2 Drugs Most Commonly Associated with the Onset of Pure Red Cell Aplasia
Carbamazepine
Chloramphenicol
Chlorpropamide
Erythropoietin (recombinant)
Mycophenolate mofetil
Phenytoin
Trimethoprim-sulfamethoxazole
Zidovudine

KEY POINTS

- Up to 80% of patients with aplastic anemia respond to immunosuppressive therapy with antithymocyte globulin, corticosteroids, and cyclosporine.
- Hematopoietic stem cell transplantation is first-line therapy for very young patients with aplastic anemia but is associated with high mortality rates in older patients.
- Patients with pure red cell aplasia may have associated parvovirus B19 infection.
- Immunosuppressive therapy with corticosteroids, cyclophosphamide, or cyclosporine is indicated when the cause of pure red cell aplasia is unknown.

Myelodysplastic Syndromes

The myelodysplastic syndromes are stem cell clonal disorders characterized by ineffective hematopoiesis and various peripheral cytopenias. Patients have signs and symptoms referable to a specific cytopenia (most often megaloblastic anemia) and bone marrow findings showing a hypercellular marrow with dyserythropoiesis. Alcohol abuse and nutritional deficiencies, especially vitamin B_{12} and folate deficiencies, may be associated with similar findings and therefore must be excluded.

Myelodysplastic syndromes are classified according to morphologic findings and clinical features. The natural history varies, depending on the number of blasts in the bone marrow (ranging from 5% to 19%) and the chromosomal aberrations. Patients with refractory anemia and less than 5% blasts have a relatively indolent course with a mean survival of about 7 years. Patients with aggressive refractory anemia with excess blasts and 11% to 19% blasts have an expected survival of less than 1 year. The International Prognosis Scoring System uses these findings to predict survival. Death usually occurs because of infection and bleeding as a result of bone marrow failure, although this may also be due to progression to acute myeloid leukemia.

Many chromosomal abnormalities are associated with myelodysplastic syndromes, including abnormal numbers of chromosomes, translocations, and structural abnormalities. In contrast to patients with a complex karyotype, patients with a normal karyotype are unlikely to develop acute myeloid leukemia. Patients with a deletion of the long arm of chromosome 5 (5q- syndrome) have a unique presentation. These patients are usually first seen at an advanced age with a mild refractory anemia and increased platelets. Women outnumber men by a ratio of 7:1.

Treatment of myelodysplastic syndromes is varied and reflects the heterogeneity of these disorders. The type of therapy depends on the age of the patient and the aggressiveness and subclassification of the disease. Many patients with anemia require long-term transfusions, and iron overload with secondary hemochromatosis may subsequently occur. Chelation therapy is indicated once a patient has received more than 30 units of erythrocytes or the serum ferritin level exceeds 1000 ng/mL (1000 mg/L). An oral chelator, deferasirox, was recently approved by the U.S. Food and Drug Administration (FDA) that is much easier to administer than parenteral preparations. However, treatment is expensive, and although chelation therapy may prevent secondary hemochromatosis, it has not been shown to prolong survival.

Growth factors have been used to treat myelodysplastic syndromes but have variable response rates. Between 20% and 55% of patients with anemia will respond to recombinant erythropoietin (at least 40,000 units/week) if their baseline serum erythropoietin level is less than 500 mU/mL (500

U/L). The response can be increased by adding granulocyte colony-stimulating factor, which acts synergistically in some patients. Azacitidine (given subcutaneously daily for 7 days on an outpatient basis) and decitabine (given intravenously for 3 consecutive days every 6 weeks) are two pyrimidine nucleoside agents that cause hypomethylation of DNA and have response rates ranging from 23% to 64%. Since responses can be delayed, both agents require treatment for at least four cycles to determine efficacy. Lenalidomide has been approved by the FDA for the specific treatment of 5q- syndrome, because 67% to 83% of patients with this syndrome will respond to this drug and become transfusion independent.

Patients with chronic myelomonocytic leukemia, which has features of both myelodysplastic syndromes and myeloproliferative disorders, will respond to hydroxyurea when the circulating leukocyte count is elevated and will also respond to hypomethylating agents. A subpopulation of patients with chronic myelomonocytic leukemia have a fusion gene involving platelet-derived growth factor and may respond to treatment with the tyrosine kinase inhibitor imatinib.

Hematopoietic stem cell transplantation (HSCT) is reserved for young patients with a myelodysplastic syndrome who have an HLA-matched sibling donor. Because these syndromes tend to occur in older age groups, few patients are eligible for HSCT. In addition, HSCT is associated with high transplant-related mortality rates and high relapse rates in this group of patients.

KEY POINTS

- Azacitidine and decitabine are pyrimidine nucleoside agents that may induce a complete remission in some patients with myelodysplastic syndromes.
- Lenalidomide is intended for the specific treatment of 5q- syndrome, with most treated patients becoming transfusion independent.
- Hematopoietic stem cell transplantation is reserved for young patients with a myelodysplastic syndrome who have an HLA-matched sibling donor.

Myeloproliferative Disorders

The myeloproliferative disorders are a group of clonal stem cell disorders characterized by aberrant regulation of proliferation that results in excess production of myeloid elements in the bone marrow. These include essential thrombocythemia and disorders of erythrocytes (polycythemia vera), granulocytes (chronic myeloid leukemia), and fibroblasts (myelofibrosis).

Essential Thrombocythemia

Essential thrombocythemia is a chronic myeloproliferative disorder characterized by overproduction of platelets. Patients usually present in the fifth and sixth decades of life with a platelet count greater than 600,000/μL (600 × 10⁹/L), although at least 30% develop this disorder in the third decade. The peripheral blood smear typically shows circulating megathrombocytes, and a mild leukocytosis may be present. Approximately 40% to 50% of patients have splenomegaly, and about 20% have hepatomegaly. Hyperuricemia and hyperphosphatemia may be present, although elevated serum potassium levels are usually due to pseudohyperkalemia (potassium released from platelets that have aggregated). Approximately 50% of patients are asymptomatic, and the thrombocytosis is noted as an incidental finding during a routine examination. Most symptomatic patients present with small-vessel thrombosis that causes erythromelalgia (burning and paresthesias of the extremities that are exacerbated by heat) or central nervous system thrombosis, such as migraine headaches, transient ischemic attacks, scotomas, amaurosis fugax (transient monocular or binocular vision loss), or seizures. Large-vessel thrombosis, such as renal vein thrombosis or Budd-Chiari syndrome, may also occur. Patients with extremely elevated platelet counts (>1 million/μL [100,000 × 10⁹/L]) will occasionally present with hemorrhagic complications that are often due to an acquired von Willebrand syndrome.

The diagnosis of essential thrombocythemia is one of exclusion. A reactive thrombocytosis (such as iron deficiency, an underlying inflammatory disorder, or cancer) must be ruled out. To establish the diagnosis, the platelet count must be greater than 600,000/μL (600 × 10⁹/L) on two different occasions separated by at least 1 month, and bone marrow examination must show hypercellular marrow and morphologically abnormal megakaryocytic hyperplasia with the megakaryocytes in clusters. Approximately 50% of patients have the *JAK2* mutation (a gain-of-function mutation on chromosome 9) that may be present in all of the myeloproliferative disorders. Chronic myeloid leukemia is excluded by testing for the Philadelphia chromosome, and polycythemia vera is excluded if the hematocrit is at or above normal limits by assessing the red blood cell mass and measuring the serum erythropoietin level.

Therapy for essential thrombocythemia depends on the age of the patient, the degree of thrombocytosis, and the medical history. The platelet count must be lowered quickly in patients with life-threatening symptoms, such as a transient ischemic attack, stroke, myocardial infarction, or gastrointestinal bleeding. Platelet apheresis along with cytoreductive therapy is indicated for these patients. High-dose hydroxyurea is the myelosuppressive agent of choice in this setting because of its rapid onset of action. For patients with less urgent symptoms, myelosuppression is instituted with lower doses of hydroxyurea, anagrelide, or interferon alfa plus low-dose aspirin. Since smoking can increase the risk of thrombosis, patients should be encouraged to stop. Erythromelalgia responds rapidly to low-dose aspirin, and a single dose can relieve symptoms for several days. Asymptomatic patients can be followed with observation alone or with observation plus low-dose aspirin, taking care to rule out any acquired platelet dysfunction that might increase the risk for bleeding. There is no absolute platelet count that dictates the need for intervention, and each patient must be assessed according to age, thrombotic or bleeding risk, and treatment risks.

The prognosis is good for patients with essential thrombocythemia. A large Spanish study published in 1991 showed no significant difference in longevity between patients with this disorder and controls. Transformation to other myeloproliferative disorders does occur, however, and 8% of patients will develop myelofibrosis over a 10-year period. A smaller number of patients will develop polycythemia vera or acute myeloid leukemia.

Polycythemia Vera

Polycythemia vera is a chronic myeloproliferative disorder characterized by overproduction of erythrocytes, although myeloid cells and megakaryocytes are also affected. Signs and symptoms include ruddy cyanosis, hypertension, splenomegaly, headache, sweating, weight loss, paresthesias, and dizziness. Generalized pruritus occurs in up to 50% of patients and is exacerbated by exposure to hot water (typically a hot bath or shower). Thrombotic disorders (erythromelalgia, transient ischemic attacks, myocardial infarction or stroke, deep venous thrombosis, and Budd-Chiari syndrome) are the most serious presenting signs of the disease and occur in about two thirds of patients with polycythemia vera. Thrombosis is due to the elevated red blood cell mass and increased whole blood viscosity and is aggravated by concomitant thrombocytosis in 50% of patients and leukocytosis in 75% of patients. The risk of thrombosis increases with increasing age, although even young patients can present with life-threatening thrombotic events. Patients who require surgery are at high risk for both thrombosis and hemorrhage in the postoperative period.

The diagnosis is suspected when the hematocrit level is repeatedly elevated. Determination of the red blood cell mass is not needed for patients with a hematocrit level greater than 60% in men and 56% in women. However, patients who have a slightly elevated hematocrit level and all patients with the Budd-Chiari syndrome should be evaluated for polycythemia vera with a nuclear medicine measurement of the red blood cell mass and plasma volume measurement to monitor for a depressed serum erythropoietin level. *JAK2 V617F* mutation testing should also be done because polycythemia vera is diagnosed in up to 40% of patients with Budd-Chiari syndrome. Because iron deficiency is common, the peripheral blood smear will often show hypochromic microcytic erythrocytes, and the bone marrow will be hypercellular with increased reticulin fibrosis. Platelet function abnormalities similar to those in patients with essential thrombocythemia may also occur.

The *JAK2* mutation is present in 90% to 95% of patients, which helps establish the diagnosis. Secondary causes of polycythemia must be excluded by measurement of the baseline serum erythropoietin level, carboxyhemoglobin level, arterial oxygen saturation, and $P_{50}O_2$ (oxygen partial pressure at which 50% hemoglobin is saturated with oxygen) (**Table 3**).

Treatment of polycythemia vera is directed toward reducing the red blood cell mass and preventing thrombosis. Therapeutic phlebotomy should be instituted with the goal of lowering the hematocrit level to less than 42% in women and less than 45% in men. Low-dose aspirin is indicated unless the patient has symptoms of easy bruising and an acquired platelet disorder. Hyperuricemia is treated with allopurinol, and patients with pruritus are given antihistamines. Interferon alfa, anagrelide, and/or hydroxyurea is the treatment of choice for older symptomatic patients with polycythemia vera that cannot be controlled with phlebotomy and aspirin alone.

Prognosis depends on the severity of the complications of the disease. Median survival after diagnosis ranges from less than 2 years to more than 15 years. Death is usually due to thrombosis, but patients may develop serious bleeding abnormalities, myelofibrosis, or acute myeloid leukemia.

Chronic Myeloid Leukemia

Chronic myeloid leukemia (CML) is a myeloproliferative disorder characterized by overproduction of myeloid cells and involves mature granulocytes as well as megakaryocytes and erythroid cells. Patients typically present in the sixth decade of life, but the age range is wide, and CML can occur in children. Most patients are asymptomatic at presentation, and CML is detected because of an increased leukocyte count. However, patients with more advanced disease may develop fatigue, night sweats, and weight loss. Splenomegaly may be the only abnormal finding on physical examination.

TABLE 3 Causes of Secondary Polycythemia and Elevated Erythropoietin Concentration
Tumor-related increased serum erythropoietin levels
Renal cell carcinoma
Hepatocellular carcinoma
Uterine fibroids
Hypoxemia
Chronic obstructive pulmonary disease
Sleep apnea
Massive obesity
High altitude
Increased carboxyhemoglobin levels
Cigarette smoking
Abnormal hemoglobin
High oxygen-affinity hemoglobin

CML is due to a chromosomal translocation in which the *BCR* gene from chromosome 22 is fused with the *ABL* gene on chromosome 9 to form *BCR-ABL* (Philadelphia chromosome), which induces a cytoplasmic tyrosine kinase. The diagnosis of CML requires the identification of this oncogene in a patient who has a leukoerythroblastic peripheral blood smear (increased granulocytes with a marked left shift plus early erythrocyte precursors) and hypercellular bone marrow with marked myeloid proliferation. Patients with chronic-phase CML initially have less than 10% blasts in the bone marrow and peripheral blood. As the disease progresses, the blast count increases. Patients with accelerated-phase CML have up to 20% blasts, and blast crisis may occur when the blast count is greater than 20%.

Treatment of CML has changed dramatically with the introduction of imatinib, a tyrosine kinase inhibitor. Before this drug was available, HSCT was the only curative treatment. However, only about 30% of patients with CML are candidates for HSCT because of older age at presentation or the lack of HLA-matched sibling donors. In addition, the mortality rate associated with HSCT is about 15%. Imatinib will induce a complete cytogenetic remission in the first year in up to 70% of patients treated during the chronic phase, and 85% of these patients will remain in cytogenetic remission for up to 5 years. Dasatinib and nilotinib are two more potent tyrosine kinase inhibitors that were recently approved by the FDA for treatment of patients with imatinib-resistant CML.

Myelofibrosis

Myelofibrosis with myeloid metaplasia is a chronic myeloproliferative disorder characterized by overproduction of megakaryocytes and bone marrow stromal cells. Patients have signs and symptoms of anemia plus night sweats and weight loss. The peripheral blood smear shows marked leukoerythroblastic findings with tear drop–shaped erythrocytes and megathrombocytes. The bone marrow aspirate is often "dry" (unsuccessful aspirate), and bone marrow biopsy shows marked fibrosis. The fibrosis causes decreased bone marrow reserve and extramedullary hematopoiesis with massive hepatosplenomegaly. As the disease progresses, patients experience bone marrow failure, portal hypertension (9% to 18% of patients), and pulmonary hypertension (due to ectopic myeloid metaplasia, thromboembolic disease, or pulmonary fibrosis that occurs in response to cytokines released by the circulating megakaryocytes).

Although there is no curative treatment for myelofibrosis, HSCT has been effective in a small number of patients and should be considered for patients younger than 60 years of age. HSCT has significant risks, however. The 1-year transplant-related mortality rate is as high as 25%, with a 5-year survival rate of 48%. Management of myelofibrosis consists of cytoreduction with hydroxyurea to control the elevated leukocyte and platelet counts or interferon alfa to control the thrombocytosis, splenomegaly, and bone marrow fibrosis. Hypersplenism may cause an increased plasma volume with a secondary decrease in the hematocrit level (spurious anemia), and anemia can be confirmed by measurement of the red blood cell mass. True anemia (due to decreased erythrocyte production, nutritional deficiency, or bleeding associated with iron deficiency) is treated with folate or iron as needed, along with erythrocyte transfusions. Many patients require repeated transfusions, which may lead to chronic iron overload and the need for iron chelation therapy. Androgen therapy controls hypoproliferative anemia in up to 50% of patients. Thrombocytopenia due to hypersplenism or decreased platelet production is managed with platelet transfusions. It is important to avoid alloimmunization caused by repeated transfusions by using a restrictive transfusion approach and by transfusing only leukodepleted blood products. Hyperuricemia is treated with allopurinol.

Massive hypersplenism may be managed with low-dose radiation therapy, but the response is transient and can be complicated by the loss of extramedullary hematopoiesis with resulting cytopenia. Splenectomy may not be an option, because the presence of portal hypertension increases the risk of surgery (coexisting disseminated intravascular coagulation is a contraindication). In addition, splenectomy is associated with a postoperative morbidity rate of 30% and a mortality rate of 10%.

Survival after diagnosis of myelofibrosis ranges from 1 year to over 30 years, but the median survival is only 5 years. Prognostic indicators have not been reproducible among different studies, but significant anemia at presentation is a reliably poor prognostic finding (**Table 4**).

TABLE 4 Risk Assessment for Myelofibrosis			
Number of Prognostic Factors[a]	Risk Group	Median Survival (months)	Patients (%)
0	Low	93	47
1	Intermediate	26	45
2	High	13	8

[a]Prognostic factors: Hemoglobin <10 g/dL (100 g/L), and leukocyte count <4000/μL or >30,000/μL (<4.0 × 10^9/L or >30.0 × 10^9/L).

Reprinted with permisson from Dupriez B, Morel P, Demory JL, et al. Prognostic factors in agnogenic myeloid metaplasia: a report on 195 cases with a new scoring system. Blood. 1996;88(3):1013-1018. [PMID: 8704209] Copyright 1996, American Society of Hematology.

- Essential thrombocythemia is diagnosed by a platelet count greater than 600,000/µL (600×10^9/L) on two different occasions separated by at least 1 month and bone marrow findings of hypercellular marrow and morphologically abnormal megakaryocytic hyperplasia.

- Polycythemia vera can be diagnosed when the hematocrit is greater than 60% in men and 56% in women in the absence of secondary causes of erythrocytosis and the presence of splenomegaly or a *JAK2* mutation.

- Initial therapy for polycythemia vera in asymptomatic patients is phlebotomy and aspirin; cytoreductive therapy is indicated for symptomatic patients who do not respond to initial treatment.

- The diagnosis of chronic myeloid leukemia requires the identification of the Philadelphia chromosome (*BCR-ABL* mutation) in a patient who has a leukoerythroblastic peripheral blood smear and hypercellular bone marrow with marked myeloid proliferation.

- Treatment with imatinib will induce a prolonged cytogenetic remission in up to 70% of patients with chronic-phase chronic myeloid leukemia.

Acute Myeloid Leukemia

Acute myeloid leukemia (AML) refers to a group of well-defined malignant disorders involving committed myeloid stem cells (**Table 5**). AML is characterized by maturation arrest and subsequent proliferation of myeloblasts and/or promyelocytes in the bone marrow and peripheral blood. Risk factors include previous chemotherapy (especially for lymphoma or breast cancer) and myelodysplastic syndromes, and patients with secondary AML have a poorer prognosis than do those with de novo acute leukemia.

Typical signs and symptoms include fatigue, easy bruising, mucosal bleeding, fever, and infection. A small group of patients have a migratory arthritis. Initial laboratory findings usually show leukocytosis and circulating blasts, anemia, and thrombocytopenia. Many patients report having symptoms for weeks or even months before seeking medical attention.

AML should be considered when circulating blasts are present in the peripheral blood smear. The diagnosis is confirmed by a bone marrow aspirate showing hypercellular marrow containing greater than 20% myeloblasts (according to the World Health Organization [WHO] classification) or greater than 30% myeloblasts (according to the French-American-British [FAB] classification.) The bone marrow may contain so many myeloblasts that it causes a "dry" tap. In this situation, the diagnosis is based on bone marrow biopsy findings alone.

Once the diagnosis of acute leukemia is established, the classification is based on the morphology of the immature cells. The presence of Auer rods confirms the myeloid nature of the leukemia. Excess promyelocytes support the diagnosis of promyelocytic leukemia, subtype M3. Increased monocytes in the peripheral blood and bone marrow indicate a diagnosis of myelomonocytic leukemia, subtype M4. Classification is also determined by cytochemical and immunophenotypic studies. Cytogenetic findings support the diagnosis of certain subtypes and have prognostic implications. Favorable cytogenetic findings include translocation of chromosomes 8 and 21 [t(8;21)] in subtype M2, translocation of chromosomes

TABLE 5 Classification and Incidence of Acute Myeloid Leukemia			
Type	**FAB**	**Subtype**	**Incidence**
AML	M0	Acute myeloblastic leukemia, minimally differentiated	3%-5%
	M1	Acute myeloblastic leukemia without maturation	15%-20%
	M2	Acute myeloblastic leukemia with maturation	25%-30%
APL	M3	Acute promyelocytic leukemia, hypergranular	10%-15%
	M3v	Acute promyelocytic leukemia, variant, microgranular	
AMML	M4	Acute myelomonocytic leukemia	20%-30%
	M4eo	Acute myelomonocytic leukemia with eosinophils	
AML	M5a	Acute monoblastic leukemia, poorly differentiated	2%-9%
	M5b	Acute monoblastic leukemia, differentiated	
AEL	M6	Acute erythroleukemia	3%-5%
	M7	Acute megakaryoblastic leukemia	3%-5%

FAB = French-American-British Classification.

15 and 17 [t(15;17)] in subtype M3, and inversion of chromosome 16 [inv(16)] in subtype M4 with abnormal eosinophils. Complex karyotypes, including monosomy 5 and 7, are unfavorable prognostic findings. Gene expression profiling is a recent advance in the diagnosis, classification, and prognosis of AML but is not available in all clinical settings.

Physical examination findings are very helpful in assessing patients with AML. Fever is almost always due to an underlying infection, and patients with a temperature above 38.2 °C (100.8 °F) must have complete cultures followed by empiric antibiotic therapy. Cutaneous nodules (Sweet syndrome, or acute neutrophilic dermatosis) and gum hypertrophy are unusual findings but, if present, suggest an acute myelomonocytic or monocytic leukemia. Occasionally, firm subcutaneous masses comprised of collections of blasts (chloromas) may precede the onset of frank AML (usually M1 or M2 subtype). Patients with AML do not develop lymphadenopathy or hepatosplenomegaly, and, if present, these findings suggest an alternative or concomitant diagnosis.

The initial laboratory evaluation in patients with suspected AML includes a complete blood count and peripheral blood smear and a blood chemistry panel. The chemistry panel should include measurement of serum electrolytes and plasma glucose, as profound hypokalemia can occur in patients with myelomonocytic and monocytic AML subtypes, and spurious hypoglycemia can be due to high numbers of circulating blasts. Additional laboratory studies include measurement of uric acid (hyperuricemia must be controlled before chemotherapy is started), serum calcium (calcium levels may be elevated in some patients), serum lactate dehydrogenase (a marker of disease activity), blood urea nitrogen, serum creatinine, and liver chemistry tests. Continued close monitoring of serum electrolytes, phosphorus, and calcium levels is required during the initial days of chemotherapy because tumor lysis syndrome may cause hyperkalemia, hyperphosphatemia, hyperuricemia, and hypocalcemia. Coagulation studies (prothrombin time, activated partial thromboplastin time, and plasma fibrinogen) are necessary to rule out disseminated intravascular coagulation, which is frequently present in patients with AML, M3 subtype.

AML rarely involves the central nervous system, and most patients do not require cerebrospinal fluid examination. However, patients with very high circulating blast counts (>50,000/μL) are at risk for leukostasis in the cerebral vessels, and emergency leukapheresis is required to reduce the blast count before chemotherapy is started.

Every patient should have a baseline chest radiograph because pneumonia is a common complication, and hyperleukocytosis syndrome (circulating blast count >50,000/μL) may cause pulmonary leukostasis and hemorrhage. A baseline electrocardiogram is needed before starting anthracyclines. Older patients also require determination of a baseline left ventricular ejection fraction. HLA testing should also be done before chemotherapy causes significant pancytopenia, in case HLA-matched platelets are needed at a later time.

Initial treatment of AML is the same for all subtypes, except acute promyelocytic leukemia, which is discussed below. Patients are first stabilized with intravenous hydration, allopurinol, and, if needed, antibiotics. Induction chemotherapy is begun with an anthracycline and cytarabine given intravenously over 7 days. Patients who do not go into remission require a second course of induction therapy in 2 to 3 weeks, and consolidation therapy is then planned. Consolidation protocols vary, but high-dose cytarabine has been used successfully in younger patients. Gemtuzumab ozogamicin is a targeted antineoplastic agent consisting of a monoclonal anti-CD33 antibody and a toxic antibiotic, calicheamicin. Because administration of gemtuzumab is not associated with profound myelosuppression, it has been used to treat elderly patients with relapsed AML, either alone or in combination with standard chemotherapy. Veno-occlusive disease of the liver is an uncommon, but serious, side effect of this drug.

The prognosis for patients with AML varies according to age, sex, and race as well as performance status, karyotype, and initial presenting findings. In general, the complete remission rate after chemotherapy is 50% to 80%, with 5-year event-free survival ranging from 16% to 24%.

Approximately 10% of adults with AML have acute promyelocytic leukemia, M3 subtype, with t(15;17) involving the retinoic acid receptor gene. These patients have an excellent response to therapy. Induction consists of chemotherapy with an anthracycline, along with all-*trans*-retinoic acid (ATRA), which is a differentiating agent that interferes with PML/RARa protein function. This combination has induced sustained remissions and cures in 90% of patients, although it can cause an unusual syndrome characterized by fever, volume overload, and pulmonary decompensation in 25% of patients. The "retinoic acid syndrome" responds to early recognition and administration of high-dose dexamethasone. Arsenic trioxide (ATO) is also effective for treating acute promyelocytic leukemia. ATO interacts with the PML/RARa protein and affects both apoptosis and differentiation. ATO has been used for induction therapy (alone or in combination with ATRA) and for salvage therapy in patients who relapse or do not respond to ATRA. Administration of these agents has increased the overall response rate to almost 100% for patients with acute promyelocytic leukemia.

- Acute myeloid leukemia is characterized by maturation arrests and subsequent proliferation of myeloblasts and/or promyelocytes in the bone marrow and peripheral blood.
- Induction therapy for patients with most subtypes of acute myeloid leukemia includes an anthracycline and cytarabine.
- Gemtuzumab is useful for treating elderly patients with relapsed acute myeloid leukemia because this agent is not associated with profound myelosuppression.

Acute Lymphoblastic Leukemia

Acute lymphoblastic leukemia (ALL) is a disorder of committed stem cells that is characterized by a proliferation of immature lymphoblasts. ALL constitutes less than 20% of acute leukemias in adult patients, with the highest incidence occurring in the seventh decade of life. Patients present with lymphocytosis, neutropenia, anemia, and thrombocytopenia, as well as lymphadenopathy and hepatosplenomegaly. Involvement of the central nervous system and testes is common, and cerebrospinal fluid examination is an essential part of the initial evaluation. The differential diagnosis includes Hodgkin and non-Hodgkin lymphomas, and the diagnosis is suspected when increased lymphoblasts are found on bone marrow examination. Immunophenotyping is necessary to confirm the diagnosis and determine if the lymphocytes are B cells, T cells, or biphenotypic cells with markers of both lymphoid and myeloid cells. Most adults have precursor B-cell ALL. However, the 25% of patients who have T-cell ALL have a better prognosis.

The initial treatment of ALL is the same as that of AML, and patients must be stabilized with intravenous hydration and allopurinol. Fever is aggressively managed with cultures and empiric antibiotics. Chemotherapy protocols are complicated and contain prednisone, vincristine, anthracyclines, L-asparaginase, 6-mercaptopurine, and high-dose cytarabine for induction; high-dose cytarabine for consolidation; and 6-mercaptopurine and methotrexate for maintenance therapy. Central nervous system prophylaxis consisting of intrathecal chemotherapy with or without cranial irradiation may be administered to treat a potential sanctuary site, because central nervous system recurrence may occur and is associated with a poor prognosis. However, central nervous system irradiation has not been proved to be an effective prophylactic therapy. Monoclonal antibody therapy has recently been added to chemotherapy regimens to improve response rates and long-term survival. In patients with the Philadelphia chromosome (present in 25% of young adults and 40% of elderly adults with ALL), imatinib can be added to the treatment protocol. Patients with B-cell ALL who are CD20 positive can be treated with rituximab, and new targeted monoclonal antibodies are being developed against CD19 for B-cell ALL and CD25 for T-cell ALL. Patients whose cells contain the CD33 surface marker (both B-cell and T-cell lineage) may be given alemtuzumab (Campath-1H), a monoclonal antibody directed against CD52.

The complete remission rate varies from 65% to 85%, with cure achieved in up to 50% of patients. Age older than 60 years; the presence of precursor B cells, early T cells, or mature T cells on immunophenotyping; and the presence of the Philadelphia chromosome indicate a poorer prognosis (**Table 6**).

- Acute lymphoblastic leukemia is a disorder of committed stem cells that is characterized by a proliferation of immature lymphoblasts.
- Monoclonal antibody therapy improves response rates and long-term survival in patients with acute lymphoblastic leukemia.

Additional Treatments

Hematopoietic Growth Factors

Numerous hematopoietic growth factors and cytokines are responsible for controlling the differentiation of committed progenitor cells. Four growth factors have been isolated and synthesized for clinical use. Granulocyte-macrophage colony-stimulating factor (GM-CSF) supports growth and development of myeloid cells, monocytes, and macrophages. Granulocyte colony-stimulating factor (G-CSF) maintains the growth and development of myeloid cell lines. Erythropoietin (EPO) stimulates and maintains erythroid maturation, and thrombopoietin (TPO) regulates megakaryocyte growth and platelet production.

GM-CSF and G-CSF are used for treating chemotherapy-induced neutropenia and fever in patients with non-myeloid malignancies, for treating severe chronic neutropenia, and for prophylaxis in patients receiving myelosuppressive chemotherapy regimens that have a high incidence of associated neutropenia. G-CSF is also used to mobilize stem cells for collection, to decrease the duration of neutropenia after stem cell transplantation, and to treat myelodysplastic syndromes.

TABLE 6 Prognostic Factors in Adult Acute Lymphoblastic Leukemia

Risk Factor	Note
Age	Age at diagnosis is one of the most important pretreatment risk factors, with advancing age associated with a worse prognosis. Chronic and intercurrent diseases impair tolerance to aggressive therapy; acute medical problems at diagnosis may reduce the likelihood of survival. High risk: age >60 years
Performance status	Performance status, independent of age, also influences ability to survive induction therapy and thus respond to treatment. High risk: poor performance status
Leukocyte count	A high presenting leukocyte count is an independent prognostic factor; duration of complete remission is inversely related to the presenting leukocyte count. High risk: leukocyte count >30,000/µL (30.0 × 10^9/L) in B-lineage disease and >100,000/µL (100.0 × 10^9/L) in T-lineage disease
Immunophenotype	Immunophenotype at diagnosis is an independent prognostic factor. In brief, T-lineage immunophenotype confers better outcome than B lineage and the presence of six or more T-cell markers is associated with favorable prognosis. High risk: B-lineage disease
Chromosome findings	Chromosome findings at diagnosis constitute an independent prognostic factor. In brief, t(9;22), +8, t(4;11), -7, and hypodiploid karyotypes are associated with unfavorable outcome; normal karyotype, +21 and del(9p), or t(9p) confer an intermediate outcome; and del(12p) or t(12p) and t(14q11-q13) may be associated with favorable outcome. High risk: t(9;22), +8, t(4;11), -7, and hypodiploid karyotypes
HOX11 oncogene	The expression of the *HOX11* oncogene has a favorable outcome in pediatric T-lineage ALL. Studies in adult T-lineage ALL are underway. In addition, promoter hypermethylation of cancer-related genes is a strong independent prognostic factor in ALL by multivariate analysis. High risk: lack of *HOX11* gene expression
Achievement of complete remission	In addition to pretreatment variables, achievement of complete remission correlates with prognosis in ALL. Complete remission is defined as a neutrophil count >1500/µL (1.5 × 10^9/L), a platelet count >100,000/µL (100.0 × 10^9/L), normal bone marrow cellularity (>25%) with trilineage hematopoiesis with <5% blasts, and resolution of all extramedullary disease. High risk: lack of achievement of complete remission

NOTE: Prognostic factors are important to tailor risk-adjusted treatments that would limit aggressive approaches for patients at high risk for relapse and reserve less rigorous treatments for lower-risk patients.

ALL = acute lymphoblastic leukemia.

EPO is produced in the peritubular cells of the renal cortex and is released in response to decreasing oxygen saturation in order to maintain an appropriate red blood cell mass. EPO is indicated for treating anemia due to chronic kidney disease when the hemoglobin level falls to less than 10 g/dL, for treating the anemia caused by AIDS, and for use in some chemotherapy-associated anemias. When using EPO, the hemoglobin level must not exceed 12 g/dL (120 g/L) in patients with chronic kidney disease because of the risk of thrombosis. In addition, in August 2008, the FDA mandated that EPO should not be used in patients receiving myelosuppressive therapy with intent to cure because of reports of worsening survival rates in this treatment setting.

TPO is a physiologic regulator of megakaryocytes and platelet production. Because early attempts to treat patients with TPO caused many complications, synthetic TPO receptor agonists were developed, and in August 2008, the first TPO receptor agonist, romiplostim, became available. This drug is administered subcutaneously weekly and stimulates megakaryocytes to increase platelet production. It is currently approved for the treatment of chronic immune thrombocytopenic purpura as a second-line agent for the treatment of patients unresponsive to or intolerant of first-line therapy or splenectomy and is under investigation for other indications. Three other TPO receptor agonists are in production, and at least one oral drug is awaiting FDA approval.

Hematopoietic Stem Cell Transplantation

HSCT and bone marrow transplantation are used to treat many of the previously discussed hematologic disorders. Autologous transplants use the patient's own hematopoietic stem cells, which are harvested, stored, and then reinfused after myeloablative chemotherapy. Allogeneic transplants harvest stem cells from an HLA-matched donor, and these stem cells are then infused in the recipient after myeloablative or nonmyeloablative chemotherapy. Nonmyeloablative transplants (also called reduced-intensity transplants or "mini" transplants) use less intensive chemotherapy and are therefore less toxic and easier to tolerate for patients older than 60 years of age. However, the immunosuppression that is required to allow engraftment increases the risk of graft-versus-host disease and opportunistic infections.

In general, the effectiveness of transplantation is determined by the underlying disease as well as by factors related to the transplantation process itself. For example, the optimal CD34 (stem cell) "dose" has not been determined. Engraftment requires an adequate dose of cells, but increasing doses of CD34 cells result in an increased incidence of graft-versus-host disease in patients following allogeneic transplantation. In addition, autologous stem cell transplantation may be complicated by contamination with tumor cells, and some centers therefore manipulate autologous donations to remove any tumor cells before transplantation.

Allogeneic HSCT following myeloablative high-dose chemotherapy is potentially curative for young patients (<40 years of age) with severe or very severe aplastic anemia, myelofibrosis, refractory chronic myeloid leukemia, high-risk acute myeloid leukemia in first clinical remission, acute lymphoblastic leukemia in clinical remission, high-risk myelodysplastic syndromes, and refractory non-Hodgkin lymphoma. Nonmyeloablative HSCT is effective in older patients with refractory chronic myeloid leukemia, chronic lymphocytic leukemia, multiple myeloma, and non-Hodgkin lymphoma. Autologous HSCT prolongs disease-free survival in patients with multiple myeloma and non-Hodgkin lymphoma.

KEY POINTS

- Erythropoietin should not be used in patients receiving myelosuppressive therapy with intent to cure because of reports of worsening survival rates in this treatment setting.

- Thrombopoietin is approved for the treatment of chronic idiopathic thrombocytopenic purpura.

- Allogeneic hematopoietic stem cell transplantation is potentially curative for young patients with aplastic anemia, myelofibrosis, certain types of leukemia, high-risk myelodysplastic syndromes, and refractory non-Hodgkin lymphoma.

Bibliography

Harrison CN, Campbell PJ, Buck G, et al; United Kingdom Medical Research Council Primary Thrombocythemia 1 Study. Hydroxyurea Compared with Anagrelide in High-Risk Essential Thrombocythemia. N Engl J Med. 2005;353(1):33-45. [PMID: 16000354]

Hillmen P, Young NS, Schubert J, et al. The Complement Inhibitor Eculizumab in Paroxysmal Nocturnal Hemoglobinuria. N Engl J Med. 2006;355(12):1233-1243. [PMID: 16990386]

Kantarjian H, Sawyers C, Hochhaus A, et al; The International ST1571 CML Study Group. Hematologic and cytogenetic responses to imatinib mesylate in chronic myelogenous leukemia [erratum in N Engl J Med. 2002;346(24):1923]. N Eng J Med. 2002;346:645-652. [PMID: 11870241]

Kurzrock R, Kantarjian HM, Druker BJ, Talpaz M. Philadelphia Chromosome-Positive Leukemias: From Basic Mechanisms to Molecular Therapeutics. Ann Intern Med. 2003;138(10):819-830. [PMID: 12755554]

Kuter DJ, Bussel JB, Lyons RM, et al. Efficacy of romiplostim in patients with chronic immune thrombocytopenic purpura: a double-blind randomised controlled trial. Lancet. 2008;371(9610):395-403 [PMID: 18242413]

List A, Dewald G, Bennett J, et al; Myelodysplastic Syndrome-003 Study Investigators. Lenalidomide in the myelodysplastic syndrome with chromosome 5q deletion. N Engl J Med. 2006;355(14):1456-1465. [PMID: 17021321]

Nimer, SD. Myelodysplastic syndromes. Blood. 2008;111(10):4841-4851. [PMID: 18467609]

Sanz MA, Martín G, González M, et al; Programa de Estudio y Traitmiento de las Hemopatías Malignas. Risk-adapted treatment of acute promyelocytic leukemia with all-trans-retinoic acid and anthracycline monochemotherapy: a multicenter study by the PETHEMA group. Blood. 2004;103(4):1237-1243. [PMID: 14576047]

Tallman MS, Gilliland DG, Rowe JM. Drug therapy for acute myeloid leukemia [erratum in Blood. 2005;106(7):2243]. Blood. 2005;106(4):1154-1163. [PMID: 15870183]

Young NS, Calado RT, Scheinberg P. Current concepts in the pathophysiology and treatment of aplastic anemia. Blood. 2006; 108(8):2509-2519. [PMID: 16778145]

Multiple Myeloma and Related Disorders

Introduction

Plasma cell dyscrasias are characterized by clonal proliferation of immunoglobulin-secreting differentiated B lymphocytes and plasma cells. Multiple myeloma is the most common malignant plasma cell dyscrasia. Other common plasma cell dyscrasias include monoclonal gammopathy of undetermined significance (MGUS), immunoglobulin light-chain (AL) amyloidosis, and Waldenström macroglobulinemia.

Multiple Myeloma

Multiple myeloma is caused by accumulation of neoplastic plasma cells in the bones and bone marrow. These plasma cells generally produce a homogeneous immunoglobulin protein that can be detected in the serum (paraprotein or M component) or urine (as the immunoglobulin light-chain component or Bence-Jones protein). Osteoclast activity occurs in myeloma secondary to overexpression of certain cytokines, resulting in the characteristic osteolytic lesions. Multiple myeloma occurs more commonly in men than in women and occurs rarely before the age of 40 years (median age at presentation, 60 years), with 12,500 new cases occurring yearly in the Untied States.

Clinical Manifestations and Findings

Patients with multiple myeloma may present with such nonspecific symptoms as bone pain (particularly in the back or the chest), fatigue, infections, fractures, and weight loss.

The most common physical finding is pallor. Neurologic findings may also be present. Large plasmacytomas can cause spinal cord or nerve-root compression, and neuropathy can develop because of the neuropathic effect of the paraprotein.

Laboratory findings include high concentrations of paraprotein, including positively charged M protein, which can lead to expansion of plasma volume and decreased anion gap, pseudohyponatremia, or pseudohypoglycemia. Hypercalcemia is present in 15% of patients at diagnosis and is mediated by cytokines (osteoclast-activating factor, IL-6, tumor necrosis factor β, and IL-1β) and immobilization caused by inactivity. Hematologic manifestations include rouleaux formation on peripheral blood smear, anemia, thrombocytopenia, and the coating of platelets by M protein, which causes platelet dysfunction. Abnormal serum creatinine, low potassium levels, and low serum bicarbonate levels could also occur in patients with renal manifestations of myeloma.

Suppression of normal immunoglobulin synthesis results in recurrent infections in patients with multiple myeloma. Anemia may be caused by bone marrow infiltration, deficiency of erythropoietin levels, and increased inflammatory cytokine levels. Nephropathy may be caused by renal tubular dysfunction due to tubular light-chain deposition; proximal tubular dysfunction leading to Fanconi syndrome, hypercalcemia-induced distal tubular dysfunction; amyloid fibril deposition in glomeruli, resulting in the nephrotic syndrome; urinary tract infections; contrast agents; and nephrotoxic antibiotics and drugs.

Plain radiography and MRI can detect the lytic bone lesions in multiple myeloma, whereas bone scan primarily detects osteoblastic activity (**Figure 1**).

Diagnosis and Prognosis

The International Myeloma Working Group has agreed on three simplified criteria for the diagnosis of symptomatic multiple myeloma (**Table 7**). The diagnostic criteria proposed by the World Health Organization rely on major and minor diagnostic criteria (see Table 7). The International Myeloma Working Group criteria distinguish asymptomatic myeloma from symptomatic myeloma on the basis of whether end-organ damage has occurred. Therapy is not required in asymptomatic patients; however, they should undergo follow-up monitoring every 3 to 4 months. Laboratory testing should include serum protein electrophoresis, complete blood count, and serum creatinine and calcium measurement. Bone survey should be considered annually to evaluate for asymptomatic bone lesions.

Multiple myeloma used to be staged according to the levels of monoclonal protein production, anemia, extent of bone disease, presence of hypercalcemia, and renal failure. A simpler staging scheme uses measurement of β_2 microglobulin concentration, a surrogate marker for myeloma tumor mass and renal function, and serum albumin to identify patients with good, intermediate, and poor prognosis (**Table 8**).

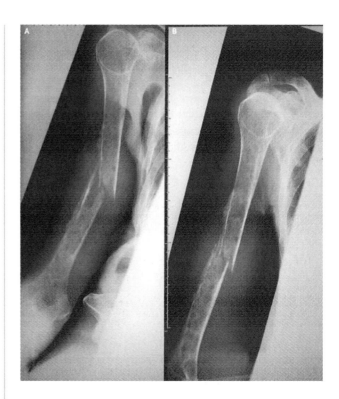

FIGURE 1.
Multiple lytic lesions and a pathologic fracture of right humerus in a patient with multiple myeloma.

Treatment

Therapy with melphalan and prednisone or combinations with additional alkylating agents or anthracyclines have yielded response rates (>50% M protein reduction) in approximately 50% of patients with multiple myeloma. Complete hematologic remission, defined as an absence of monoclonal gammopathy in serum or urine and normal bone marrow aspirate/biopsy, occurs in no more than 5% of patients. Median event-free survival and overall survival have not exceeded 18 and 30 to 36 months, respectively; cures have not been reported. The poor prognosis of patients with multiple myeloma reflects the exquisite drug resistance of even newly diagnosed multiple myeloma.

High-dose dexamethasone pulsing alone or in combination with continuous infusions of vincristine and doxorubicin represent an effective regimen for patients whose disease has progressed while receiving melphalan and prednisone. As initial therapy, vincristine and doxorubicin induce a more marked and rapid tumor cytoreduction than standard melphalan and prednisone or similar regimens. Overall survival, however, is not improved.

Interferon has been evaluated as part of remission induction and maintenance therapy as well as part of salvage therapy. Although interferon results in prolonged event-free survival, its impact on overall survival has been negligible.

TABLE 7 Criteria for the Diagnosis of Multiple Myeloma

International Myeloma Working Group Criteria for the Diagnosis of Multiple Myeloma

1. Monoclonal plasma cells in the bone marrow >10% and/or presence of a biopsy-proven plasmacytoma.

2. Monoclonal protein present in the serum and/or urine.

3. Myeloma-related organ dysfunction (1 or more):

   Calcium elevation in the blood (serum calcium >10.5 mg/L [2.63 mmol/L] or upper limit of normal)

   Renal insufficiency (serum creatinine >2 mg/dL [152.6 μmol/L])

   Anemia (hemoglobin <10 g/dL [100 g/L] or 2 g < normal)

   Lytic bone lesions or osteoporosis

WHO Criteria for the Diagnosis of Multiple Myeloma[a]

Major Criteria
   Plasmacytoma on tissue biopsy
   Bone marrow clonal plasma cells >30%
   High M protein (IgG >3.5 g/dL [35 g/L], IgA >2.0 g/dL [20 g/L], Bence-Jones proteinuria >1.0 g/24 h)
Minor Criteria
   Bone marrow clonal plasma cells 10%-30%
   M-protein less than above
   Lytic bone lesions
   Reduced normal immunoglobulins to <50% of normal

WHO = World Health Organization.

[a]Diagnostic requirements: The diagnosis of multiple myeloma requires a minimum of one major criterion and one minor criterion or three minor criteria, which must include bone marrow plasmacytosis of 10%-30% and the presence of a monoclonal protein.

TABLE 8 International Staging System for Multiple Myeloma

Stage	Criteria	Median Survival (months)
I	Serum β2-microglobulin <3.5 mg/L, serum albumin ≥3.5 g/dL (35 g/L)	62
II	Not stage I or III	44
III	Serum β2-microglobulin ≥5.5 mg/L	29

Randomized and historically controlled trials have recently demonstrated the superiority of high-dose chemotherapy and autologous stem cell transplantation over standard treatment in achieving remission rates of up to 40% to 50% and extending median event-free and overall survival to 3 years and more than 5 years, respectively.

Supportive Therapy

Erythropoietin improves multiple myeloma–associated anemia in about 75% of patients, even in the absence of kidney disease, and is especially useful when anemia persists because of irreversible renal failure. An important adjunct in treatment, especially for bone lesions, is parenteral bisphosphonate therapy, such as pamidronate or zoledronic acid, which delays the onset of skeletal-related events and seems to extend survival. Renal dysfunction and osteonecrosis of the jaw (**Figure 2**) after dental procedures are potential adverse effects of long-term parenteral bisphosphonate therapy.

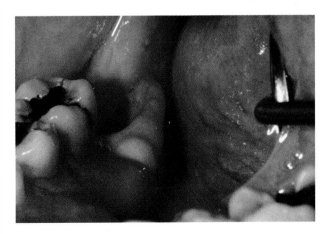

FIGURE 2.
Osteonecrosis of the jaw, a complication related to bisphosphonate therapy.

Reprinted with permission from Woo SB, Hellstein JW, Kalmar JR. Systematic Review: Bisphosphonates and Osteonecrosis of the Jaws. Ann Intern Med. 2006;144(10):753-761. [PMID: 16702591] Copyright 2006, American College of Physicians.

Hypercalcemia in patients with multiple myeloma is managed with saline hydration, corticosteroids, and bisphosphonates. Prophylactic immunizations for pneumonia and influenza are mandatory. Patients with recurrent bacterial infections may benefit from prophylactic monthly immune globulin infusion.

Novel Therapies

Thalidomide is a novel treatment in multiple myeloma that does not appear to act through a cytotoxic effect. Instead, it may inhibit the growth and survival of tumor cells, bone marrow stromal cells, or both; alter the profile of adhesion molecules and interactions between tumor cells and bone marrow stromal cells; modulate the cytokine milieu; inhibit angiogenesis; or increase the number of CD8 cells through its immunomodulatory effects. Thalidomide-based regimens have been evaluated in several trials and are being used in relapsed, refractory, and front-line settings. Therapy is generally well tolerated, and toxicities include fetal malformations, constipation, sedation, skin rash, peripheral neuropathy, fatigue, and thromboembolism. Discontinuation of thalidomide is not always required to manage toxicities. Lenalidomide, a potent analogue of thalidomide, offers great promise in myeloma. The toxicity profile is different from that of thalidomide, with less neuropathy, fatigue, and somnolence, but with increased risk for neutropenia and thrombocytopenia. Lenalidomide also can lead to thromboembolism.

Bortezomib, a proteasome inhibitor, inhibits cell growth, induces apoptosis, and allows myeloma cells in vitro to overcome drug resistance, and it has shown significant activity in myeloma. This agent was U.S. Food and Drug Administration approved as second-line therapy for myeloma in 2004. Major toxicities are fatigue, asthenia, peripheral neuropathy, and thrombocytopenia.

Novel therapies, alone and in combination regimens, have replaced oral melphalan and prednisone as well as vincristine and doxorubicin and can be used for initial treatment and in relapsed or refractory disease.

KEY POINTS

- Patients with asymptomatic multiple myeloma can be followed without therapy, until end-organ damage occurs.
- Novel therapeutic agents with promising results in the treatment of multiple myeloma include thalidomide, lenalidomide, and bortezomib.

Monoclonal Gammopathy of Undetermined Significance

Monoclonal gammopathy of undetermined significance (MGUS) is found in approximately 1% to 2% of adults. The incidence is higher in patients older than 70 years and in blacks. MGUS is defined by the criteria listed in (**Table 9**) and is characterized by a tendency towards development of

multiple myeloma or a related malignancy at the rate of 1% to 1.5% per year. Whether these associations are pathogenetically related or are merely coincidental is not clear. MGUS is always asymptomatic and is usually discovered through incidental laboratory findings, most often, hyperproteinemia. A monoclonal spike is identified on subsequent protein electrophoresis. Laboratory evaluation should include a complete blood count and measurement of serum calcium, creatinine, and electrolytes as well as immunoglobulin quantitation, serum and urine protein electrophoresis, serum and urine immunofixation electrophoresis, and a bone survey. Examination of the bone marrow is not always required, but, if done, should show less than 10% plasma cells.

IgG or IgA MGUS may progress to multiple myeloma, AL amyloidosis, or a related plasma cell disorder, whereas IgM MGUS may progress to a lymphoproliferative disorder (non-Hodgkin lymphoma, chronic lymphocytic leukemia, or Waldenström macroglobulinemia). A risk-stratification model to predict the risk of progression of MGUS uses three adverse risk factors: (1) a serum M protein level greater than or equal to 1.5 g/dL, (2) non-IgG MGUS, and (3) an abnormal serum free light-chain ratio. Using this model, the risk of disease progression over 20 years for patients with various combinations of risk factors is as follows:

- three risk factors (high-risk MGUS) — 58%
- two risk factors (high–intermediate-risk MGUS) — 37%
- one risk factor (low–intermediate-risk MGUS) — 21%
- no risk factors (low-risk MGUS) — 5%

MGUS may rarely be associated with nonmalignant disorders, such as skin diseases (scleroderma, pyoderma gangrenosum), liver diseases (cirrhosis, primary biliary cirrhosis, hepatitis), rheumatologic diseases (rheumatoid arthritis, polymyositis, polymyalgia rheumatica), and HIV infection.

Patients with MGUS should be evaluated every 3 to 6 months for symptoms suggestive of myeloma and receive repeat laboratory tests every 6 to 12 months. Repeat bone marrow evaluation should be done only if other laboratory features suggest progression to multiple myeloma. Although there is no treatment to prevent progression of MGUS to multiple myeloma, monitoring for plasma cell dyscrasias is important because early recognition and treatment favorably affect outcome.

KEY POINTS

- Non-IgG monoclonal gammopathy of undetermined significance, abnormal serum free light-chain ratio, and an M spike greater than 1.5 g/dL are predictive of progression to a plasma cell proliferative disorder over 20 years.
- Monitoring for plasma cell dyscrasias is important in patients with monoclonal gammopathy of undetermined significance because early recognition and treatment favorably affect outcome.

TABLE 9 Monoclonal Gammopathy of Undetermined Significance
The presence of a serum monoclonal protein (M-protein, whether IgA, IgG, or IgM), at a concentration ≤3 g/dL (30 g/L)
Bone marrow plasma cells <10%
The absence of lytic bone lesions, anemia, hypercalcemia, and renal insufficiency related to the plasma cell proliferative process or related B-cell lymphoproliferative disorder

Immunoglobulin Light-Chain (AL) Amyloidosis

The amyloidoses are a group of diseases that share a common feature of extracelluar deposition of pathologic, insoluble fibrils in various tissues and organs. Classification of the amyloidoses is based on the precursor protein that forms the amyloid fibrils and the distribution of amyloid deposition, systemic or localized.

AL amyloidosis is the most common systemic amyloidosis associated with an underlying clonal plasma cell dyscrasia. The precursor protein in AL amyloidosis is an immunoglobulin light chain or a fragment of a light chain, produced by the clonal plasma cell population in the bone marrow. The plasma cell burden in this disorder is usually low, at 5% to 10%, although AL amyloidosis is associated with overt multiple myeloma in 10% to 15% of cases.

AL amyloidosis most frequently affects the kidneys and the heart. Kidney involvement usually is manifested by nephrotic syndrome with progressive worsening of renal function. Amyloid deposition in the heart results in rapidly progressive heart failure caused by restrictive cardiomyopathy. Low voltage on electrocardiography is found in many patients with AL amyloidosis and often is associated with a pseudoinfarct pattern. Splenomegaly occurs rarely, whereas hepatomegaly occurs commonly and is caused by congestion from right heart failure or by amyloid infiltration. Profound elevation of the serum alkaline phosphatase concentration with only a mild elevation of aminotransferases is characteristic of hepatic amyloidosis. Autonomic nervous system involvement can lead to orthostatic hypotension, early satiety caused by delayed gastric emptying, erectile dysfunction, and intestinal dysmotility. A painful, bilateral, symmetric, distal, sensory neuropathy that progresses to motor neuropathy is the usual neurologic manifestation in AL amyloidosis. Soft-tissue involvement is characterized by macroglossia (**Figure 3**), carpal tunnel syndrome, skin nodules, arthropathy, alopecia, nail dystrophy, submandibular gland enlargement, periorbital purpura (**Figure 4**), and hoarseness. Endocrinopathy occurs rarely but may develop owing to amyloid infiltration of the glands.

The diagnosis of amyloidosis requires a tissue biopsy that demonstrates apple-green birefringence when stained with Congo red and viewed under a polarizing microscope. The site of the biopsy may reflect underlying organ dysfunction. If the clinical syndrome suggests amyloidosis, less-invasive biopsy of an abdominal fat pad may be diagnostic.

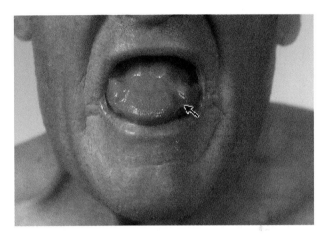

FIGURE 3.
Macroglossia.
A hallmark feature of AL amyloidosis.

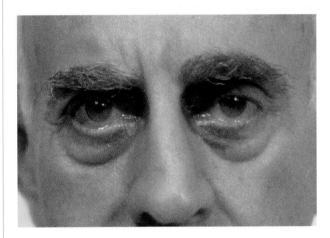

FIGURE 4.
Periorbital ecchymoses.
Raccoon eyes in a patient with AL amyloidosis.

Confirmation of AL amyloidosis requires detection of a plasma cell dyscrasia by serum and urine immunofixation electrophoresis, serum free light-chain assay, and immunohistochemistry studies of the bone marrow biopsy specimen.

Treatment of AL amyloidosis with standard melphalan plus prednisone regimens used to treat multiple myeloma is associated with a short-lived response rate and a poor prognosis. High-dose melphalan and stem cell transplantation induces hematologic remission and prolongs survival, with reversal of amyloid-related organ dysfunction; however, patients who do not meet predefined criteria, such as age, cardiac status, performance status, and others, are not eligible for this aggressive therapy.

Specific chemotherapy is directed towards the underlying plasma cell dyscrasia to eradicate the production of the precursor protein. Novel treatments for myeloma are also being used for AL amyloidosis in clinical trials. Supportive organ-specific treatment may include diuretics, midodrine, or defibrillation.

KEY POINTS

- Detection of monoclonal gammopathy in serum and urine by immunofixation electrophoresis, abnormal serum free light-chain ratio, or clonal plasmacytosis (5% to 10%) with the presence of Congo red–staining amyloid deposits in the tissues support the diagnosis of AL amyloidosis.

- Selected patients with AL amyloidosis who qualify for treatment with high-dose melphalan and stem cell transplantation experience hematologic remission and prolonged survival, with reversal of amyloid-related organ dysfunction.

Waldenström Macroglobulinemia

Waldenström macroglobulinemia results from the proliferation of B lymphocytes that show maturation to plasma cells and is characterized by a lymphoplasmacytic infiltrate of the bone marrow, lymphadenopathy, anemia, neuropathy, organomegaly, IgM monoclonal gammopathy, and hyperviscosity syndrome. Hyperviscosity syndrome, which is related to the physicochemical properties of IgM, is identified by blurred vision; fatigue; mucosal bleeding caused by impaired platelet function; heart failure; headache; and altered mentation. Funduscopic examination in these patients may show engorged retinal veins. Plasmapheresis temporarily relieves acute symptoms and should be combined with specific treatment that may include chlorambucil, rituximab, and fludarabine or cladribine.

KEY POINTS

- The hyperviscosity syndrome of Waldenström macroglobulinemia is characterized by blurred vision, fatigue, mucosal bleeding, headache, heart failure, and altered mentation.

- Hyperviscosity syndrome should be treated with plasmapheresis and specific treatment for Waldenström macroglobulinemia including chlorambucil, rituximab, and fludarabine or cladribine.

Bibliography

Barlogie B, Shaughnessy J, Tricot G, et al. Treatment of multiple myeloma. Blood. 2004;103(1):20-32. [PMID: 12969978]

Blade J. Clinical practice. Monoclonal gammopathy of undetermined significance. N Engl J Med. 2006;355(26):2765-2770. [PMID: 17192542]

Dimopoulos MA, Kyle RA, Anagnostopoulos A, Treon SP. Diagnosis and management of Waldenstrom's macroglobulinemia. J Clin Oncol. 2005;23(7):1564-1577. [PMID: 15735132]

Falk RH, Comenzo RL, Skinner M. The systemic amyloidoses. N Engl J Med. 1997;337(13):898-909. [PMID: 9302305]

Greipp PR, San Miguel J, Durie BG, et al. International staging system for multiple myeloma. J Clin Oncol. 2005;23(15):3412-3420. [PMID: 15809451]

International Myeloma Working Group. Criteria for the classification of monoclonal gammopathies, multiple myeloma and related disorders: a report of the International Myeloma Working Group. Br J Haematol. 2003;121(5):749-757. [PMID: 12780789]

Kyle RA, Rajkumar SV. Multiple myeloma [erratum in N Engl J Med. 2005;352(11):1163]. N Engl J Med. 2004;351(18):1860-1873. [PMID: 15509819]

Rajkumar SV, Kyle RA, Therneau TM, et al. Serum free light chain ratio is an independent risk factor for progression in monoclonal gammopathy of undetermined significance. Blood. 2005;106(3):812-817. [PMID: 15855274]

Sanchorawala V. Light-chain (AL) amyloidosis: diagnosis and treatment. Clin J Am Soc Nephrol. 2006;1(6):1331-1341. [PMID: 17699366]

Treon SP, Gertz MA, Dimopoulos M, et al. Update on treatment recommendations from the Third International Workshop on Waldenstrom's macroglobulinemia. Blood. 2006;107(9):3442-3446. [PMID: 16410453]

Approach to Anemia

Overview

Anemia is defined as a reduction in the oxygen-carrying capacity of the blood caused by a diminished erythrocyte mass. It can be divided into three general categories: blood loss, diminished erythrocyte production, and increased erythrocyte destruction (hemolysis). Underproduction anemias can be further divided into those associated with erythropoietin deficiency and those associated with diminished marrow response to erythropoietin. Erythropoietin, a 165–amino acid glycoprotein normally produced by the kidney, stimulates proliferation and maturation of erythroid cells. Erythropoietin production is regulated at the level of transcription and is increased in response to hypoxia. In addition to erythroid precursors in the marrow and erythropoietin, elemental iron, vitamins, cytokines, and a suitable microenvironment are essential for normal erythrocyte production.

In the evaluation of patients with anemia, the first steps, after obtaining the history and performing the physical examination, are to review the peripheral blood film and to check the reticulocyte count. The reticulocyte count is a reflection of the marrow's response to anemia. As such, a high reticulocyte count reflects adequate marrow response to anemia as typically occurs in patients with hemolytic anemia. An inappropriately low reticulocyte count is indicative of an underproduction anemia. The reticulocyte count is typically reported as a percentage of total erythrocytes. In the presence of anemia, the percentage may be increased artificially because of a decrease in the total number of erythrocytes. In addition, excess erythropoietin production during marrow stress can cause a doubling in the half-life of circulating reticulocytes. Therefore, in the evaluation of the patient with anemia, the reticulocyte count is often corrected as the reticulocyte index, which is represented by:

$$\text{reticulocyte index} = \text{percentage of reticulocytes} \times \text{patient's hematocrit}/45 \times 0.5.$$

Alternatively, using flow cytometry, the reticulocyte count can be determined in absolute numbers, with a normal value ranging from 31.7 to $104.6 \times 10^9/L$. Values higher than $110 \times 10^9/L$ are indicative of marrow that is responding normally to anemia. The flow cytometric reticulocyte count is currently the most commonly used, and least awkward, representation of reticulocyte response.

The peripheral blood smear and red cell indices provide information on erythrocyte size, morphology, and distribution. Microcytic anemia is usually caused by iron deficiency or thalassemia. Normocytic anemia typically occurs in inflammatory anemia or kidney disease, although the former may also be mildly microcytic. Macrocytic anemia is typical of cobalamin or folate deficiency, induced by the use of drugs affecting cellular differentiation, such as antimetabolites; excessive alcohol consumption; or myelodysplasia. Reviewing the peripheral blood film can provide information on erythrocyte-shape abnormalities in addition to providing information on platelet or leukocyte morphology, which is not available from a typical complete blood count report.

An algorithm for the basic workup of anemia is illustrated in **Figure 5**. Examination of bone marrow histology may also be useful in the evaluation of some patients with anemia whose diagnosis is not readily apparent from review of the peripheral blood film. For example, Prussian blue staining can be helpful in determining iron stores. Wright stain also is useful in identifying abnormalities in cellular differentiation as found in patients with leukemia or myelodysplasia.

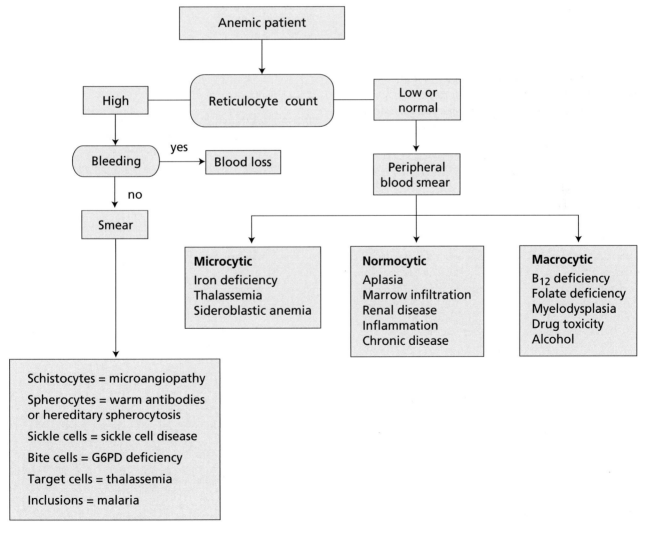

FIGURE 5.
Diagnostic workup for the patient with anemia.

Anemia Due to Erythrocyte Underproduction or Maturation Defects

Iron Deficiency

Iron deficiency is a worldwide problem that is exacerbated in women by pregnancy and lactation. Iron is required for DNA synthesis, oxygen transport, and cellular respiration. Most total body iron is stored in erythrocytes. Each milliliter of packed erythrocytes contains about 1 mg of iron. Iron absorption is closely modulated by the small polypeptide hepcidin, which inhibits iron absorption in the enterocyte and iron release from the macrophages by causing internalization and proteolysis of the iron transport protein, ferroportin. In iron-deficient states, hepcidin levels are depressed, facilitating iron absorption (**Figure 6**).

In addition to pregnancy and lactation, iron deficiency may also be the result of normal growth, blood loss, intravascular hemolysis, gastric bypass procedures, and malabsorption; however in the adult male and nonmenstruating female, gastrointestinal blood loss must be the presumed cause until proved otherwise. Iron absorption from the gut is tightly regulated, such that the daily amount of iron absorbed is approximately equal to the daily amount of iron lost (1 mg/d for men and 1.5 mg/d for women). Iron is absorbed mostly in the proximal small bowel, and malabsorption states, such as celiac disease and inflammatory bowel disease, can lead to iron deficiency. Most adults consume about 5 mg of iron per 1000 calories. Meats and liver are rich sources of iron, legumes contain moderate amounts of iron, and most other vegetables contain some iron that is often chelated by phytates or oxalates, making absorption difficult.

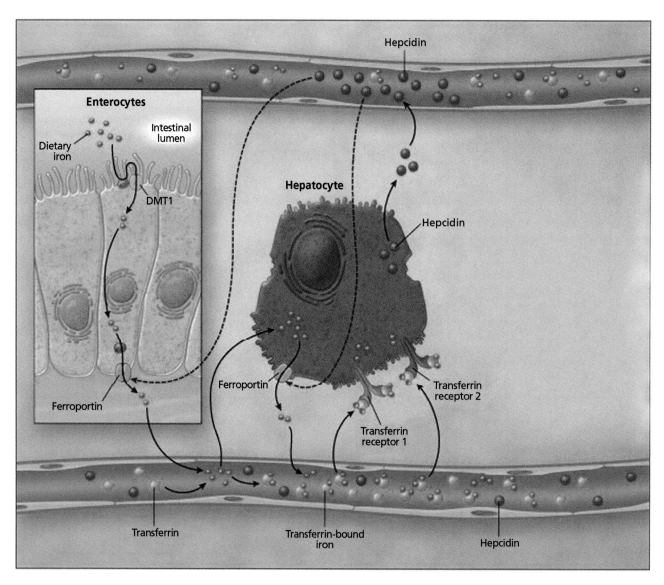

FIGURE 6.
Regulation of iron absorption.

Patients with mild iron deficiency may complain of fatigue, irritability, decreased exercise tolerance, and headaches before they become anemic. Occasionally, patients with advanced iron deficiency exhibit the tendency to eat ice, clay, starch, and crunchy materials (pica).

The physical examination in iron-deficient patients is typically normal. More severe deficiency includes findings of pallor, glossitis, and stomatitis. Conjunctival pallor is a sensitive physical finding in iron deficiency. In patients with severe iron deficiency, spooning of the nails (koilonychia) is noted.

The first step in the evaluation of patients with suspected iron deficiency is review of the peripheral blood smear, followed by measurement of serum iron concentration, total iron-binding capacity (TIBC), and serum ferritin concentration. The peripheral blood smear in patients with iron deficiency (**Figure 7**) is remarkable for microcytic, hypochromic erythrocytes, with marked anisopoikilocytosis (that is, abnormalities in erythrocyte size and shape). Thrombocytosis is noted frequently in patients with iron deficiency.

The serum iron concentration, a poor reflection of iron stores, is usually low in patients with iron deficiency; the TIBC is high; the percentage of transferrin saturation (iron/TIBC) is low; and the serum ferritin concentration is low. Because the serum ferritin concentration can increase in inflammatory states, ferritin may be normal or elevated in patients with iron deficiency, but a ferritin concentration of more than 100 ng/mL (100 mg/L) effectively rules out iron deficiency, and a ferritin of less than 15 ng/mL (15 mg/L) rules in iron deficiency. Elevated concentrations of soluble transferrin receptor and zinc protoporphyrin have been used to establish a diagnosis of iron deficiency, but there is significant overlap between levels found in iron-deficient patients and normal control patients. As such, iron deficiency should be suspected in an anemic patient with hypochromia and microcytosis regardless of the serum ferritin level. A bone marrow biopsy can be used to establish a diagnosis of iron

deficiency but is indicated only if results of the tests described above are not confirmatory.

Iron deficiency is best treated by using oral iron salts, with ferrous sulfate, 325 mg three times daily, as the least-expensive preparation. Each 325-mg tablet of ferrous sulfate contains 66 mg of iron, 1% to 2% of which is absorbed. Although ascorbic acid has been shown to augment oral iron absorption, there are no convincing data suggesting that the addition of this agent is worth the cost or increase in gastrointestinal side effects. Although there are alternative preparations of oral iron, none of these has conclusively been shown to increase oral tolerability. Iron absorption is inhibited by antacids, antibiotics, and many foods, including cereals and dietary fiber. Optimally, iron should not be taken with meals. Most patients tolerate oral ferrous sulfate with minimal side effects, which tend to be gastrointestinal in nature. For those intolerant of full-dose oral iron, the dosage can be reduced to 325 mg daily for several days with increasing dosing over time. Iron therapy is typically continued several months following normalization of the hemoglobin level. Patients who are unable to absorb iron orally (for example, patients with Crohn disease, celiac disease, or small bowel resection) instead may receive parenteral iron. Although iron dextran has been used in the past for this purpose, ferric gluconate and iron sucrose preparations appear less apt to cause anaphylaxis-like reactions and are safer to administer.

After iron therapy is initiated, symptoms such as headache, fatigue, and burning of the tongue resolve within days. Reticulocytosis occurs several days after therapy is begun and reaches its peak within 7 to 12 days of initiation of therapy. Noticeable increases in hemoglobin concentration usually occur within several weeks.

KEY POINTS

- Gastrointestinal blood loss or malabsorption states such as celiac disease and inflammatory bowel disease can lead to iron deficiency.

- Patients with iron deficiency may present with fatigue, irritability, decreased exercise tolerance, and headaches before anemia is confirmed.

- Review of the peripheral blood smear, followed by measurement of serum iron and ferritin concentrations and assessment of total iron-binding capacity, are the first steps in the evaluation of suspected iron deficiency.

- A ferritin concentration of higher than 100 ng/mL (100 mg/L) effectively rules out iron deficiency.

- Iron deficiency is best treated by using oral iron salts, with ferrous sulfate as the least-expensive preparation.

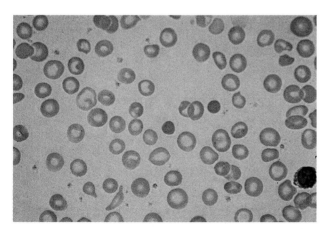

FIGURE 7.
Hypochromia and microcytosis with anisopoikilocytosis in a patient with iron deficiency.

Reprinted with permission from the ASH Image Bank. Copyright 2009 American Society of Hematology; www.ashimagebank.org.

Cobalamin (Vitamin B$_{12}$) Deficiency

Cobalamin is necessary for DNA synthesis. Unlike some microorganisms, humans must consume cobalamin to survive.

Upon ingestion, cobalamin is released from food by gastric peptidases. In the acidic stomach, cobalamin is bound to R-binders released by saliva and the stomach. In the alkaline small bowel, cobalamin is bound to intrinsic factor, which is necessary for intestinal absorption in the terminal ileum. It then becomes bound to transcobalamin for storage. Because cobalamin has a large enterohepatic circulation and large reserves in the liver, cobalamin deficiency from decreased oral intake takes years to develop.

Cobalamin deficiency results from malabsorption, or, very rarely, decreased intake in vegans. Such malabsorption may be selective for cobalamin in patients with pernicious anemia who lack intrinsic factor or may be part of a broader malabsorptive process in patients with inflammatory bowel disease affecting the terminal ileum or resulting from pancreatic insufficiency or bacterial overgrowth. Cobalamin deficiency has been reported as a result of metformin therapy. This may be related to decreased calcium-mediated absorption of cobalamin in the ileum.

Typical physical examination findings in patients with cobalamin deficiency include glossitis, weight loss, and pale yellow skin caused by the combination of anemia and hemolysis of abnormal erythrocytes. Patients with cobalamin deficiency also may have neurologic findings, including loss of position and vibratory sense, which can progress to spastic ataxia. In patients with cobalamin deficiency, neuropsychiatric findings, including dementia or psychosis, may occur in the absence of significant anemia.

The diagnostic approach to patients with cobalamin deficiency is two-pronged, consisting of establishing the diagnosis and determining the cause of the deficiency. In addition to being characterized by neurologic findings on physical examination, cobalamin deficiency should be suspected in patients who are elderly, abuse alcohol, and have malnutrition. The next step in establishing a diagnosis is review of the peripheral blood smear, followed by measurement of serum cobalamin and folate concentrations. In the event of equivocal results in these values, methylmalonic acid and total homocysteine levels can be measured.

The peripheral blood smear in cobalamin deficiency is identical to that found in folate deficiency or other types of megaloblastic anemia, showing macro-ovalocytes and hypersegmented polymorphonuclear cells (**Figure 8**). Affected patients may have thrombocytopenia and leukopenia as well as anemia. Macrocytic red blood cell indices and megaloblastic marrow changes may also be present in patients with cobalamin deficiency, and basophilic stippling may occur. Because cobalamin deficiency leads to ineffective hematopoiesis, serum lactate dehydrogenase, unconjugated bilirubin, and uric acid levels may all be increased. Although very low levels of cobalamin (<200 pg/mL) are indicative of cobalamin deficiency, some patients may have significant cobalamin deficiency with serum cobalamin levels in the low-normal range (200 to 400 pg/mL). Serum methylmalonic acid and

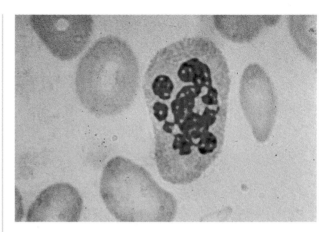

FIGURE 8.
Hypersegmented polymorphonuclear cell in a patient with pernicious anemia.

homocysteine levels increase before cobalamin levels decrease below the normal range and are the most reliable indicators of tissue cobalamin deficiency (**Figure 9**); however, these tests are expensive and should be ordered only when the diagnosis is suspected and the serum vitamin B_{12} level has been measured and is in the equivocal low-normal range (200 to 400 pg/mL [147.6 pmol/L to 295.2 pmol/L]).

Pernicious anemia is a specific etiology of cobalamin deficiency resulting from a deficiency in intrinsic factor that is caused by an antibody response directed against hydrogen-potassium adenosine triphosphatase (H-K-ATPase) in the membrane of parietal cells; this mechanism leads to parietal cell atrophy. Antiparietal cell antibodies are found in 90% of patients with pernicious anemia compared with 5% of the general population, and antibodies to intrinsic factor are found in 70% of patients with this disorder. Although antibody testing is often used to establish a diagnosis of pernicious anemia, the poor sensitivity and specificity of such testing hinder its utility. However, testing for anti–intrinsic factor antibodies may be confirmatory for pernicious anemia (sensitivity, 50% to 84%) in the setting of a low serum cobalamin concentration and megaloblastic anemia. In the past, the Schilling test was used in the diagnosis of pernicious anemia, but this test is seldom performed currently because it uses radioactive cobalamin and is unavailable in many laboratories in the United States.

Because the anemia of cobalamin deficiency can be reversed with folate therapy, it is important to rule out cobalamin deficiency before treating patients with folate. Otherwise, neurologic status may deteriorate in such patients despite improvement in anemia. Cobalamin deficiency has typically been treated with parenteral replacement (1000 µg intramuscularly/mo). However, oral replacement of cobalamin, 1000 to 2000 µg daily, has been shown to be as effective as and less expensive than parenteral therapy. Oral replacement of cobalamin can be accomplished with a tablet or gel formulation. Patients deficient in cobalamin typically

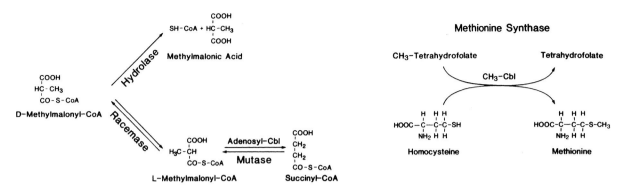

FIGURE 9.
The two vitamin B_{12}-dependent enzymes, L-methylmalonyl-CoA mutase (left) and methionine synthase (right).

respond with a decrease in serum bilirubin and lactate dehydrogenase levels within days. Within 12 hours of initiation of therapy, improvement is shown in the megaloblastic changes of the bone marrow, and within 3 to 5 days of start of therapy, reticulocytosis occurs. Hemoglobin levels usually normalize within several months of initiation of therapy in patients with cobalamin deficiency. If normalization of hemoglobin does not occur, an alternative diagnosis must be considered, including myelodysplasia or concurrent iron deficiency.

> **KEY POINTS**
>
> - Cobalamin deficiency is characterized by elevations in serum homocysteine and methylmalonic acid levels, and those markers may be useful for diagnosis in patients with low-normal levels of serum cobalamin.
> - Oral replacement of cobalamin is as effective as parenteral replacement in treating cobalamin deficiency.
> - Folate replacement can improve the anemia in cobalamin-deficient patients but will not improve neurologic abnormalities.

Folate Deficiency

Foodborne folate is normally conjugated with glutamic acid residues. For folate to be absorbed in the duodenum and proximal jejunum, it must be deconjugated to a monoglutamate form to facilitate uptake by cells as methyltetrahydrofolate. Folate is found in greens, vegetables, and fruits, such as lemons, bananas, and melons. Grains in the United States are also fortified with folate. The recommended allowance of folate is 400 µg daily.

Folate deficiency can occur with decreased oral intake, increased utilization, or impaired absorption. Because the body's stores of folate can be depleted in weeks to months, persons whose diets are folate deficient become anemic within several months. Patients who abuse alcohol may not consume folate-rich food but also do not absorb folate well because the enzyme responsible for deglutamation is partially inhibited by

alcohol. Excessive cooking of vegetables can also lead to folate deficiency due to heat destruction. Patients with celiac disease, Crohn disease, amyloidosis, or other diseases of the small bowel may have folate malabsorption. Pregnant women and patients with desquamating skin disorders such as psoriasis, sickle cell disease, other types of chronic hemolytic anemia, and conditions associated with rapid cell division and turnover also have increased folate needs. Drugs such as triamterene or phenytoin can accelerate folate metabolism.

The peripheral blood smear in folate deficiency is identical to that in cobalamin deficiency and other megaloblastic conditions. Erythrocyte folate levels may be more reliable than serum folate levels in establishing folate deficiency but may also be increased in cobalamin deficiency. Because the serum homocysteine level is increased in patients with folate deficiency but the methylmalonic acid level is normal, measurement of the serum homocysteine level is a reasonable test for detecting folate deficiency (sensitivity ~90%; specificity, 86% to 99%). Overall, if the diagnosis of cobalamin deficiency is reliably excluded, a therapeutic trial of folate in presumed deficient patients may be the most cost-effective way of pursuing the diagnosis.

Folate-deficient persons and pregnant women are treated with 1 to 5 mg of daily oral folate. Care must be taken to firmly exclude cobalamin deficiency in patients with folate deficiency because supplemental folate can improve the anemia of cobalamin deficiency but not the associated neurologic sequelae.

> **KEY POINTS**
>
> - Alcohol abuse, excessive cooking of vegetables, small bowel diseases, pregnancy, and desquamatory skin diseases are associated with folate deficiency.
> - Folate deficiency is treated with daily oral folate supplementation.
> - Folate replacement can improve the anemia in patients with cobalamin deficiency but will not improve neurologic complications.

Inflammatory Anemia

Patients with chronic inflammatory conditions, such as collagen vascular diseases, malignancy, or chronic infections, including tuberculosis or osteomyelitis, are frequently anemic. This contributed to the previous terminology for inflammatory anemia, the anemia of chronic disease. Patients with inflammatory anemia have decreased secretion of erythropoietin in response to anemia and decreased responsiveness of erythroid precursors to erythropoietin. Levels of inflammatory cytokines, such as tumor necrosis factor α, IL-6, IL-1, and interferon, are elevated and may be implicated in the altered erythropoietin responsiveness in these patients. A small peptide, hepcidin, has recently been identified as being principally responsible for the anemia occurring in inflammatory states. Hepcidin is synthesized in the liver, and levels are increased in response to IL-6. Hepcidin leads to decreased iron absorption from the gut and decreased release of iron from macrophages, two physiologic conditions occurring in inflammatory anemia. There is not yet a commercial test available for hepcidin measurement.

Inflammatory anemia typically results in mild to moderate anemia, with a hemoglobin level usually greater than 8 g/dL (80 g/L). This type of anemia is initially normocytic and normochromic but can become hypochromic and microcytic over time. The reticulocyte count is typically low in inflammatory anemia as are the serum iron concentration and total iron-binding capacity, but the serum ferritin level is normal or elevated. Although generally unnecessary in patients with inflammatory anemia, examination of bone marrow reveals ample stainable iron. **Table 10** lists the laboratory features of inflammatory anemia, iron deficiency, and iron deficiency with inflammation. Inflammatory anemia may also occur in patients with chronic heart failure or diabetes mellitus. Although these conditions are not typically associated with chronic inflammation, these patients may nonetheless have elevations in inflammatory cytokine levels. Some patients with inflammatory anemia have no clear underlying chronic disease and do not require evaluation for occult malignancy or infection.

Inflammatory anemia usually does not require specific therapy. Importantly, iron replacement is not necessary in inflammatory anemia and will not lead to improvement in erythropoiesis. Treating the underlying inflammatory disorder in patients with inflammatory anemia can improve the anemia itself. When absolutely necessary, patients with inflammatory anemia who have symptomatic anemia and low serum erythropoietin levels may benefit from erythropoietin supplementation. Erythropoietin must be used with caution because of the risk of hypertension and thrombosis.

KEY POINTS

- Inflammatory anemia is characterized by a low serum iron level and total iron-binding capacity and increased ferritin level.
- Inflammatory anemia typically results in mild to moderate anemia, with a hemoglobin level usually greater than 8 g/dL (80 g/L), and usually does not require treatment.

Anemia of Kidney Disease

Because erythropoietin is produced in the kidney, kidney disease is associated with an underproduction anemia caused by renal cortical loss. The anemia of kidney disease is usually normochromic and normocytic with a low reticulocyte count. Additionally, patients with kidney disease are prone to ulcer disease and angiodysplasia-induced gastrointestinal blood loss, resulting in a microcytic anemia. Patients with minor increases in serum creatinine levels may have reduced erythropoietin

| Finding | Type of Anemia | | |
	Inflammatory Anemia	IDA	IDA with Inflammation
MCV	72-100 fL	<85 fL	<100 fL
MCHC	<36 g/dL (360 g/L)	<32 g/dL (320 g/L)	<32 g/dL (320 g/L)
Serum iron	<60 µg/dL (10.7 µmol/L)	<60 µg/dL (10.7 µmol/L)	<60 µg/dL (10.6 µmol/L)
TIBC	<250 µg/dL (44.8 µmol/L)	>400 µg/dL (71.6 µmol/L)	<400 µg/dL (71.6 µmol/L)
TIBC saturation	2%-20%	<15% (usually <10%)	<15%
Ferritin	>35 ng/mL (35 mg/L)	<15 ng/mL (15 mg/L)	<100 ng/mL (100 mg/L)
Serum soluble transferrin receptor concentration	Normal	Increased	Increased
Stainable iron in bone marrow	Present	Absent	Absent

TABLE 10 Laboratory Characteristics of Inflammatory Anemia, Iron Deficiency Anemia (IDA), and IDA with inflammation

MCV = mean corpuscular volume; MCHC = mean corpuscular hemoglobin concentration; TIBC = total iron-binding capacity.

levels. Measurement of the serum erythropoietin level may be useful in confirming a diagnosis of underproduction anemia in patients with minimally elevated creatinine levels in whom the origin of anemia is uncertain. The peripheral blood smear in patients with uremia frequently shows "burr cells" or echinocytes (**Figure 10**).

National groups currently recommend a target hemoglobin level of 11 to 12 g/dL (110 to 120 g/L) for patients receiving dialysis. Recent evidence has shown an increase in morbidity and mortality in patients whose hemoglobin is maintained at a level higher than 12 g/dL (120 g/L). Most patients who receive dialysis will require supplemental erythropoietin as do many patients with anemia and less advanced renal disease.

The principal side effects of erythropoietin therapy include hypertension and thrombosis of arteriovenous fistulas. Additionally, an increase in cardiovascular events, including stroke and myocardial infarction, has been associated with hemoglobin increases of more than 1 g/dL (10 g/L) in a 2-week period. For erythropoietin to be effective, iron stores must be adequate. Current recommendations are to maintain a serum ferritin level of more than 100 ng/mL (100 mg/L), with an iron saturation of at least 20%. Patients with kidney disease have increased iron needs because of chronic blood loss and the need for freely available iron to achieve an adequate response to erythropoietin. Most patients receiving hemodialysis require intravenous iron to reach these target values. Although iron dextran has been used in the past as a form of parenteral iron, newer parenteral iron preparations, such as iron sucrose or ferric gluconate, are currently used instead. Although more than 95% of patients with anemia of chronic kidney disease respond to erythropoietin therapy, erythropoietin failure can result from folate deficiency, aluminum toxicity, inflammation, ongoing blood loss, or even iron overload. Patients with iron overload who are receiving

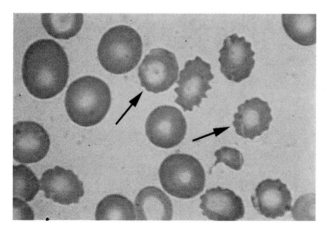

FIGURE 10.
Uremia with echinocytes.

dialysis can achieve better responses to erythropoietin if supplemental vitamin C is provided.

Darbepoetin, a newer U.S. Food and Drug Administration–approved erythropoiesis-stimulating protein, can be used in kidney disease as an alternative to erythropoietin. Darbepoetin has the potential advantage that it has a longer half-life than erythropoietin. Current guidelines suggest initiating darbepoetin weekly, with adjustments in dosage based on erythropoietic responses. There are insufficient data to recommend darbepoetin instead of erythropoietin or vice versa.

KEY POINTS

- The anemia associated with kidney disease is typically normochromic and normocytic.
- Supplemental erythropoietin corrects the anemia of kidney disease in more than 95% of patients.
- Darbepoetin, a newer U.S. Food and Drug Administration–approved erythropoiesis-stimulating protein with a longer half-life than erythropoietin, can be used in kidney disease as an alternative to erythropoietin.

Anemia Due to Peripheral Destruction of Erythrocytes or Blood Loss

Blood Loss

Severe acute blood loss not only decreases the ability to deliver oxygen to tissues, but it also results in blood volume loss, which can lead to circulatory failure and death. Circulatory compromise occurs when there is a loss of more than 20% of the blood volume, and a sudden loss of 50% of blood volume confers a significant risk for shock and death. Blood products and volume replacement are discussed in the Transfusion Medicine section.

Erythrocyte Destruction (Hemolytic Anemia)

Hemolysis may result from congenital hemoglobin abnormalities (hemoglobinopathies or thalassemia), erythrocyte membrane abnormalities (hereditary spherocytosis), or abnormalities of the enzymes required for erythrocyte metabolism (glucose-6-phosphate dehydrogenase deficiency [G6PD] deficiency). It may also be acquired as an immune process or through infection. Regardless of the cause, hemolytic anemia is characterized by increased destruction of erythrocytes that is usually, but not inevitably, associated with a bone marrow response (reticulocytosis). Elevated levels of unconjugated bilirubin, lactate dehydrogenase, and uric acid and depressed levels of haptoglobin are characteristic of hemolysis. The peripheral blood smear can help in evaluating erythrocyte shape to elucidate the cause of the hemolytic process. Patients with chronic hemolysis require supplemental folate. Patients with hemolytic anemia may have a worsening of anemia if infected with parvovirus B19 because of the suppression of erythrocyte production.

Microangiopathic Hemolytic Anemia

Microangiopathic hemolytic anemia is characterized by erythrocyte fragmentation that results from mechanical destruction by fibrin strands (see schistocytes as depicted in **Figure 11**). Thrombotic thrombocytopenic purpura (TTP) and hemolytic uremic syndrome (HUS) are two common causes of microangiopathic anemia that will be discussed below. Microangiopathic hemolysis also occurs in eclampsia and preeclampsia, with the presence of elevated liver chemistry tests representing the HELLP syndrome (defined as hemolysis with a microangiopathic blood smear, elevated liver enzymes, and a low platelet count). Microangiopathic hemolytic anemia is associated with diffuse intravascular coagulation, malignancy, snake envenomation, and exposure to some drugs, including ticlopidine and cyclosporine. This disorder may also occur in patients with mechanical heart valves, especially if the valve has become dysfunctional. Patients with microangiopathic hemolytic anemia or other forms of more pure intravascular hemolysis may become iron deficient, because the erythrocyte hemoglobin is excreted into the genitourinary tract as either hemoglobinuria or hemosiderinuria. These patients may also lack the elevated unconjugated bilirubin levels present in other forms of hemolysis.

Treatment of microangiopathic hemolytic anemia is specific to the underlying disorder and may involve cessation of the offending drugs or initiation of plasmapheresis in the case of TTP.

Autoimmune Hemolytic Anemia

Autoimmune hemolytic anemia (AIHA) may result from drugs, lymphoproliferative disorders, collagen vascular diseases, or malignancy; it is also frequently idiopathic. This condition occurs when autoantibodies of IgG, IgM, or, rarely, IgA, bind to erythrocyte antigens (**Table 11**).

The most common type of AIHA is warm antibody–mediated. In this condition, antibodies of the IgG class bind to Rh-type antigens on the erythrocyte surface at 37.0°C (98.6°F). Although these antibodies may fix complement, they more commonly bind to the erythrocyte surface and facilitate Fc-receptor–mediated erythrocyte destruction by splenic macrophages. Patients with warm antibody hemolytic anemia have microspherocytes on peripheral blood smear (**Figure 12**) and an increased reticulocyte count. Warm antibodies are diagnosed by the direct antiglobulin test (Coombs test), which detects IgG or complement on the erythrocyte surface. However, results of direct antiglobulin testing in 5% to 10% of patients with warm antibody AIHA may be normal. In these patients, the diagnosis is based on a high degree of clinical suspicion.

Drug-induced warm antibody hemolytic anemia is caused by the drug itself, the drug's metabolites, or an interaction between the drug and the erythrocyte membrane. These reactions are characterized by a positive direct antiglobulin test result; however, not all positive direct antiglobulin test results are indicative of hemolytic anemia, with positive results reported in approximately 1 in 10,000 healthy blood donors.

Warm antibody hemolytic anemia is typically treated initially with corticosteroids to decrease antibody production and the ability of the splenic macrophage to clear IgG- or complement-coated erythrocytes. The typical dosage consists of prednisone, 1 mg/kg/d, followed by a tapering dose. Approximately two thirds of patients with warm antibody hemolytic anemia respond to corticosteroids, with 20% achieving long-term remission. Splenectomy is considered for patients with recurrent disease or for those in whom hemolysis cannot be controlled with corticosteroids. This procedure results in increased hemoglobin levels in two thirds of patients with warm antibody hemolytic anemia, half of whom achieve a normal hemoglobin level. For patients unresponsive to corticosteroids and splenectomy, immunosuppressive therapy with chemotherapeutic agents, such as cyclophosphamide or azathioprine; the monoclonal antibody rituximab; danazol; and intravenous immune globulin; have been used with varying efficacy.

Cold agglutinin disease occurs as a result of IgM binding to erythrocytes at temperatures below 37.0 °C (98.6 °F). IgM antibodies recognize the carbohydrate I-antigen system and cause complement fixation, with the potential for intravascular hemolysis. In addition, Kupffer cells in the liver can clear complement-coated erythrocytes. The peripheral blood smear typically shows erythrocyte clumping and agglutination in cold agglutinin disease (**Figure 13**). As a result, spurious elevations in mean corpuscular volume and mean corpuscular hemoglobin concentration occur. Cold

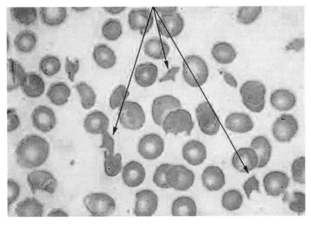

FIGURE 11.
Schistocytes in microangiopathic hemolytic anemia.

Reprinted with permission from the ASH Image Bank. Copyright 2009 American Society of Hematology; www.ashimagebank.org.

TABLE 11 Diagnosis and Management of Type of Autoimmune Hemolytic Anemia

Type of Anemia	Antibody	Antigen	Smear	Steroid Responsive	Splenectomy Appropriate
Warm Antibody	IgG	Rh	Spherocytes	Yes	Yes
Cold Agglutinin	IgM	I,i	Agglutination	No	No
PCH	IgG	P	Agglutination	Yes	No

PCH = paroxysmal cold hemoglobinuria.

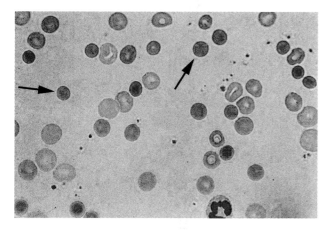

FIGURE 12.
Microspherocytes in a patient with warm antibody–induced hemolysis.

Reprinted with permission from the ASH Image Bank. Copyright 2009 American Society of Hematology; www.ashimagebank.org.

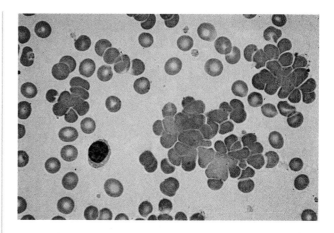

FIGURE 13.
Cold agglutinin disease.
Notice the red cell agglutination on the slide, which can lead to a spuriously large mean corpuscular volume on automated counters.

Reprinted with permission from the ASH Image Bank. Copyright 2009 American Society of Hematology; www.ashimagebank.org.

agglutinin disease does not respond to corticosteroids or splenectomy. Usually, the anemia in patients with cold agglutinin disease is mild. If hemolysis is severe, other immunosuppressive modalities, including alkylating agents such as cyclophosphamide or rituximab, may be helpful. Pheresis has also been suggested as a means to transiently decrease cold agglutinin titers, with varied responses described.

The least common type of AIHA in adults is paroxysmal cold hemoglobinuria, which occurs more commonly in children than adults. This disorder usually results from viral infection or syphilis. The Donath-Landsteiner antibody is an IgG antibody that binds to the erythrocyte P-antigen at temperatures less than 37.0 °C (98.6 °F) but causes complement-mediated hemolysis at body temperature. Special testing using paroxysmal nocturnal hemoglobinuria erythrocytes, with increased complement sensitivity, is required to establish this diagnosis. Paroxysmal cold hemoglobinuria usually responds to corticosteroid therapy.

Hereditary Spherocytosis
Hereditary spherocytosis, hereditary elliptocytosis, hereditary stomatocytosis, and pyropoikilocytosis are examples of congenital hemolytic anemias caused by abnormalities in erythrocyte membrane proteins. Of these conditions, hereditary spherocytosis is the most common, characterized by

spherocytic erythrocytes (**Figure 14**) with increased osmotic fragility owing to their large volume-to-surface–area ratio.

The clinical spectrum in patients with hereditary spherocytosis varies widely, ranging from the presence of no symptoms to significant hemolysis. Affected patients have splenomegaly and may develop leg ulcers and gallstones. Folate supplementation is important in patients with this

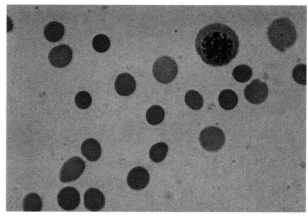

FIGURE 14.
Spherocytes in a patient with hereditary spherocytosis.

Reprinted with permission from the ASH Image Bank. Copyright 2009 American Society of Hematology; www.ashimagebank.org.

disorder as it is in patients with other types of hemolysis. Splenectomy can reduce the amount of hemolysis occurring in hereditary spherocytosis.

Other Causes of Hemolysis

Glucose-6-phosphate dehydrogenase (G6PD) deficiency is the most common enzyme erythrocyte defect. Various mutations in the gene coding for G6PD, carried on the X chromosome, have been described, including some with a severe dysfunctional G6PD enzyme and lifelong hemolysis. Patients with the more common G6PD mutation, found most commonly in blacks, functions adequately under normal conditions but may be unable to deal with additional oxidative stress caused by certain medications or some acute illnesses. Typically, patients with a G6PD deficiency present with anemia and signs of jaundice. The peripheral blood smear in these patients is remarkable for "bite cells," which are characterized by eccentrically located hemoglobin confined to one side of the cell (**Figure 15**). To confirm a diagnosis of G6PD deficiency, it is best to check G6PD levels 2 to 3 months after the hemolytic event occurs, rather than checking these levels immediately following the onset of hemolysis because reticulocytes tend to have increased G6PD activity when compared with older cells.

Paroxysmal nocturnal hemoglobinuria (PNH) is characterized by episodic hemolysis, bone marrow aplasia, and thrombosis. Erythrocytes from patients with PNH have increased susceptibility to complement-mediated lysis because of a lack of CD55 and CD59, two surface proteins that regulate the destructive effect of complement on circulating erythrocytes. Both of these proteins are anchored to the cell surface by glycosylphosphatidylinositol (GPI). Mutations in the *PIGA* gene, which encodes the enzyme involved in the first step of the synthesis of the GPI anchor, are associated with

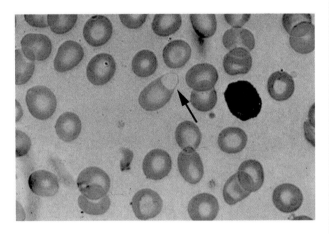

FIGURE 15.
Bite cells in a patient with glucose-6-phosphate dehydrogenase (G6PD) deficiency.

Reprinted with permission from the ASH Image Bank. Copyright 2009 American Society of Hematology; www.ashimagebank.org.

PNH. Because anemia is the major manifestation of PNH, corticosteroids are frequently used in these patients to reduce complement activation. More recently, eculizumab, a humanized monoclonal antibody to the C5 terminal complement component, has been shown to decrease transfusion requirements and improve the quality of life in patients with PNH. Thrombosis, especially in unusual locations such as the mesentery or portal vein, is another major problem for patients with PNH. A prospective study has suggested that patients with a large PNH clone (>50% PNH granulocytes) and no contraindications to anticoagulation have marked reduction in spontaneous thrombosis when treated with warfarin. Immunosuppressive therapy and bone marrow transplantation have both been used in younger patients with severe complications of PNH, such as aplastic anemia or unrelenting hemolysis.

KEY POINTS

- Microangiopathic hemolytic anemia is characterized by erythrocyte fragmentation.
- Warm antibody–mediated hemolytic anemia is characterized by microspherocytes on the peripheral blood smear and a positive Coombs test.
- Splenectomy is helpful in reducing hemolytic episodes in patients with hereditary spherocytosis.
- Paroxysmal nocturnal hemoglobinuria is characterized by hemolysis, thrombosis, and bone marrow aplasia.

Hemoglobin Disorders

Thalassemia

Hemoglobin is a tetrameric molecule encoded by genes on chromosomes 16 and 11. The two α-globin chains and two β-globin chains are linked to heme (iron and protoporphyrin) and reversibly bind one molecule of oxygen. The thalassemic syndromes result from defects in synthesis of the α or β chains and lead to ineffective erythropoiesis and intramedullary hemolysis. Patients with homozygous β-thalassemia have severe, lifelong anemia and require specialized care. Those with heterozygous thalassemia have milder anemia than those with homozygous thalassemia and may enter adult life without diagnosis. These gene defects are varied and include point gene mutations, unstable mRNA, gene-promoter region mutations, and gene deletions. These patients have splenomegaly and may develop pigment gallstones due to hemolysis. A low mean cellular volume and target cells on peripheral blood smear are also found in patients with thalassemia (**Figure 16**).

α-Thalassemia is prevalent in Africa, the Mediterranean, the Middle East, and Asia. Because there are four genes representing the α chain, several genotypes of α-thalassemia are possible. A single gene deletion (— α/αα) results in a silent

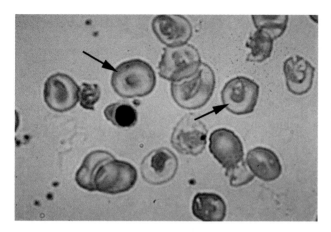

FIGURE 16.
Target cells in a patient with β-thalassemia major.

Reprinted with permission from the ASH Image Bank. Copyright 2009 American Society of Hematology; www.ashimagebank.org.

carrier state that is clinically normal. α-Thalassemia trait, characterized by the absence of two genes (— —/αα or —α/—α), leads to a mild microcytic anemia with a preserved or increased erythrocyte count. Because there is no substitution gene for an α gene, results of hemoglobin electrophoresis are normal in patients with the α-thalassemia trait. Hemoglobin H disease (γ_4) arises from a three-gene defect (— —/— α) and causes severe anemia and inadequate oxygen release, leading to hypoxia, heart failure, and death early in life. Hydrops fetalis results from homozygous inheritance of a double gene deletion (— —/— —) and is associated with fetal demise occurring at 30 to 40 weeks' gestation.

β-Thalassemia occurs most commonly among individuals from the Mediterranean, Southeast Asia, India, and Pakistan. This disorder is uncommon among Africans. β-Thalassemia is caused by various abnormalities in the β-gene complex. Decreased β-chain synthesis leads to impaired production of hemoglobin A ($\alpha_2\beta_2$) and resultant increased synthesis of hemoglobin A2 ($\alpha_2\delta_2$) and/or hemoglobin F ($\alpha_2\gamma_2$). Thalassemia major (Cooley anemia) is caused by the near absence of β-chain synthesis in homozygotes or compound heterozygotes, resulting in severe β-chain defects (β°). These patients experience severe growth retardation unless they receive blood transfusions early in life, in addition to skeletal complications and iron overload from facilitated iron absorption in the gut. Allogeneic bone marrow transplantation is a successful therapy for patients with thalassemia major. Patients with β-thalassemia intermedia (β+) have at least one partially functional β gene. These patients have anemia but usually do not require transfusions. Even without transfusion, iron overload can be a problem in thalassemic patients. Administration of inappropriate iron therapy in the mistaken belief that microcytic anemia is caused by iron deficiency compounds this problem. Patients with β-thalassemia trait (wt/β+) are asymptomatic despite a mild microcytic anemia.

Sickle Cell Syndromes

Hemoglobin S results from a single base substitution of the β gene. Patients homozygous for hemoglobin S have clinical manifestations relating to the ability of hemoglobin S to polymerize when deoxygenated. Patients with sickle cell trait are asymptomatic except for the presence of hematuria when they are dehydrated. Diagnosis of the sickle cell syndromes can be established by hemoglobin electrophoresis (**Table 12**). Most clinical findings in homozygous sickle cell disease (SS) are related to vasoocclusion from deformed sickled erythrocytes (**Figure 17**). Patients with vasoocclusive crisis present with severe pain in the arms, legs, chest, abdomen, and back and are managed with hydration, supplemental oxygen in the setting of hypoxia, and opiate analgesics. Complications of sickle cell anemia are listed in **Table 13**.

Meperidine is to be avoided in patients with sickle cell disease because it leads to the toxic buildup of the metabolite, normeperidine, which can lead to seizures. This mechanism

TABLE 12 Hemoglobin Electrophoresis Patterns For Various Sickle Cell Hemoglobinopathies

Disease	A (%)	A2 (%)	F (%)	S (%)	MCV
Normal	>97	<3.5	0	0	>80 fL
S trait	>50	<3.5	0	<50	>80 fL
SS	0	<3.5	<10	>90	>80 fL
Sβ+thal	10-30	>3.5	<20	>60	<75 fL
Sβ°thal	0	>3.5	<20	>80	<80 fL
SSαthal	0	<3.5	<10	>90	<75 fL
SC	0	50[a]	<5	50	<80 fL

MCV = mean corpuscular volume.

[a]Hemoglobin C runs as Hemoglobin A2 on alkaline electrophoresis gel.

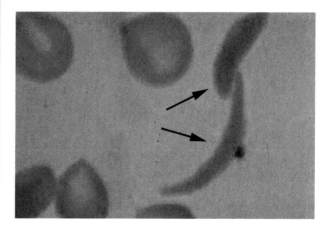

FIGURE 17.
Sickled erythrocytes.

Reprinted with permission from the ASH Image Bank. Copyright 2009 American Society of Hematology; www.ashimagebank.org.

TABLE 13 Major Complications of Sickle Cell Anemia

Complication	Notes
Acute chest syndrome (ACS) vs. pneumonia, fat embolism, VTE (venous thromboembolism)	ACS correlates with risk of pulmonary hypertension and is the most frequent cause of death. Associated with chlamydia, mycoplasma, respiratory syncytial virus, coagulase-positive *S. aureus*, *S. pneumoniae*, *Mycoplasma hominis*, parvovirus, and rhinovirus infections (in decreasing order of frequency). Pneumonia is usually a localized infiltration, whereas ACS is usually characterized by diffuse pulmonary infiltrates. Cultures of bronchial washings or deep sputum are usually positive in pneumonia. Fat embolism presents with chest pain, fever, dyspnea, hypoxia, thrombocytopenia, and multiorgan failure. Fat embolism is also a component of the ACS, and it is usually associated with acute painful episodes. It is best differentiated by the presence of fat bodies in bronchial washings or in deep sputum and by multiorgan involvement (e.g., stroke, renal failure). Presence of lower extremity thrombophlebitis may differentiate VTE from ACS, but in some cases pulmonary arteriography may be needed. Newer contrast agents may be safer than hypertonic contrast agents, which precipitate intravascular sickling.
Avascular necrosis	Involving hips and shoulders; may require surgery. More common in sickle-α-thalassemia than in other sickle cell syndromes.
Cerebrovascular accidents	Occurs in 8%-17% of patients. Infarction is most common in children and hemorrhage is most common in adults. Brain imaging and lumbar puncture establish the diagnosis.
Cholecystitis vs. hepatic crisis	Chronic hemolysis may result in gallstones and acute cholecystitis. Fever, right upper quadrant pain and elevated aminotransferase levels may also be due to sickle cell–related ischemic hepatic crisis; abdominal ultrasonography can help differentiate.
Dactylitis vs. osteomyelitis	A painful, usually symmetrical, swelling of hands or feet, erythema, and low-grade fever. More common in children before age 5. Osteomyelitis usually involves one bone.
Heart failure	Related to pulmonary and systemic hypertension and ischemia.
Infection	Related to functional asplenia.
Leg ulcers	Most common in HbS disease.
Liver disease	Viral hepatitis and/or iron overload from transfusions and ischemic–induced hepatic crisis.
Pain syndrome vs. myocardial infarction (MI), appendicitis	Sickle pain crisis involving the chest may suggest acute MI. The quality of pain of MI (central pressure) is different from that of sickle cell pain (sharp, pleuritic). Serial determination of cardiac enzymes will differentiate the two. Abdominal pain, fever, and leukocytosis may suggest appendicitis. A high level of lactate dehydrogenase and normal bowel sounds support sickle cell pain syndrome.
Priapism	Prolonged or repeated episodes may cause impotence.
Proteinuria and renal failure	Prevalence of proteinuria and renal failure is approximately 25% and 5%, respectively.
Pulmonary hypertension	Risk of development correlates with increasing age and history of acute chest syndrome.
Retinopathy	More common in patients with compound heterozygosity for HbSC.
Sickle anemia vs. aplastic crisis, hyperhemolysis	Anemia that decreases by ≥2 g/dL during a painful crisis could be due to aplastic crisis or hyperhemolysis. Aplastic crisis could be due to coexistent infection (e.g., parvovirus B19), cytotoxic drugs, or could be idiopathic. Hyperhemolysis could be due to infection (i.e., mycoplasma), transfusion reaction, or coexistent glucose-6-phosphate dehydrogenase deficiency. The reticulocyte count is decreased with aplastic crisis and increased with hyperhemolysis. Bilirubin, lactic dehydrogenase, and aminotransferase levels are elevated in hyperhemolysis.
Splenomegaly and splenic sequestration	Common in children <5 years who afterwards manifest asplenia from splenic infarction. Patients with HbSC often have splenomegaly persisting into adulthood.

HbS = hemoglobin S; HbSC = hemoglobin SC.

is due in part to decreased renal clearance of normeperidine in patients with sickle cell disease. Some patients with SS have a chronic pain syndrome that can be managed with long-acting opiate analgesics.

Patients with sickle cell disease are at increased risk for stroke. Acute stroke is managed with erythrocyte exchange to reduce the percentage of hemoglobin S to less than 30%, with a target hemoglobin concentration of 10 g/dL (100 g/L).

Patients with a history of stroke have a high incidence of recurrent stroke, which can be reduced with monthly simple blood transfusions. However, monthly transfusions may be complicated by iron overload, alloimmunization, and issues of compliance.

Sickle chest syndrome is characterized by hypoxia, pulmonary infiltrates on chest radiograph, pain, and dyspnea in a patient with a sickling disorder. Acute chest syndrome may be caused by infection, in situ thrombosis, fat emboli, or a combination of these events. Management of patients with acute chest syndrome includes exchange transfusion to decrease the percentage of hemoglobin S. In addition, antibiotics, supplemental oxygen, and intravenous hydration may be necessary as clinically indicated. Incentive spirometry may be useful in patients with sickle cell crisis to prevent the sickle chest syndrome.

Pulmonary hypertension has been described as a major cause of morbidity and mortality in patients with SS. These patients present with signs and symptoms of right heart failure. There is no consensus as to the proper management of patients with sickle cell disease and pulmonary hypertension, other than to treat the resultant heart failure.

Severe anemia from aplastic crisis in a patient with SS is usually caused by infection with parvovirus B19. This virus is usually a self-limited infection in patients with normal immune function, lasting several days. The classic symptoms of parvovirus B19 infection include rash or arthralgia, occurring in 25% of infected patients. Half of patients with this infection have nonspecific flu-like symptoms, whereas one quarter of patients are asymptomatic during infection.

Because of the long erythrocyte life span in healthy persons (120 days), anemia is not typical of patients with parvovirus B19 infection. However, owing to the shortened erythrocyte life span in patients with hemolytic disorders, anemia in such patients can be profound and may require transfusion support. In patients with sickle cell disease who are not taking supplemental folate therapeutic regimens, severe anemia may also result from folate deficiency.

Nearly a decade ago, hydroxyurea was shown to decrease the number of painful crises in sickle cell disease by increasing levels of fetal hemoglobin. More recently, hydroxyurea also has been shown to improve mortality in patients with SS. Hydroxyurea therapy at 35 mg/kg/d may also help to prevent stroke in patients who are not candidates for monthly erythrocyte transfusions. Hydroxyurea is generally well tolerated, but care should be used in women of childbearing age owing to its potential teratogenicity. However, its role in preventing pulmonary hypertension is unclear.

Patients with sickle cell disease need routine medical follow up plus annual influenza vaccinations, periodic pneumococcal vaccines, and annual eye examinations. Although guidelines have not been firmly established, it is not unreasonable to also vaccinate these patients against other encapsulated organisms, including *Haemophilus influenzae* and *Neisseria meningitidis*.

Erythrocyte transfusions must be given with care in patients with sickle cell disease. These transfusions are associated with iron overload; in some patients, "hyperhemolysis" occurs due to alloimmune responses to erythrocyte antigens, which leads to a delayed transfusion reaction characterized by hyperbilirubinemia and anemia. Patients typically present with jaundice and signs and symptoms of anemia. In addition, erythrocyte transfusions that result in a hemoglobin level of 10 g/dL (100 g/L) can increase blood viscosity and potentially cause thrombotic complications. If needed, transfused blood should be sickle-trait negative and does not need to be irradiated.

In addition to homozygosity for hemoglobin S, patients with sickle cell disease may possess compound heterozygosity for hemoglobin C, hemoglobin E, or the thalassemias. In general, these patients have less-severe disease than patients who are homozygous for hemoglobin S. However, patients with hemoglobin SC disease have greater ophthalmologic and orthopedic complications, including avascular necrosis of the hip, than patients with SS.

KEY POINTS

- Results of hemoglobin electrophoresis are normal in patients with α-thalassemia trait.
- Patients with β-thalassemia have increased levels of hemoglobin A2 and fetal hemoglobin.
- Administration of inappropriate iron therapy in the mistaken belief that microcytic anemia in thalassemic patients is caused by iron deficiency compounds iron overload issues.
- Hydroxyurea improves mortality and decreases painful crisis in patients with SS disease.

Iron Overload Syndromes

Hemochromatosis

Hemochromatosis is a genetic disease characterized by increased absorption of iron from the gut. It is an autosomal-recessive disease occurring in 1 of 200 persons of Northern European descent. The major gene responsible for most inherited cases of hemochromatosis, *HFE*, has been cloned. The HFE protein interacts with the transferrin receptor, bone morphogenic protein, and other proteins to modulate hepcidin production, which regulates the amount of iron absorbed from the gut. A G→A mutation in HFE at nucleotide 845, leading to a substitution of tyrosine for cysteine at residue 282 (C282Y); and a G→C mutation at nucleotide 187, leading to a substitution of aspartic acid for histidine at residue 63 (H63D), are the two most common mutations associated with hemochromatosis.

Ninety percent of patients with clinical hemochromatosis are homozygous for *C282Y*. In contrast, evidence of iron overload develops in few patients who are heterozygous for *C282Y*. Some patients who are homozygous for *H63D* develop clinical iron overload, and those with compound heterozygosity for *C282Y* and *H63D* develop mild iron overload. Other iron-related genes, including those for hepcidin, ferroportin, transferrin receptor 2, and hemojuvelin, may influence the penetrance of hemochromatosis.

Clinically, hemochromatosis is associated with skin bronzing, hepatomegaly, liver failure, heart failure, and iron overload–induced diabetes mellitus. Early signs and symptoms, including myalgia and arthralgia, chronic fatigue, abdominal pain, and mild elevation of liver enzymes, should prompt evaluation for hemochromatosis. Typically, early hemochromatosis is characterized by a mild elevation in aminotransferase levels. Therefore, hemochromatosis should be considered in patients with a family history of cirrhosis and aminotransferase elevations. In addition to liver failure, cirrhosis from iron overload carries a significant risk for hepatocellular carcinoma. Patients with untreated hemochromatosis may also die of heart failure–related complications. Arthropathy, most commonly affecting the wrists and metacarpal joints, may also occur (see MKSAP 15 Rheumatology).

The initial step in the evaluation of patients in whom hemochromatosis is suspected is measurement of serum transferrin saturation, the most sensitive measure for detecting this disease. Levels higher than 60% for men and 50% for women increase the clinical suspicion for this disease. Serum ferritin levels are a surrogate for tissue iron stores, and values greater than 1000 ng/mL (1000 mg/L) are suggestive of iron overload in the absence of inflammation. Establishing a definitive diagnosis of iron overload requires liver biopsy to obtain quantitative iron measurements. Newer technologies, such as MRI and superconductive quantum interference device (SQUID) measurements, are being investigated as techniques less invasive than liver biopsy in the diagnosis of iron overload. Genetic testing may be useful to confirm the diagnosis of hemochromatosis and for family screening. The role of population-based screening for hemochromatosis remains unclear. In 2005, the American College of Physicians published guidelines for hemochromatosis screening (www.acponline.org/ clinical/guidelines). These guidelines are summarized as follows:

1. There is insufficient evidence to recommend for or against screening for hereditary hemochromatosis in the general population.

2. In case-finding for hereditary hemochromatosis, serum ferritin and transferrin saturation tests should be performed.

3. Physicians should discuss the risks, benefits, and limitations of genetic testing in patients with a positive family history of hereditary hemochromatosis or those with an elevated serum ferritin or transferrin saturation level.

Secondary Iron Overload

Initial treatment of patients with hemochromatosis consists of phlebotomy to remove excess iron. Each unit of blood contains 200 to 250 milligrams of iron. Phlebotomy can initially be performed weekly or twice weekly and should continue until serum ferritin levels are less than 50 ng/mL (50 mg/ L). Phlebotomy in patients with hemochromatosis who have not yet developed cardiomyopathy or cirrhosis will prevent these complications. Conversely, this therapy is much less effective when performed after end organ damage has occurred.

Secondary iron overload occurs in heavily transfused patients and, occasionally, in patients with thalassemia in the absence of transfusion. Management of these patients is difficult because iron overload typically occurs in the setting of anemia. Deferoxamine is a parenteral iron chelator that is administered by nightly continuous infusion (25 to 50 mg/ kg). Recently, deferasirox, an oral iron chelator, has become available for the treatment of secondary iron overload. Deferasirox is generally well tolerated. Serious, but rare, side effects include renal failure and agranulocytosis.

KEY POINTS

- The most common gene abnormalities in hemochromatosis are *C282Y* and *H63D*, two mutations in the *HFE* gene.
- Early hemochromatosis is typically characterized by a mild elevation in aminotransferase levels.
- Phlebotomy is the initial treatment of patients with hemochromatosis.
- Iron chelation is indicated for patients with secondary iron overload.

Erythrocytosis

Erythrocytosis may be induced by polycythemia vera, discussed elsewhere (see Hematopoietic Stem Cells and Their Disorders chapter), in addition to other causes (**Table 14**). In the past, determination of the red blood cell mass has been recommended in the diagnosis of polycythemia vera. This test is difficult to obtain, expensive to perform, and inaccurate in inexperienced hands. An appropriate first step in establishing the cause of erythrocytosis is to measure the serum erythropoietin level.

Erythropoietin is regulated at the level of transcription by hypoxic induction factor-1α (HIF-1α). HIF-1α is normally degraded in the proteosome through its interaction with the von Hippel-Lindau (VHL) protein. Erythropoietin levels may be elevated in patients with renal tumors that produce mutated VHL proteins, which are unable to bind to HIF-1α and result in HIF-1α degradation. Less commonly, erythropoietin may be elevated in patients with renovascular disease, polycystic kidney disease, or other renal disease and will be suppressed in polycythemia vera.

Polycythemia vera is the likely diagnosis in patients with erythrocytosis and an erythropoietin level of less than 5 mU/mL (5 U/L), leukocytosis, thrombocytosis, and splenomegaly. Although the presence of the *JAK2* mutation would further corroborate the diagnosis, testing for this

TABLE 14 Causes of Secondary Erythrocytosis

Cause	Symptoms or Findings
Gaisbock syndrome	Hypertension, plethora, decreased plasma volume
Tumors	Pheochromocytoma, hepatic, uterine leiomyoma, cerebellar hemangiomas, kidney
High altitude	Relative hypoxia
Pulmonary and cardiac disease	Relative hypoxia
Mutant high-affinity hemoglobin	Shift in oxygen saturation curve
Congenital polycythemia	VHL mutations
von Hippel-Lindau syndrome	VHL mutations
Post renal transplantation	Increased angiotensin II concentration

VHL = von Hippel-Lindau syndrome.

mutation is expensive and of uncertain value if the diagnosis is already established. If the erythropoietin level is low, no *JAK2* mutation is identified, and a family history of erythrocytosis exists, a mutation in the erythropoietin receptor that renders it constitutively active may be present. In contrast, in patients in whom the erythropoietin level is greater than 5 mU/mL (5 U/L) decreased arterial pulse oxygen saturation should lead to a presumptive diagnosis of cardiac or pulmonary disease. Some patients with chronic pulmonary conditions such as sleep apnea may have intermittent oxygen desaturation that is significant enough to prompt erythrocytosis. Otherwise, erythropoietin-producing tumors, or a high-affinity hemoglobinopathy, should be suspected, the latter of which is likely to occur in young, otherwise-healthy patients with erythrocytosis. At least half of these hemoglobin mutations have a normal electrical charge and, therefore, are represented by normal results on hemoglobin electrophoresis. Of particular note is erythrocytosis occurring after renal transplantation, which is believed to be secondary to increased erythroid sensitivity to angiotensin II and increased production of erythropoietin in the native kidney. Postrenal transplant erythrocytosis usually responds to angiotensin-converting enzyme inhibitor therapy. Mild erythrocytosis has been described in the setting of reduced plasma volume. "Relative" erythrocytosis occurs in patients who typically are obese, hypertensive, and smoke cigarettes. Whether such erythrocytosis is related to tobacco smoke–induced elevations in carboxyhemoglobin levels, which leads to increased hemoglobin oxygen avidity, is uncertain.

Patients with erythrocytosis caused by ectopic erythropoietin production, like patients with polycythemia vera, should undergo phlebotomy, with a target hemoglobin concentration of 15 g/dL (150 g/L), in preparation for definitive treatment to eliminate the cause of excess erythropoietin, or as maintenance therapy if no other treatment is feasible. Deciding whether to perform phlebotomy is more complicated in patients with secondary erythrocytosis caused by hypoxic pulmonary disease or cyanotic heart disease, but this procedure should only be performed in patients whose hemoglobin level is significantly elevated (>18 g/dL [180 g/L]) and in those with heart failure and volume overload. Patients with erythrocytosis caused by an oxygen-avid hemoglobinopathy or with erythrocytosis who live at high altitude do not seem to have any adverse risk and require no treatment.

KEY POINTS

- Low serum erythropoietin levels help to distinguish polycythemia vera from secondary forms of erythrocytosis.
- Postrenal transplant erythrocytosis responds to angiotensin-converting enzyme inhibitor therapy.
- Patients with erythrocytosis caused by ectopic erythropoietin production should undergo phlebotomy.

Bibliography

Andrews NC. Anemia of inflammation: the cytokine-hepcidin link. J Clin Invest. 2004;113:1251-1253. [PMID: 15124013]

Brissot P, de Bels F. Current approaches to the management of hemochromatosis. Hematology Am Soc Hematol Educ Program. 2006:36-41. [PMID: 17124037]

Charache S, Terrin ML, Moore RD, et. al. Effect of hydroxyurea on the painful crisis in sickle cell anemia. Investigators of the Multicenter Study of Hydroxyurea in Sickle Cell Anemia. N Engl J Med. 1995;332:1317-22. [PMID: 7715639]

Cohen AR. New advances in iron chelation therapy. Hematology Am Soc Hematol Educ Program. 2006:42-47. [PMID: 17124038]

Eussen SJ, de Groot LC, Clarke R, et al. Oral cyanocobalamin supplementation in older people with vitamin B12 deficiency: a dose-finding trial. Arch Intern Med. 2005;165:1167-1172. [PMID: 15911731]

Ganz T. Hepcidin and its role in regulating systemic iron metabolism. Hematology An Soc Hematol Educ Program. 2006;29-35,507. [PMID: 17124036]

Ganz T. Molecular pathogenesis of anemia of chronic disease. Pediatr Blood Cancer. 2006;46(5):554-557. [PMID: 16261603]

Hall C, Richards S, Hillmen P. Primary prophylaxis with warfarin prevents thrombosis in paroxysmal nocturnal hemoglobinuria (PNH). Blood. 2002;102:3587-3591. [PMID: 12893760]

Hill A, Hillmen P, Richards SJ, et al. Sustained response and long-term safety of eculizumab in paroxysmal nocturnal hemoglobinuria. Blood. 2005;106:2559-2565. [PMID: 15985537]

Keven K, Kutlay S, Nergizoglu G, Erturk S. Randomized crossover study of the effect of vitamin C on EPO response in hemodialysis patients. Am J Kidney Dis 2003;41(6):1233-9. [PMID: 12776276]

Pakasama S, Hongeng S, Chaisiripoomkere W, Chuansumrit A, Sirachainun N, Jootar S. Allogeneic peripheral blood stem cell transplantation in children with homozygous beta-thalassemia and severe beta-thalassemia/hemoglobin E disease. J Pediatr Hematol Oncol 2004;26(4):248-252. [PMID: 15087953]

Qaseem A, Aronson M, Fitterman N, Snow V, Weiss KB, Owens DK; Clinical Efficacy Assessment Subcommittee of the American College of Physicians. Screening for Hereditary Hemochromatosis: A Clinical Practice Guideline from the American College of Physicians. Ann Intern Med. 2005;143(7):517-521. [PMID: 16204164]

Silverstein SB, Rodgers SM. Parenteral iron therapy options. Am J Hematol. 2004;76(1):74-78. [PMID: 15114602]

Solomon LR. Disorders of cobalamin (vitamin B12) metabolism: emerging concepts in pathophysiology, diagnosis, and treatment. Blood Rev. 2007;21(3):113-130. [PMID: 16814909]

Ting RZ, Szeto CC, Chan MH, Ma KK, Chow KM. Risk factors of vitamin B(12) deficiency in patients receiving metformin. Arch Intern Med. 2006;166(18):1975-1979. [PMID: 17030830]

Transfusion Medicine

Antigens and Alloimmunization in Blood Transfusion

More than 20 blood group systems have been identified to date. The most important groups in determining transfusion compatibility are the ABO group and the Rh group. ABO antibodies develop after infancy and are mostly IgM, which binds complement and may lead to intravascular hemolysis. An individual's erythrocytes express A antigen only (group A), B antigen only (group B), neither antigen (group O), or both A and B antigens (group AB). An individual's plasma contains antibodies against the A or B antigen that are not present on his/her erythrocytes. Rh antigens are transmembrane proteins that are present on erythrocytes. One of these antigens, the Rh(D) antigen, is highly immunogenic and induces IgG anti-D antibody formation in most Rh(D)-negative individuals exposed either from pregnancy or the transfusion of Rh(D)-positive erythrocytes.

Alloimmunization (the development of antibodies to foreign erythrocyte antigens) develops in about 10% of transfused patients. The frequency of alloimmunization increases with the number of units transfused. The prevalence may be as high as 30% to 40% in patients who require chronic transfusions. The consequences of alloimmunization range from a delay in finding compatible blood for transfusion to development of delayed hemolytic transfusion reactions.

Transfusion Compatibility

Pretransfusion compatibility testing begins with typing (ABO/Rh determination) and screening (detection of non-ABO antibodies). If an erythrocyte transfusion is needed, the crossmatch can be done quickly by using the patient's serum or plasma and a representative sample from an ABO/Rh-compatible donor unit. Verification of patient identity at the bedside prior to administration is a critical final step in safe transfusion.

If a patient needs an emergency transfusion, group O erythrocyte units and group AB plasma units are used until the ABO/Rh type can be determined. Group O erythrocytes can be transfused to anyone, because there are no A or B antigens on these cells to react with anti-A or anti-B hemagglutinins. Similarly, group AB plasma can be transfused to anyone because it contains no hemagglutinins to react with A or B antigens. Rh-positive patients can safely receive either Rh(D)-positive or Rh(D)-negative blood, but Rh-negative patients must receive Rh(D)-negative blood to avoid alloimmunization. This is especially a concern for women of childbearing potential in order to prevent formation of anti-D antibodies, leading to severe hemolytic disease of the newborn.

Platelets are generally transfused without regard to ABO compatibility, but, rarely, hemagglutinins in platelet-rich plasma may cause self-limited hemolysis. Because Rh-negative platelets are in short supply, Rh immunoprophylaxis should be considered in Rh-negative women of childbearing age who are transfused with Rh-positive platelets if the platelets contain more than 2 mL of donor erythrocytes. Certain patients have a higher risk for alloimmunization. Patients with sickle cell disease can form multiple alloantibodies. Providing donor units that are matched for the patient's Rh and other blood group antigens helps to prevent alloimmunization. Patients with warm autoimmune hemolytic anemia often have positive crossmatches because the autoantibody reacts with both the donor's and the patient's erythrocytes. "Incompatible" transfusion for these patients can provide critically needed oxygen-carrying capacity until medical therapy becomes effective or splenectomy is performed.

KEY POINTS

- Alloimmunization (the development of antibodies to foreign erythrocyte antigens) is common in transfused patients.
- Rh-positive patients can safely receive Rh(D)–positive or Rh(D)–negative blood, but Rh-negative patients must receive Rh(D)–negative blood to avoid alloimmunization.
- Compatibility testing may be deferred by using group O erythrocytes and group AB plasma for patients with emergent massive bleeding, and "incompatible" blood may be life-saving when transfused in patients with autoimmune hemolysis and severe anemia.

Blood Products

Erythrocytes, platelets, plasma, and cryoprecipitate may be transfused. Before being transfused, donor erythrocytes and platelets can be modified to make the blood safer for the recipient. Leukoreduction involves removal of greater than 99% of leukocytes by filtration or platelet apheresis to reduce the incidence of febrile reactions, cytomegalovirus transmission, and HLA alloimmunization. Irradiation is required to prevent transfusion-associated graft-versus-host disease, and washing removes plasma and is useful when transfusing patients who have recurrent allergic reactions.

Transfusion of one unit of packed erythrocytes should raise the hemoglobin level by 1 g/dL (10 g/L) in a non-bleeding average-sized adult. Transfusion is rarely needed for patients with a hemoglobin level above 10 g/dL (100 g/L). In a randomized controlled study of threshold hemoglobin levels in patients in intensive care units, patients who did not have acute bleeding or coronary ischemia did as well after transfusion at a threshold hemoglobin level of 7 g/dL (70 g/L) as those transfused at a threshold level of 10 g/dL (100 g/L). Patients with a hemoglobin level of 8 to 10 g/dL (80 to 100 g/L) who do not have active coronary ischemia generally tolerate anemia, and the decision to transfuse these patients should be individualized.

Platelets can be obtained from a whole blood donation or collected by apheresis. Randomized studies of patients with cancer have shown that a prophylactic transfusion for a platelet threshold count of 10,000/µL (10 × 10^9/L) is as safe as a count of 20,000/µL (20 × 10^9/L) if the patient is not febrile or bleeding. A platelet count of 50,000/µL (50 × 10^9/L) is generally considered adequate for patients undergoing most surgical procedures, although a count of 100,000/µL (100 × 10^9/L) is recommended for those who require central nervous system surgery. A bag of apheresis platelets provides a platelet dose that is equivalent to four to six units of platelet concentrate and raises the platelet count of an average-sized adult by 20,000 to 25,000/µL (20 to 25 × 10^9/L). An inadequate platelet increment after platelet transfusion may point to conditions that cause increased platelet consumption, such as fever and sepsis, or may indicate the development of antibodies to antigens expressed on platelets.

Plasma should be transfused only to replace coagulation factor proteins. Common indications for plasma transfusion include warfarin reversal in anticoagulated patients with serious or life-threatening bleeding and correction of dilutional coagulopathy in patients requiring massive transfusion.

Cryoprecipitate is a fraction of plasma that contains mostly fibrinogen. For adult patients who require fibrinogen replacement (usually patients with disseminated intravascular coagulation), 8 to 10 units of cryoprecipitate obtained from multiple donors are pooled to obtain an effective dose. Although cryoprecipitate contains von Willebrand factor and factor VIII, patients who need replacement of these factors should receive specific factor concentrates if at all possible.

KEY POINTS

- Erythrocyte transfusion is rarely needed for patients with a hemoglobin level above 10 g/dL (100 g/L).
- The need for erythrocyte transfusion should be individualized for patients with a hemoglobin level of 8 to 10 g/dL (80 to 100 g/L) because the risk of organ ischemia is low in these patients.
- Platelet transfusion is seldom needed for surgical patients with a platelet count greater than 50,000/µL (50 × 10^9/L).

Adverse Transfusion-related Events

Acute and Delayed Hemolytic Transfusion Reactions

The incidence of acute hemolytic transfusion reactions (within 24 hours of transfusion) is about 1/18,000 units transfused, and the mortality rate is approximately 1/600,000 units transfused. The leading cause of fatal transfusion reactions is inadvertent transfusion of ABO-incompatible erythrocytes, which is almost always due to a breakdown in safeguard systems rather than to an incompatible antibody that was not detected during laboratory testing. In an acute reaction, complement activation and cytokine generation cause hypotension, renal failure, and disseminated intravascular coagulation. Supportive treatment includes intravenous hydration and inotropic support as needed.

The incidence of delayed hemolytic transfusion reactions (within 7 to 14 days of transfusion) is about 1/5000 units transfused. A delayed reaction is characterized by fever, jaundice, and an unexplained decrease in the hemoglobin level. Results of laboratory studies are consistent with hemolysis. A delayed hemolytic transfusion reaction can mimic a sickle cell crisis in patients with sickle cell disease. The reaction is generally self-limited, but the identification of the implicated alloantibody is important to avoid future reactions.

Transfusion-related Acute Lung Injury

Transfusion-related acute lung injury (TRALI) is characterized by dyspnea, hypoxemia, and diffuse pulmonary infiltrates on chest radiographs that occur within 6 hours of transfusion in the absence of circulatory overload. The incidence is approximately 1/5000 units transfused, and the mortality rate is approximately 5%. Plasma is the blood component that is most often implicated in TRALI. Donor leukocyte antibodies bind to the corresponding antigens on recipient neutrophils, which then sequester in the lungs. This binding process can take several weeks, and the diagnosis of TRALI is therefore usually made on clinical grounds.

TRALI must be differentiated from acute respiratory distress syndrome (ARDS) and circulatory overload. Although the clinical features of TRALI are consistent with features of ARDS, recovery occurs more quickly in patients with TRALI than those with ARDS. Differentiating between TRALI and transfusion-associated circulatory overload can sometimes be difficult. However, a serum B-natriuretic peptide level was useful in one study as a diagnostic marker of circulatory overload. Patients at the extremes of age are particularly at risk for circulatory overload; diuretic treatment is indicated if this complication is suspected. Patients with TRALI generally recover after 3 or 4 days of ventilatory support.

Sepsis

Platelets, which are stored at room temperature, are especially susceptible to bacterial contamination from inadequate donor skin disinfection or unrecognized donor bacteremia. Screening for bacterial contamination of platelets has been standard practice in the United States since 2004. If bacterial contamination is suspected, both the patient's blood and the implicated component should be cultured. Erythrocyte units may rarely be contaminated with gram-negative bacteria such as *Yersinia* species. These bacteria may be present in very dilute concentration in the blood of asymptomatic donors but can readily proliferate in an iron-rich medium at cold temperatures and result in transfusion-related sepsis.

Febrile Nonhemolytic Transfusion Reactions

Fever during or immediately after a transfusion occurs in 0.3% of transfusions and can be the only sign of a hemolytic transfusion reaction. Therefore, if a patient becomes febrile during a transfusion, the transfusion must be stopped until a hemolytic reaction can be ruled out. If hemolysis is excluded, the most likely cause is the presence of donor leukocytes or cytokines in donor plasma. The treatment consists of antipyretics and consideration of leukoreduced components for future transfusions.

Allergic Reactions and Anaphylaxis

Allergic reactions occur in 1% of transfusions and range from the appearance of limited wheals to the development of diffuse urticaria with or without bronchospasm. Mild allergic reactions typically develop when patients receive plasma-rich blood components and generally do not recur during subsequent transfusions. Giving an antihistamine before a transfusion is reasonable for patients who have already had one or two mild allergic reactions. Patients with multiple recurrent allergic reactions should be transfused with washed erythrocytes or platelets, although washing reduces the effectiveness of platelet transfusions.

Anaphylaxis after transfusion occurs in 1/50,000 transfusions and is often attributable to IgA deficiency in the recipient. If anti-IgA antibody is present in the context of severe IgA deficiency in a patient requiring a transfusion, using blood components from IgA-deficient donors may prevent anaphylaxis.

Transfusion-associated Graft-Versus-Host Disease

Transfusion-associated graft-versus-host disease (GVHD) is a rare but fatal complication in which donor lymphocytes in erythrocytes or platelets engraft in an immunocompromised recipient and cause reactions that affect the bone marrow, skin, liver, and gastrointestinal tract. At-risk patients include those undergoing chemotherapy, recipients of blood components from first-degree relatives, and premature infants. Transfusion-associated GVHD is prevented by gamma irradiation of cellular blood components in at-risk populations. Immunodeficient patients require irradiated cellular blood components indefinitely whenever transfusions are needed.

KEY POINTS

- Erythrocyte alloantibodies (other than ABO antibodies) may cause a delayed hemolytic reaction that typically occurs 7 to 14 days after transfusion.
- Bacterial contamination of donor platelets is the most common cause of transfusion-related sepsis.
- If a patient develops a fever during a transfusion, the transfusion must be stopped until a hemolytic reaction can be ruled out.
- Fatal transfusion-associated graft-versus-host disease is prevented by gamma irradiation of cellular blood components.

Massive Transfusion

Massive transfusion consists of one total blood volume, which is equivalent to 8 to 10 units of blood, within a 24-hour period. Massive transfusion is required in trauma, ruptured aortic aneurysm, and severe gastrointestinal bleeding. When whole blood is lost and replaced with crystalloid and packed erythrocytes, a dilutional coagulopathy may develop that is often exacerbated by hypotension, hypothermia, and acidosis. The platelet count, prothrombin time, and activated partial thromboplastin time should be monitored in patients receiving massive transfusion, and additional transfusions of platelets or fresh frozen plasma should be given if bleeding persists and coagulopathy is documented. As patients are resuscitated, they need to be monitored for electrolyte disturbances such as hypocalcemia, hyperkalemia, or hypokalemia, and metabolic alkalosis.

- Transfusion of 8 to 10 units of blood within a 24-hour period may result in a dilutional coagulopathy that is often exacerbated by hypotension, hypothermia, and acidosis.

Strategies to Minimize Allogeneic Transfusions

Donor Screening

Allogeneic blood donors in the United States undergo screening to provide a history of any high-risk behaviors and to test for transfusion-transmissible diseases. Testing is done for hepatitis B and C, HIV infection, human T-lymphotropic virus (HTLV) infection, West Nile virus infection, and syphilis. The estimated risk for viral disease transmission is 1 in 2 million transfusion units for HIV, 1 in 1.5 million units for hepatitis C, and 1 in 100,000 units for hepatitis B. Donor testing for *Trypanosoma cruzi* (the protozoan causing Chagas disease) has also recently become available.

Recombinant Erythropoietin

The use of recombinant erythropoietin for patients with chronic renal failure who require dialysis has virtually eliminated the need for transfusion in these patients. Erythropoietin may also be used to treat patients in earlier stages of chronic kidney disease, who typically have less severe anemia. A recent study showed that the hemoglobin level in these patients should be maintained at no higher than 11 to 12 g/dL (110 to 120 g/L).

Recombinant erythropoietin has also reduced the need for transfusion in cancer patients undergoing chemotherapy. However, several recent randomized clinical trials have reported that patients with head and neck cancer and metastatic breast cancer who received erythropoietin had decreased survival compared with controls.

Autologous Blood Transfusion

The need for allogeneic blood transfusions in patients undergoing elective surgery can be minimized by optimizing preoperative hemoglobin levels and using autologous blood donations. Achieving optimal hemoglobin levels should be part of an overall strategy to minimize the need for allogeneic transfusion. Preoperative autologous blood donation has been used for many years to reduce the risks associated with allogeneic transfusion. However, clerical errors, volume overload, and bacterial contamination may still occur. In addition, patients who donate autologous blood have an increased risk of developing perioperative anemia and an increased need for additional blood transfusions.

Therapeutic Apheresis

Therapeutic apheresis is a continuous-flow process that separates whole blood into its components, removes abnormal components, and administers an appropriate replacement fluid. Plasma exchange is the most common therapeutic apheresis procedure in which plasma containing abnormal proteins and antibodies is removed and replaced with albumin solution or fresh frozen plasma. Plasma exchange is considered standard therapy for patients with acute and chronic inflammatory demyelinating polyneuropathy, myasthenia gravis, Goodpasture syndrome, cryoglobulinemia, hyperviscosity in patients with monoclonal gammopathies, and thrombotic thrombocytopenic purpura.

Adverse events associated with therapeutic apheresis are uncommon and are generally due to bleeding or infection from central venous access catheters or hypocalcemia from the use of citrate anticoagulant in the extracorporeal circuit. Using plasma as the replacement fluid, such as for treatment of thrombotic thrombocytopenic purpura, confers the additional risks associated with plasma transfusion, such as allergic reactions and transfusion-related acute lung injury.

KEY POINTS

- In patients with chronic kidney disease, the hemoglobin level should be maintained at no higher than 11 to 12 g/dL (110 to 120 g/L) to reduce the incidence of cardiovascular events.
- Plasma exchange is used for patients with acute and chronic inflammatory demyelinating polyneuropathy, myasthenia gravis, Goodpasture syndrome, cryoglobulinemia, hyperviscosity, and thrombotic thrombocytopenic purpura.

Bibliography

Blajchman M, Vamvakas E. The continuing risk of transfusion-transmitted infections. N Engl J Med. 2006;355(13):1303-1305. [PMID: 17005947]

Goodnough LT, Shander A. Blood management. Arch Pathol Lab Med. 2007;131(5):695-701. [PMID: 17488154]

Khuri FR. Weighing the hazards of erythropoiesis stimulation in patients with cancer. N Engl J Med. 2007;356(24):2445-2446. [PMID: 17568023]

Klein HG, Spahn DR, Carson JL. Red blood cell transfusion in clinical practice. Lancet 2007;370(9585):415-426. [PMID: 17679019]

O'Shaughnessy D, Atterbury C, Bolton Maggs P, et al; British Committee for Standards in Haemotology, Blood Transfusion Task Force. Guidelines for the use of fresh-frozen plasma, cryoprecipitate and cryosupernatant. Br J Haematol. 2004;126(1):11-28. [PMID: 15198728]

Schonewille H, van de Watering LM, Loomans DS, and Brand A. Red blood cell alloantibodies after transfusion: factors influencing incidence and specificity. Transfusion. 2006;46:250-256. [PMID: 16441603]

Singh AK, Szczech L, Tang K, et al; CHOIR Investigators. Correction of anemia with epoetin alfa in chronic kidney disease. N Engl J Med. 2006;355(20):2085-2098. [PMID: 17108343]

Stroncek DF, Rebulla P. Platelet transfusions. Lancet. 2007;370(9585):427-438. [PMID: 17679020]

Szczepiorkowski ZM, Bandarenko N, Kim HC, et al; American Society for Apheresis; Apheresis Applications Committee of the American Society for Apheresis. Guidelines on the use of therapeutic apheresis in clinical practice. J Clin Apheresis. 2007;22(3):106-175. [PMID: 17394188]

Toy P, Popovsky, MA, Abraham E, et al; National Heart, Lung and Blood Institute Working Group on TRALI. Transfusion-related acute lung injury: definition and review. Crit Care Med. 2005;33(4):721-726. [PMID: 15818095]

Zhou L, Giacherio D, Cooling L, Davenport RD. Use of B-natriuretic peptide as a diagnostic marker in the differential diagnosis of transfusion-associated circulatory overload. Transfusion 2005;45(7):1056-1063. [PMID: 15987348]

Hemostasis Disorders

Normal Hemostasis

The control of bleeding by coagulation and vasoconstriction involves the vascular system, platelets, and coagulation proteins. Primary hemostasis occurs when platelets are activated following injury to a blood vessel. Platelet activation involves adhesion, release or secretion, and aggregation. Adhesion is mediated by von Willebrand factor, which binds to platelet glycoprotein Ib and subendothelial collagen. Subsequent activation of platelets involves the prostaglandin cascade and other mediators, which results in a change in the shape of the platelets and release or secretion of granule contents that further enhances platelet activation. Aggregation of platelets is mediated by binding of fibrin(ogen) to platelet glycoprotein IIb/IIIa receptors that are exposed when platelets are activated. The result is a primary hemostatic plug. Each of these processes can be associated with hereditary or acquired defects that result in impaired primary hemostasis.

Coagulation activation (secondary hemostasis) is enhanced as the platelet phospholipid membrane interacts with coagulation proteins, resulting in a definitive hemostatic plug. Coagulation proceeds principally by means of activated factor VII (factor VIIa), which binds to exposed tissue factor (TF) on endothelial cells at the site of injury (**Figure 18**).

Factor VIIa/TF directly activates factor X and also activates factor IX in the intrinsic cascade. Factor IX, along with factor VIII, also activates factor X. Factor Xa and factor V next convert prothrombin to thrombin. Thrombin then cleaves two small peptides from the fibrinogen molecule and leaves the remaining protein (fibrin monomer), which polymerizes with other fibrin monomers by means of hydrostatic forces. This unstable fibrin thrombus is stabilized by the action of factor XIIIa, which introduces disulfide bonds between fibrin monomers. Intrinsic coagulation can also be initiated by contact activation of factor XII, which first activates factor XI and then factor IX. However, this initial pathway is less important

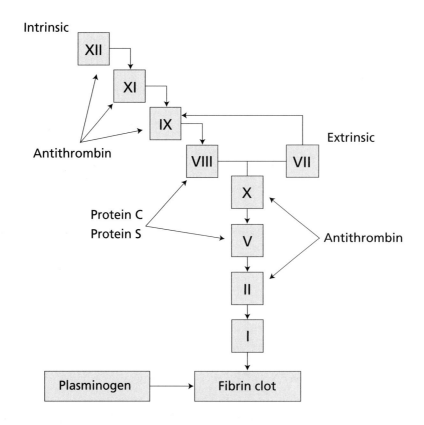

FIGURE 18.
The coagulation cascade.
Antithrombin, protein C, and protein S are natural inhibitors of the coagulation factors indicated.

than originally believed, considering that patients with deficiencies of factor XII or factor XI generally do not have a bleeding disorder.

A cell-based model of coagulation may define the coagulation processes more accurately. This model involves three phases: initiation, amplification, and propagation. During the initiation phase, small amounts of thrombin are generated in an area of subendothelial injury. Thrombin generation occurs by activation of factor VII after contact with TF and by limited generation of factor Xa. Thrombin then activates surrounding platelets, as well as factor VIII and factor V (amplification phase). The platelet membrane then becomes the site for an explosive burst of additional thrombin formation (propagation phase) by means of additional activation of factor X by factor VIIa/TF and factor IXa.

> ### KEY POINT
> - The control of bleeding by coagulation and vasoconstriction involves an interplay between the vascular system, platelets, and coagulation proteins.

Approach to the Bleeding Patient

History and Physical Examination

The clinical history should focus on the presence of any systemic illnesses; the severity of bleeding; whether the bleeding is spontaneous or is an excessive response to normal bleeding following injury, surgery, or dental procedures; whether the bleeding pattern is lifelong or recently acquired; and whether the bleeding suggests a platelet or a coagulation defect. Platelet-related bleeding tends to occur immediately after injury and often affects the skin in the form of petechiae or the mucous membranes. Coagulation-related bleeding may be delayed in onset, is manifested more by deep tissue bruises (ecchymoses), and may produce hemarthroses in patients with congenital deficiencies. Women should be asked about the pattern of menstrual bleeding or, if postmenopausal, about whether any abnormal bleeding has occurred. Obtaining a detailed medication history and a family history of any bleeding disorders is imperative. Physical examination may reveal petechiae, ecchymoses, or the site of bleeding, which may help determine whether there is a platelet or a coagulation disorder.

Laboratory Testing

Platelets are assessed quantitatively by a direct platelet count. Platelet function is determined by a platelet aggregation assay and, occasionally, by a bleeding time. The coagulation cascade is assessed by measurement of the prothrombin time and activated partial thromboplastin time (**Figure 19**). The thrombin time measures the time to convert fibrinogen to fibrin. If results of any of these assays are prolonged, an inhibitor

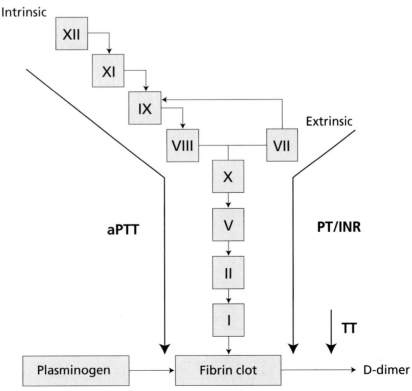

FIGURE 19.
The coagulation cascade illustrating the pathways assessed by the prothrombin time/International Normalized Ratio (PT/INR), activated partial thromboplastin time (aPTT), and the thrombin time (TT).
The D-dimer results from the breakdown of fibrin by plasmin.

mixing study should be done. This involves repeating the abnormal assay with a 1:1 mixture of the patient's plasma and normal plasma to detect either a factor deficiency or the presence of an inhibitor (that is, an antibody directed against a factor). The results of the mixing study will normalize in a patient with a factor deficiency but will remain abnormal if an inhibitor is present. Additional assays can be obtained to determine which factor is deficient, or more specialized tests can be performed to identify the inhibitor and its target. A D-dimer assay detects fragments of fibrin and is helpful in the diagnosis of disseminated intravascular coagulation (see Figure 19).

KEY POINTS

- Platelets are assessed quantitatively by a direct platelet count; platelet function is determined by a platelet aggregation assay or a bleeding time.
- If results of either the prothrombin time or the activated partial thromboplastin time are abnormal, a mixing study can detect either a factor deficiency or the presence of an inhibitor.

Diagnosis and Management of Bleeding Disorders

Hereditary Factor Deficiencies

The three most common inherited factor deficiencies are factor VIII deficiency (hemophilia A), factor IX deficiency (hemophilia B), and von Willebrand factor deficiency (which is discussed under Platelet Disorders). Factor VIII and factor IX deficiency are both X-linked recessive disorders. Females are carriers (with one defective X chromosome), and males are fully affected. Both deficiencies cause spontaneous and excessive trauma-related bleeding that begins several months after birth. Bleeding is typically intramuscular or intra-articular, but fatal intracranial hemorrhage can occur.

Most patients today are treated with self-administered factor VIII or factor IX concentrate on a scheduled prophylactic basis or at the first sign or symptom of potential bleeding. The goal of therapy is to increase the deficient factor level from 50% to 100%. Treatment with these factors has reduced the number of intra-articular hemorrhages and subsequent joint contractures and immobility. Infectious complications have been significantly reduced by the development of recombinant human factor IX concentrate and better purification and virus inactivation of factor VIII concentrates.

Hereditary deficiencies of factors other than factor VIII and factor IX are rare. Factor XI deficiency is most prevalent in Ashkenazi Jews; affected patients, including those with severe forms of this disorder, typically do not have excessive bleeding. They have a prolonged activated partial thromboplastin time but a normal prothrombin time, thrombin time, and bleeding time. Inherited factor XII deficiency also usually does not cause excessive bleeding and is also associated with a prolonged activated partial thromboplastin time.

Acquired Bleeding Disorders

Disorders Associated with Liver Disease

All coagulation factors are synthesized in the liver, and severe hepatic impairment leads to various factor deficiencies. The vitamin K–dependent factors (II, VII, IX, and X) may be the most sensitive, and vitamin K deficiency may further increase the risk for deficient coagulation factors. Patients with liver disease, especially cirrhosis, have an enlarged spleen and a moderate reduction in the platelet count (50,000 to 100,000/µL) caused by splenic sequestration (hypersplenism), which may increase the risk for bleeding. In addition, cirrhosis is often associated with esophageal varices, which also cause gastrointestinal bleeding. Coagulation usually does not become impaired until the cirrhosis is advanced, and the prothrombin time, activated partial thromboplastin time, and thrombin time are all prolonged (**Table 15**).

A coagulopathy may occur in patients with acute hepatic failure or acute hepatic necrosis, and coagulopathy with a prolonged prothrombin time may be the first laboratory sign of acute liver injury in these patients. Levels of most coagulation factors are decreased, and D-dimer concentrations are elevated because of reduced hepatic clearance of D-dimer and variable degrees of coagulation activation. Choice of treatment is guided by the presence of bleeding or the need for prophylaxis before an invasive procedure. Fresh frozen plasma is most often administered to increase the levels of deficient factors. Occasionally, concentrates of the vitamin K–dependent factors (prothrombin concentrates) are given to quickly replace deficient factors without the need to infuse the large volumes of plasma required when fresh frozen plasma is used. Large infusions of fresh frozen plasma are also contraindicated in patients with incipient hepatic encephalopathy because such infusions may precipitate full-blown encephalopathy.

Vitamin K Deficiency

Vitamin K deficiency results in a reduction of factors II, VII, IX, and X and is associated with an initial prolongation of the prothrombin time followed by a prolonged activated partial thromboplastin time. Vitamin K deficiency occurs most often in chronically ill patients, especially those in intensive care units, and in malnourished patients who are taking antibiotics. Vitamin K, 5 to 10 mg orally, provides adequate treatment. Acute bleeding due to vitamin K deficiency requires administration of fresh frozen plasma to replace the missing factors more quickly.

Disseminated Intravascular Coagulation

Disseminated intravascular coagulation (DIC) involves the widespread activation of coagulation that leads to formation of fibrin clots. Some patients have a thrombotic disorder characterized by deep venous thrombosis or pulmonary

TABLE 15 Constellation of Coagulation and Platelet Function Test Results Found in Various Coagulation and Platelet Disorders

Coagulation or Platelet Disorder	PT/INR	aPTT	Mixing Study[a]	TT	Fibrinogen	D-dimer	Platelet Count	Bleeding Time	Platelet Aggregation	Blood Smear[b]	Comment
Liver disease	↑	↑	Corrects	↑	↓	↑	↓	↑ or →	Nl	Target cells	Findings are often variable and most prominent in advanced liver disease with cirrhosis
Vitamin K deficiency	↑	↑	Corrects	→	→	→	→	→	→	Normal	PT/INR rises before aPTT because of short half-life of factor VII
Disseminated intravascular coagulation	↑	↑	Corrects	↑	↓	↑	↓	↑	Nl	Schistocytes	Results vary depending on severity; some tests may be normal
Thrombocytopenia	→	→	NI	→	→	→	↓	↑	Abnormal	Large platelets	Bleeding time and platelet size depend on cause of thrombocytopenia
Qualitative platelet defect	→	→	NI	→	→	→	→	↑	Abnormal	Normal	Platelet aggregation patterns vary, depending on defect
von Willebrand disease	→	↑ or → Corrects		→	→	→	→	↑	Normal	Normal	aPTT dependent on factor VIIIc activity; platelet aggregation does not detect abnormal adhesion; vWF level and ristocetin cofactor are abnormal. Ristocetin cofactor is a platelet aggregation study measuring the function of vWF. The structure of vWF can be determined by a vWF multimer assay.

PT = prothrombin time; INR = International Normalized Ratio; aPTT = activated partial thromboplastin time; TT = thrombin time; NI = not indicated; vWF = von Willebrand factor; ↑ = increased; ↓ = decreased; → = normal.

[a]Mixing study is performed on PT or aPTT, depending on which is prolonged.

[b]Findings on blood smear are variable, depending on severity of disorder and may not be present.

embolism. Arterial thrombi and infarction may also rarely occur. In most patients, secondary fibrinolysis dissolves the fibrin clot, and consumption of platelets and coagulation factors causes thrombocytopenia, clotting factor deficiencies, bleeding, and vascular injuries. Erythrocyte consumption is manifested by a microangiopathic hemolytic anemia with fragmented erythrocytes seen on a peripheral blood smear (see Figure 11 from the Approach to Anemia section).

However, patients with mild DIC may be asymptomatic. DIC most commonly occurs in patients with infections, cancer (typically mucin-producing adenocarcinomas), and obstetrical complications. Gram-negative sepsis is the most common infection associated with DIC, although infection due to gram-positive organisms and viruses, including HIV, may also be causative. Patients with head trauma or other extensive injuries are also at risk. In addition, most patients with DIC have an acute or a chronic underlying liver disease.

The diagnosis of DIC is based on the presence of a prolonged prothrombin time, activated partial thromboplastin time, and thrombin time; a high D-dimer titer; a reduced serum fibrinogen level and platelet count; and the presence of microangiopathic hemolytic anemia. The degree of these abnormalities depends on the extent of consumption of platelets and coagulation factors and the ability of the patient to compensate for these findings. A scoring system to aid in diagnosing DIC has been studied prospectively and was found to have a sensitivity of 91% and specificity of 97% for establishing the diagnosis.

Treatment of DIC is focused on correcting the underlying cause. Patients may require fresh frozen plasma to replace coagulation factors or transfusion of platelets or erythrocytes. Cryoprecipitate may also be given. Antithrombin III and activated protein C concentrates have been used with some effectiveness. Unfractionated heparin and low-molecular-weight heparin, which were once thought to interrupt the consumptive process, are rarely used today because these formulations may increase the bleeding risk and do not improve outcome.

Acquired Factor VIII Inhibitors

Acquired factor VIII inhibitors are a rare cause of an acquired bleeding disorder. Most commonly, factor VIII inhibitors occur in hemophiliacs. However, they may rarely occur spontaneously, especially in older patients, and in patients with autoimmune disease, cancer, lymphoproliferative diseases, and pregnant woman, especially in the postpartum period. Acquired factor VIII inhibitors are associated with severe bleeding, which is controlled with various factor concentrates or desmopressin. The long-term goal is to eradicate the antibody by immunosuppressive therapy and treat the underlying disease.

KEY POINTS

- Factor VIII and factor IX deficiencies are the two most common inherited coagulation factor deficiencies.
- Liver disease, vitamin K deficiency, and disseminated intravascular coagulation are the three most common acquired coagulation factor deficiencies.
- In patients with liver disease, coagulation usually does not become impaired until the cirrhosis is advanced, and the prothrombin time, activated partial thromboplastin time, and thrombin time are all prolonged.

Bibliography

Bakhtiari K, Meijers JC, de Jonge E, Levi M. Prospective validation of the International Society of Thrombosis and Haemostasis scoring system for disseminated intravascular coagulation. Crit Care Med. 2004;32(12):2416-2421. [PMID: 15599145]

Berntorp E, Michiels JJ. A healthy hemophilic patient without arthropathy: From concept to clinical reality. Semin Thromb Hemost. 2003;29(1):5-10. [PMID: 12640559]

Dahlback B. Blood coagulation and its regulation by anticoagulant pathways: genetic pathogenesis of bleeding and thrombotic diseases. J Intern Med. 2005;257(3):209-223. [PMID: 15715678]

Franchini M. Veneri D. Lippi G. Inherited factor XI deficiency: a concise review. Hematology. 2006;11(5):307-309. [PMID: 17607578]

Hoffman M, Monroe DM. Rethinking the coagulation cascade. Current Hematol Rep. 2005;4(5):391-396. [PMID: 16131441]

Kamal AH, Tefferi A, Pruthi RK. How to interpret and pursue an abnormal prothrombin time, activated partial thromboplastin time, and bleeding time in adults. Mayo Clin Proc. 2007;82(7):864-873. [PMID: 17605969]

Kessler GM, Khokhar N, Liu M. A systematic approach to the bleeding patient: Correlation of clinical symptoms and signs with laboratory testing. In: C Kitchens, B Alving, C Kessler. eds. Consultative Hemostasis and Thrombosis. 2nd ed. Philadelphia, PA: Saunders; 2007:17-33.

Levi M. Disseminated intravascular coagulation. Crit Care Med. 2007;35:2191-2195. [PMID: 17855836]

Lisman T, Leebeek FW, de Groot PG. Haemostatic abnormalities in patients with liver disease. J Hepatol. 2002;37(2):280-287. [PMID: 12127437]

Platelet Disorders

Approach to the Patient with Thrombocytopenia

Thrombocytopenia (a platelet count <150,000/μL [150 × 10^9/L]) is due to reduced bone marrow production that may be associated with increased peripheral destruction, hemodilution, or splenic pooling of platelets. Platelet disorders can be both quantitative and qualitative. Specific causes are listed in **Table 16**.

Medical history can help determine whether the process is chronic or acute, whether systemic diseases associated with thrombocytopenia are present, and whether medications known to cause thrombocytopenia are being used. A complete

TABLE 16 Differential Diagnosis of Thrombocytopenia (Common Causes)

Increased Platelet Destruction

Immune-mediated	
ITP	Isolated thrombocytopenia; usually a diagnosis of exclusion; antibody often directed against platelet GP IIb/IIIa; increased megakaryocytes in bone marrow, but bone marrow examination not usually needed for diagnosis.
Infection	Antibodies against pathogens adsorbed to platelets, resulting in increased destruction. Seen in HIV, hepatitis B and C, EBV, and other viral and bacterial infections.
Drug-induced	
HIT	Most common drug-induced thrombocytopenia; about 5% with unfractionated heparin after 5 to 7 days of treatment; associated with thromboses in 20% to 50% of cases; must use alternative, nonheparin, anticoagulant in affected patients.
Sulfa drugs, quinine/quinidine, penicillin	Drugs bind to different platelet membrane receptors (e.g., GP Ib/IX or IIb/IIIa) with varying degrees of reversibility, depending on drug. Platelet reductions can be acute and severe as with quinine, or more mild.
Nonimmune-mediated	
DIC	Coagulation activation leading to consumption of platelets with thrombosis in milder cases or bleeding in severe cases. Commonly associated with gram-negative sepsis, cancer, or obstetric complications.
TTP/HUS	Most commonly due to secretion of large molecular complexes of vWF not cleaved into smaller units by ADAMTS13, a metalloproteinase, which is deficient on a congenital basis or owing to antibodies. vWF's binding to platelets leads to platelet consumption, characterized by thrombocytopenia, microangiopathic hemolytic anemia, neurologic deficits, fever, and renal failure. Renal failure predominates in HUS, more often occurring in children.
Hypersplenism	Sequestration/removal of platelets in the presence of splenic hypertrophy, resulting in mild to moderate thrombocytopenia.
Adhesion to foreign surfaces	Extracorporeal circulation; dialysis.

Decreased Platelet Production

Bone Marrow Disorder	
Leukemia, myeloproliferative disease, myelodysplasia, aplastic anemia, bone marrow infiltration with cancer	Decreased platelet production due either to a stem cell defect or dysplasia or bone marrow replacement with other cells, such as in cancer infiltration or myelofibrosis.
Drug-induced	
Chemotherapy and radiotherapy	Direct toxic effect on cell division via various mechanisms depending on class of chemotherapeutic agent or site of radiation therapy.
Alcohol	Direct toxic effect on megakaryocyte development; hypersplenism may play a role if advanced liver disease is present. Thrombocytopenia in affected patients is usually mild to moderate.
Infectious (viral)	
HIV, CMV	Direct toxic effect on megakaryocyte development.
Nutritional	
Folate/B_{12}	Defect in DNA maturation, resulting in reduced platelet production.

ITP = Immune thrombocytopenic purpura; HIT = heparin-induced thrombocytopenia; DIC = disseminated intravascular coagulation; GB = glycoprotein; EBV = Epstein-Barr virus; TTP/HUS = thrombotic thrombocytopenic purpura/hemolytic uremic syndrome; vWF = von Willebrand factor; CMV = cytomegalovirus.

blood count is required because other cell lines (leukocytes, erythrocytes) may also be abnormal in a patient with a bone marrow or stem cell disorder. The peripheral blood smear may show large platelets when platelet turnover is increased, although giant platelets may also occur in some hereditary syndromes. The presence of fragmented erythrocytes suggests a thrombotic microangiopathy (disseminated intravascular coagulation, thrombotic thrombocytopenic purpura, hemolytic-uremic syndrome, HELLP syndrome), and nucleated erythrocytes may indicate an invasive bone marrow process (**Figure 20**).

Immature leukocytes on the peripheral blood smear may be associated with a bone marrow stem cell disorder such as leukemia. Although a bone marrow aspirate or biopsy may be helpful in assessing platelet production, this procedure is not done as often today because less invasive studies may be equally effective in making a presumptive diagnosis.

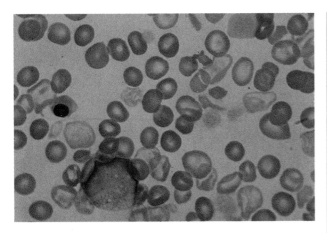

FIGURE 20.
Fragmented erythrocytes and nucleated erythrocytes suggestive of a thrombotic microangiopathy.

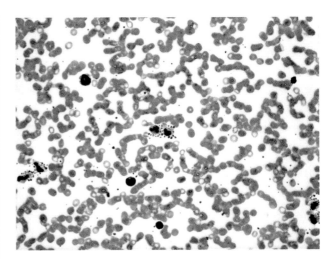

FIGURE 21.
A peripheral blood smear depicting platelet clumping characteristic of pseudothrombocytopenia.

Pseudothrombocytopenia (a falsely low platelet count) may occasionally occur and is caused by platelet clumping or aggregation around leukocytes in the collection tube (**Figure 21**).

This process is mediated by use of EDTA as the anticoagulant and results in a reduced count when electronic counting instruments are used. Pseudothrombocytopenia can be confirmed when the platelet count normalizes after the count is repeated in a tube containing citrate or heparin as the anticoagulant.

KEY POINTS

- The most common causes of thrombocytopenia are decreased production, increased destruction, and splenic pooling of platelets.
- Pseudothrombocytopenia is caused by platelet clumping or aggregation around leukocytes when EDTA is used in the collection tube.

Quantitative Platelet Disorders

Immune Thrombocytopenic Purpura

Immune thrombocytopenic purpura (ITP) may be autoimmune mediated (previously called idiopathic ITP) or drug-induced. ITP is a relatively common disorder (approximately 20,000 cases per year in the United States) and occurs in both children and adults. In adults, younger women are affected more often than younger men, but the sex-related differences in prevalence diminish in older patients.

ITP may be acute or chronic. Acute ITP occurs most often in children (approximately 90% of cases) and usually resolves within 6 months with or without treatment. Chronic ITP occurs most often in adults. Adult patients with ITP may present with new-onset bleeding and thrombocytopenia, suggesting an acute disorder. However, thrombocytopenia is often found coincidentally when a complete blood count is done for another indication, suggesting a more chronic onset.

The autoantibody causing ITP is most often targeted to platelet glycoprotein IIb/IIIa or platelet glycoprotein Ib/IX, although other antigen targets have been identified on the platelet surface. Bound antibody leads to platelet removal by binding to Fc receptors on the membrane of macrophages. The spleen is the major site of removal. Assays for specific antibodies to platelet glycoprotein IIb/IIIa are not readily available, and measuring nonspecific platelet-associated immunoglobulin concentrations is not helpful in diagnosing ITP.

The clinical manifestations of ITP range from mild bleeding (epistaxis, gingival bleeding, petechiae, and ecchymoses) to severe gastrointestinal or intracranial hemorrhage. The diagnosis is based on excluding other causes of thrombocytopenia, other systemic illnesses, and medications. Petechiae are usually the only finding on physical examination; splenomegaly is typically absent. The peripheral blood smear shows large platelets decreased in number. The complete blood count is generally normal except for thrombocytopenia. As discussed above, pseudothrombocytopenia must be excluded as the cause for a decreased platelet count. Bone marrow aspirate or biopsy is usually not needed if the complete blood count is otherwise normal.

Prolonged treatment is usually needed to increase and stabilize the platelet count, and ITP never resolves completely in some patients. Initial treatment includes high-dose corticosteroids (approximately 1 mg/kg daily for 2 to 4 weeks). The platelet count initially improves in most patients following corticosteroid administration, but it will subsequently decline in many as the dose is tapered or even if the high dose is maintained. As many as 70% of adult patients will not have an adequate sustained response to corticosteroids and will require additional therapy.

Splenectomy, traditionally the next treatment intervention, results in a sustained increased platelet count in approximately 50% to 75% of patients. However, fewer patients undergo splenectomy today because of the availability of other equally effective treatments. Those who do have surgery should receive polyvalent pneumococcal vaccine, *Haemophilus influenzae* vaccine, and quadrivalent meningococcal polysaccharide vaccine at least 2 weeks preoperatively.

Intravenous immune globulin (IVIG) may increase very low platelet counts in patients with ITP. However, the effect is transient (days to weeks). IVIG is therefore often used only for patients before splenectomy or as a temporizing measure until more definitive treatment is tried. It may also be used as an option to quickly elevate the platelet count while corticosteroids are taking effect. In patients who might have difficulty with corticosteroids (for example, patients with diabetes mellitus), IVIG may be preferred until longer-term solutions can be applied. Intravenous anti-D immune globulin may sometimes be effective in patients with an intact spleen. Anti-D immune globulin can be administered in a smaller-volume infusion than that required for IVIG and can also be given over a shorter duration.

Other therapeutic options for treatment of ITP include danazol, which is an attenuated androgen, and the cytotoxic agents cyclophosphamide and azathioprine. Several recent case reports have confirmed the effectiveness of rituximab, a monoclonal antibody directed against CD20 (B lymphocyte membrane receptor), in treating ITP. Rituximab decreases antibody-producing B cells, including those responsible for the autoimmune antibody. The result may last for 6 to 12 months, but repeat courses of rituximab are often needed. Because of its immune-suppressing effects, rituximab can cause adverse events. Investigators have also recently confirmed an association between ITP and *Helicobacter pylori* infection, suggesting that eradication of *H. pylori* can result in remission of ITP. However, this finding seems to be most prominent in selected Asian populations and does not appear to be a factor in treating patients with ITP in the United States. Most recently, clinical trials have reported that thrombopoietin or thrombopoietin receptor agonists have been successful in treating patients with ITP. Recombinant human thrombopoietin has been tried, but because of antibody formation and the development of thrombocytopenia, it has not proved useful. The rationale behind using a growth factor for treatment when megakaryocyte development is already stimulated in patients with ITP is that megakaryocyte growth is actually depressed in some patients, presumably from the antiplatelet antibody that effects megakaryocyte development, and that growth factors may counter this effect. The two agents recently approved by the U.S. Food and Drug Administration are romiplostim, given subcutaneously once weekly, or eltrombopag, given orally on a daily basis. Both agents have shown good response in patients with refractory ITP, with few serious side effects. There have been a few cases of thrombosis and an increase in bone marrow reticulin reported with the use of these agents.

ITP is well characterized in other conditions such as systemic lupus erythematosus (SLE), in which it may occur in 10% to 15% of patients, sometimes as the earliest manifestation of SLE. ITP is not an uncommon cause of thrombocytopenia in HIV, although decreased platelet production also occurs in HIV and must be differentiated from peripheral platelet destruction. ITP is also found in patients with lymphoproliferative disorders such as chronic lymphocytic leukemia, occurring in less than 5% of patients.

Because the treatment of ITP after corticosteroid failure is complex, and splenectomy no longer is the automatic next therapeutic step, consultation with a hematologist is appropriate in the management of such patients.

KEY POINTS

- The clinical manifestations of immune thrombocytopenic purpura range from mild bleeding to severe gastrointestinal or intracranial hemorrhage.
- High-dose corticosteroids are the initial treatment of immune thrombocytopenic purpura in adults.
- Because immune thrombocytopenic purpura often does not respond completely to corticosteroids, treatment with immunosuppressive agents or splenectomy may be required.
- New thrombopoietin receptor agonists are available for the treatment of refractory immune thrombocytopenic purpura.

Heparin-induced Thrombocytopenia

Heparin-induced thrombocytopenia (HIT), the most common drug-induced immune thrombocytopenia, is caused by antibodies directed against a complex of heparin and platelet factor 4 (PF4), a protein released from platelets. Antibodies bind to the heparin-PF4 complex and then bind to Fcγ receptors on platelets, which results in additional platelet activation and release of prothrombotic platelet microparticles. The antibody-heparin-PF4 complex may also bind to endothelial cells, resulting in endothelial injury.

HIT occurs in approximately 5% of patients treated with unfractionated heparin for 5 or more days. It develops in only about 1% of patients treated with low-molecular-weight heparin and is almost nonexistent in patients taking fondaparinux, although fondaparinux is associated with antibody production, and one case of thrombocytopenia has been described. HIT occurs more commonly after full-dose intravenous administration of unfractionated heparin. The risk of developing HIT is highest in surgical patients, especially in those undergoing open heart surgery. Medical patients and pregnant women who require heparin have a lower risk for developing HIT. Platelet monitoring includes a baseline count and periodic platelet counts during the first 7 to

10 days of therapy. HIT may occur after discontinuing unfractionated heparin, primarily within the first 3 months of recent treatment. Therefore, HIT should be suspected in patients who were recently hospitalized and develop either thrombocytopenia or a thrombotic event.

The criteria for diagnosing HIT include (1) thrombocytopenia (defined as a platelet count <150,000/μL [150 × 10^9/L] or a 50% decrease in platelet count from baseline, in which case the platelet count may still be within the normal range) in the presence of heparin or its use over the past 3 months; (2) exclusion of other causes of thrombocytopenia; (3) reversal of thrombocytopenia on cessation of heparin; and (4) positive laboratory test results.

The diagnosis is often made on clinical grounds with confirmation by a specific antibody assay, such as the enzyme-linked immunosorbent assay (ELISA) or the serotonin-release assay, the results of which generally take several days to become available. The ELISA is highly sensitive but less specific than the serotonin-release assay for detecting antibodies that may cause thrombocytopenia. A heparin-induced platelet aggregation assay is not very sensitive or specific.

The most serious complication of HIT is a thrombotic event. Venous thromboses are more common (about two thirds of events), but arterial thromboses also occur and can be life-threatening. Once HIT is detected or even suspected, heparin must be stopped immediately and an alternative rapidly acting anticoagulant begun even if thrombosis has not occurred. A new thrombotic event develops in 20% to 50% of patients who do not receive subsequent antithrombotic prophylaxis. Alternative agents include the direct thrombin inhibitors lepirudin and argatroban. Bivalirudin may also be used in selected patients, usually those undergoing cardiac interventions. These agents require intravenous administration and close monitoring. Once the platelet count is greater than 100,000/μL (100 × 10^9/L), transition to warfarin can be started, if considered necessary. Platelet transfusions are indicated only if life-threatening bleeding is present. Patients with a confirmed history of HIT should not receive unfractionated heparin or low-molecular-weight heparin within the next 3 to 6 months because of the persistence of antibodies and recurrence of HIT. After a longer duration, however, many patients have no evidence of antibodies and do not have an amnestic response to repeat exposure. However, each patient responds differently, and great caution must be used in patients in whom subsequent heparin is absolutely required.

KEY POINTS

- A diagnosis of heparin-induced thrombocytopenia requires immediate discontinuation of heparin and initiation of an alternative rapidly acting anticoagulant.
- Heparin-induced thrombocytopenia is associated with a high risk for thrombotic events.

Other Immune Thrombocytopenias

Other drugs implicated as the cause of immune thrombocytopenia include NSAIDs followed by anticonvulsants, antibiotics, gold salts, cinchona alkaloids (quinine/quinidine), diuretics, penicillamine, analgesics, and vaccines. If drug-induced thrombocytopenia is suspected, other diagnoses must be excluded, and the causative drug should be discontinued. Platelet transfusions are required only for patients with significant bleeding.

Thrombotic Microangiopathies

The two thrombotic microangiopathies are thrombotic thrombocytopenic purpura (TTP) and hemolytic uremic syndrome (HUS). TTP is primarily a disorder of the systemic circulation caused by microvascular aggregation of platelets in the brain and other organs. HUS mainly affects the kidneys as a result of intrarenal platelet-fibrin thrombi. The two syndromes overlap, and it is often difficult to distinguish which syndrome predominates. Patients with TTP have been found to have unusually large multimers of von Willebrand factor (vWF) in their plasma. This led to the discovery of the role of ADAMTS13 (a disintegrin and metalloprotease with thrombospondin type 1 repeats, member 13) in the pathogenesis of TTP. ADAMTS13 cleaves large multimers of vWF released from endothelial cells. Familial deficiencies of, or antibodies to, ADAMTS13 lead to increased concentrations of large vWF multimers that bind to platelets, resulting in platelet aggregates in the microvasculature. TTP can also occur by other mechanisms in patients with cancer, in transplant recipients, and following administration of chemotherapeutic agents and other drugs.

HUS primarily affects children and is not associated with ADAMTS13. The two most common causes are infection by Shiga toxin–producing *Escherichia coli* (*E. coli* O157:H7 and other serotypes) and familial deficiency of factor H. The toxin causes bloody diarrhea and enters the circulation and binds to platelets, glomerular capillary endothelial cells, mesangial cells, and glomerular and tubular epithelial cells. Shiga toxin binds to platelets by means of globotriaosylceramide receptors, which leads to platelet aggregation. Shiga toxin may also stimulate endothelial cells to release large vWF multimers, which can further enhance platelet aggregation. Factor H, a protein in the complement pathway, normally protects cells from damage by the alternative complement pathway. A deficiency of factor H allows C3 to potentiate autoantibody-mediated or immune complex–mediated injury to glomerular cells, leading to exposure of subendothelium and activation of both platelets and coagulation.

The pentad of findings in TTP includes thrombocytopenia, microangiopathic hemolytic anemia, neurologic deficits, renal impairment, and fever. All five findings do not need to be present for the diagnosis to be established, but TTP should always be considered in all patients with both thrombocytopenia and microangiopathic hemolytic anemia (**Figure 22**). Rare cases of familial TTP occur.

Patients may also have fatigue, nausea, vomiting, and abdominal pain. Since patients with disseminated intravascular coagulation (DIC) may have similar signs and symptoms, including thrombocytopenia and microangiopathic hemolytic anemia, DIC must be excluded before a diagnosis of TTP can be confirmed. Although ADAMTS13 assays or antibody studies are available, their accuracy has not been established.

Plasma exchange transfusion is the treatment of choice for TTP. The procedure removes ADAMTS13 antibodies or replaces ADAMTS13 in patients with a deficiency of this compound. However, such therapy is recommended even without demonstrable ADAMTS13 antibodies or deficiency. Daily exchanges are usually required to replace 1.0 to 1.5 times the predicted plasma volume with each exchange. The effectiveness of treatment is assessed by improvement in the platelet count, hematocrit value, and serum lactate dehydrogenase level. Some patients with TTP also require corticosteroids and sometimes with more potent immunosuppressive agents. Rituximab has recently been used with some success. Splenectomy may also be considered.

KEY POINTS

- Thrombotic thrombocytopenic purpura is most often caused by antibodies to or a deficiency of ADAMTS13, an enzyme that cleaves large multimers of von Willebrand factor.

- Thrombotic thrombocytopenic purpura should always be considered in any patient with both thrombocytopenia and microangiopathic hemolytic anemia.

- Patients with thrombotic thrombocytopenic purpura are treated with plasma exchange transfusions.

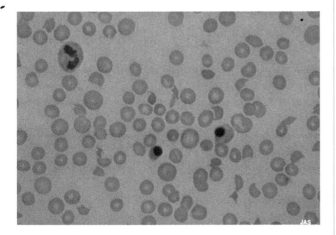

FIGURE 22.
A peripheral blood smear showing thrombocytopenia and schistocytes in a patient with thrombotic thrombocytopenic purpura.

Acquired Thrombocytopenia Due to Inadequate Platelet Production

Reduced platelet production resulting in thrombocytopenia can be caused by stem cell disorders; leukemia or aplastic anemia; nutritional disorders (for example, folic acid or vitamin B_{12} deficiency); or, rarely, advanced iron deficiency, viral infections, drug-induced disorders, and infiltration of the bone marrow by cancer or a granulomatous process. In most of these disorders, the thrombocytopenia is associated with anemia and less frequently with leukopenia. Some causes, such as nutritional deficiencies or drug-induced disorders, are easily reversible, whereas others, such as stem cell disorders, are difficult to correct. The risk of bleeding begins to increase when the platelet count drops below $50,000/\mu L$ ($50 \times 10^9/L$) and increases significantly when the count decreases to $10,000/\mu L$ ($10 \times 10^9/L$) to $20,000/\mu L$ ($20 \times 10^9/L$). Platelet transfusions are indicated if bleeding is present, but prophylactic platelet transfusions are usually not given until the platelet count drops below $10,000/\mu L$ ($10 \times 10^9/L$) .

KEY POINT

- In patients with thrombocytopenia, the risk of bleeding begins to increase when the platelet count drops below $50,000/\mu L$ ($50 \times 10^9/L$) and increases significantly when the count decreases to $10,000/\mu L$ ($10 \times 10^9/L$) to $20,000/\mu L$ ($20 \times 10^9/L$).

Qualitative Platelet Disorders

Platelet-related bleeding can be due to a qualitative defect in platelet function even though the platelet count is normal. Qualitative platelet defects can be acquired (for example, drug-induced disorders) or congenital (for example, von Willebrand disease). Acquired defects are quite common, and congenital defects are rare.

Platelet Function Testing

Only a limited number of platelet function tests are available. The bleeding time assesses primary platelet plug formation but is used only in selected patients, such as in the evaluation of von Willebrand disease. This study is inaccurate for determining the risk of bleeding in patients scheduled to undergo surgical procedures.

A platelet aggregation assay assesses the release reaction or secretion of platelets and their ability to aggregate. It does not assess platelet adhesion.

The Platelet Function Analyzer-100® (PFA-100®), an instrument designed specifically to measure platelet function, may be useful as a screening device, especially for assessing the effect of platelet inhibitor drugs. The Ultegra Rapid Platelet Function Analyzer® is a bedside instrument designed to monitor platelet inhibition by platelet glycoprotein IIb/IIIa antagonists.

Congenital Qualitative Platelet Disorders

Disorders of platelet adhesion, secretion, and aggregation can be congenital. Examples include absence of platelet membrane receptors involved in adhesion (platelet glycoprotein Ib or giant platelet syndrome); defects in aggregation (platelet glycoprotein IIb/IIIa or Glanzmann thrombasthenia); or defects in prostaglandins or platelet storage granules (absence of α or δ granules). The most common inherited qualitative platelet defect is von Willebrand disease.

Although usually referred to as a platelet defect, von Willebrand disease (vWD) is actually a deficiency or defect in the plasma protein von Willebrand factor (vWF). This factor is important for platelet adhesion and serves as the bridge between platelets and subendothelial collagen at sites of injury by binding to platelet membrane glycoprotein Ib and collagen. vWF is also a carrier for the coagulant protein factor VIII (factor VIIIc). When factor VIIIc is unable to bind to defective or deficient vWF, the half-life and concentration of this factor are reduced, which may result in a coagulation defect.

vWD is classified according to the type of mutation. The two principal types are type 1 (a deficiency of vWF) and type 2 (a defect in the polymerization of vWF subunits). vWD can be either inherited or acquired. It is the most common hereditary bleeding disorder and occurs in approximately 1/1000 persons in the United States. Type 1 vWD is inherited as an autosomal dominant trait. Depending on the concentration of vWF, bleeding can occur spontaneously (severe form) or after minor trauma. Symptoms and signs include ecchymoses, menorrhagia, and bleeding from the oral or nasal mucosa and gastrointestinal tract. The activated partial thromboplastin time may be prolonged because of a concomitant factor VIIIc deficiency. A prolonged bleeding time is also common. However, a definitive diagnosis is made by finding low or variable levels of vWF, ristocetin cofactor (a measure of the role of vWF in platelet function), and a multimeric analysis of the von Willebrand protein.

The goal of treatment is to increase vWF levels by administration of desmopressin (DDAVP) or infusions of cryoprecipitate or factor concentrates that contain vWF.

The acquired form of vWD is rare. Over 50% of patients with acquired vWD have an associated lymphoproliferative or myeloproliferative disorder. Other associations include nonhematologic malignancies, aortic stenosis and other cardiac defects, and administration of certain drugs (for example, valproic acid). Treatment of acquired vWD is similar to that for inherited disease, but treatment of the underlying associated disease is of paramount importance.

Acquired Qualitative Platelet Disorders

Acquired qualitative platelet disorders are most commonly caused by drugs, especially aspirin. Aspirin (acetylsalicylic acid) neutralizes platelet cyclooxygenase and impairs platelet secretion. Platelet transfusion is indicated for the treatment of serious aspirin-related bleeding. NSAIDs may also cause a transient qualitative platelet disorder, which remits once the drug is stopped.

Several other antiplatelet agents used to treat cardiovascular disease may also cause platelet disorders. These include platelet glycoprotein IIb/IIIa inhibitors (for example, abciximab and eptifibitide) and thienopyridine adenosine diphosphate receptor antagonists (for example, clopidogrel).

Uremia is another common cause of a qualitative platelet disorder. The platelet defect in uremia has been attributed to toxic effects of uremic plasma, impaired platelet–vessel wall adhesion, and increased production of nitric oxide. Treatment includes dialysis and administration of DDAVP. Conjugated estrogens may be helpful in reducing bleeding. Platelet transfusions are ineffective.

Qualitative platelet defects may also occur in patients with myeloproliferative and myelodysplastic disorders, in which case platelet transfusions are indicated if bleeding occurs.

KEY POINTS

- von Willebrand disease, a qualitative platelet disorder, is the most common inherited bleeding disorder.
- Treatment of von Willebrand disease includes administration of desmopressin (DDAVP) or infusion of cryoprecipitates or factor concentrates that contain von Willebrand factor.
- Drugs, especially aspirin and NSAIDs, are the most common cause of acquired qualitative platelet disorders.

Bibliography

Arnold DM, Dentali F, Crowther MA, et al. Systematic review: Efficacy and safety of rituximab for adults with idiopathic thrombocytopenic purpura. Ann Intern Med. 2007;146(1):25-33. [PMID: 17200219]

Bussel JB, Kuter DJ, George JN, et al. AMG 531, a thrombopoiesis-stimulating protein, for chronic ITP [erratum in N Engl J Med. 2006;355(19):2054]. N Engl J Med. 2006;355:1672-1681. [PMID: 17050891]

Cines DB, Bussel JB. How I treat idiopathic thrombocytopenic purpura (ITP). Blood. 2005;106(7):2244-2251. [PMID: 15941913]

Federici AB. Diagnosis of inherited von Willebrand disease: A clinical perspective. Semin Thromb Hemost. 2006;32(6):555-565. [PMID: 16977566]

Federici AB. Management of inherited von Willebrand disease in 2006. Semin Thromb Hemost. 2006;32:616-620. [PMID: 16977571]

Franchini M, Lippi G. Acquired von Willebrand syndrome: An update. Amer J Hematol. 2007;82(5):368-375. [PMID: 17133419]

Greinacher A, Warkentin TE. Recognition, treatment, and prevention of heparin-induced thrombocytopenia: Review and update. Thromb Res. 2006(2);118:165-176. [PMID: 16139874]

Hirsh J, Heddle N, Kelton JG. Treatment of heparin-induced thrombocytopenia: A critical review. Arch Intern Med. 2004;164(4):361-369. [PMID: 14980986]

Lubenow N, Eichler P, Lietz T, Farner B, Greinacher A. Lepirudin for prophylaxis of thrombosis in patients with acute isolated heparin-induced thrombocytopenia: an analysis of 3 prospective studies. Blood. 2004;104(10):3072-3077. [PMID: 15280202]

Moake JL. Thrombotic microangiopathies. N Engl J Med. 2002; 347(8):589-600. [PMID: 12192020]

Patrono C, Coller B, FitzGerald GA, Hirsh J, Roth G. Platelet-active drugs: the relationships among dose, effectiveness, and side effects: the Seventh ACCP Conference on Antithrombotic and Thrombolytic Therapy. Chest. 2004;126:234S-264S [PMID: 15383474].

Pedersen-Bjergaard U, Andersen M, Hansen PB. Thrombocytopenia induced by noncytotoxic drugs in Denmark 1968-1991. J Intern Med 1996;239(3 Suppl):509-515. [PMID: 8656144]

Rice L, Attisha WK, Drexler A, Francis JL. Delayed-onset heparin-induced thrombocytopenia. Ann Intern Med. 2002;136(3):210-215. [PMID: 11827497]

Starke R, Machin S, Scully M, Purdy G, Mackie I. The clinical utility of ADAMTS13 activity, antigen and autoantibody assays in thrombotic thrombocytopenic purpura. Brit J Haematol. 2006;136(4):649-655. [PMID: 17367414]

Vesely SK, Perdue JJ, Rizvi MA, Terrell DR, George JN. Management of adult patients with persistent idiopathic thrombocytopenic purpura following splenectomy. A systematic review. Ann Intern Med. 2004;140(2):112-120. [PMID: 14734334]

Thrombotic Disorders

Pathophysiology of Thrombosis and Thrombophilia

Thrombosis may represent a positive normal response to injury or an unwanted response to an inciting factor. Platelet-rich thrombi are found in high-flow, high-shear environments, such as in the arterial circulation, whereas fibrin-rich thrombi predominate in the venous or low-flow circulatory environments. The latter will be the focus of this section.

Rudolph Virchow, the 19th century pathologist, postulated that thrombosis involved disorders of the blood vessels, blood flow, or factors intrinsic to the blood. Today, individuals with multiple risk factors are known to be at the highest risk for thrombotic disorders, and Virchow triad is best thought of as a Venn diagram with overlapping and cumulative areas of risk (**Figure 23**).

Factors limiting thrombosis or coagulation include rapid blood flow and dilution of activated factors, a nonthrombogenic endothelium, inhibitors to coagulation factors, and a fibrinolytic system that degrades fibrin clots (see Figure 19 from Hemostasis section). Thus, venous stasis limits blood flow and allows activated factors to accumulate, vascular injury disrupts the endothelium and exposes platelet and coagulation-active surfaces, and a defect or deficiency of inhibitors or lytic factors allows coagulation activation to go unchecked. Thrombophilia refers to an increased risk for thrombosis typically attributed to an acquired or inherited inhibitor deficiency, or to another process in the blood. **Table 17** lists several acquired and inherited risk factors for thrombosis.

Congenital Causes of Thrombophilia

Of the inherited thrombophilic conditions, factor V Leiden is the most common. A single mutation in the factor V gene results in an amino acid substitution (Arg to Gln at position 506), rendering factor V more resistant to cleavage by

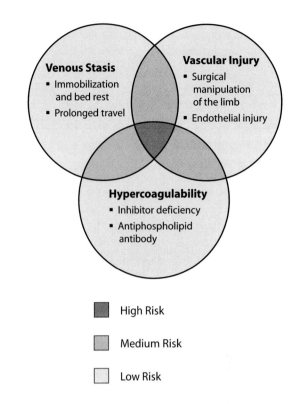

High Risk

Medium Risk

Low Risk

FIGURE 23.

Venn diagram depicting Virchow's triad, with overlapping and cumulative areas of risk for thromboses.

Adapted with permission from Hirsh J, Hoak J. Management of deep vein thrombosis and pulmonary embolism. A statement for healthcare professionals. Council on Thrombosis (in consultation with the Council on Cardiovascular Radiology), American Heart Association. Circulation. 1996;93(12):2212-2245. [PMID: 8925592] Copyright 1996, The American Heart Association.

activated protein C. This mutation can be detected by genetic analysis or by a coagulation assay (that is, the activated protein C resistance assay), results for the latter of which may also be abnormal because of other circumstances. In the United States, the factor V Leiden mutation occurs in approximately 6% of the white population and less frequently in other ethnic populations (**Table 18**). This mutation is found in approximately 20% of all individuals with a deep venous thrombosis (DVT) and occurs much more frequently in those with idiopathic DVT; it is also associated with DVT in women who take oral contraceptive pills.

Another common genetic thrombophilia is a G→A mutation in the prothrombin gene at position 20210 ($PT^{G20210A}$), resulting in higher prothrombin levels in affected individuals. This condition occurs in approximately 3% of white individuals in the United States and confers a three- to fourfold increased risk for venous thromboembolism (VTE). Surprisingly, neither the heterozygote factor V Leiden nor the $PT^{G20210A}$ phenotypes are associated with a significantly increased risk for recurrent VTE, possibly because patients with an initial episode of thrombosis or pulmonary embolism have an alternative predisposing risk or, perhaps, because the venous damage from the initial thrombophlebitis itself predisposes to recurrent thrombosis.

TABLE 17 Major Risk Factors for Thrombosis

Acquired		Inherited	Unknown
Prior thrombosis	Prolonged air travel	Antithrombin deficiency	Hyperhomocysteinemia
Advancing age	Antiphospholipid antibody syndrome	Protein C deficiency	High levels of factor VIII
Obesity	Myeloproliferative disorders (especially polycythemia vera and essential thrombocythemia)	Protein S deficiency	APC-resistance in the absence of Factor V Leiden
Immobilization	Paroxysmal nocturnal hemoglobinuria	Factor V Leiden	High levels of factor IX
Major surgery	Heparin-induced thrombocytopenia	Prothrombin 20210A	High levels of factor XI
Estrogens (includes OCPs, HRT, SERMs)	Inflammatory bowel disease	Dysfibrinogenemias (rare)	High levels of TAFI
Malignancy	Nephrotic syndrome		Low levels of free TFPI Decreased fibrinolytic potential

APC = activated protein C; OCP = oral contraceptive pills; HRT = hormone replacement therapy; SERM = selective estrogen receptor modulator; TAFI = thrombin-activatable fibrinolysis; TFPI = tissue factor pathway inhibitor.

TABLE 18 Familial or Acquired Thrombophilia: Estimated Prevalence by Population, and Incidence and Relative Risk of Incident or Recurrent Venous Thromboembolism by Thrombophilia

	Prevalence			Incident VTE		Recurrent VTE	
	Normal	Incident VTE	Recurrent (1.0-3.3)	Incidence[a] (95% CI)	Relative Risk (95% CI)	Incidence[a] (95% CI)	Relative Risk (95% CI)
Antithrombin deficiency	0.02-0.04	1-2	2-5	500 (320,730)	17.5 (9.1,33.8)	10,500 (3800,2300)	2.5
Protein C deficiency	0.02-0.05	2-5	5-10	310 (530,930)	11.3 (5.7,22.3)	5100 (2500,9400)	2.5
Protein S deficiency	0.01-1	1-3	5-10	710 (530,930)	32.4 (16.7-62.9)	6500 (2800-11,800)	2.5
Factor V leiden[b,c]	3-7	12-20	50-50	150 (80,260)	4.3‡ (1.9,9.7)	3500 (1900,6100)	1.3 (1.0-3.3)
Prothrombin 20210[b]	1-3	3-8	15-20	350	1.9 (0.9-4.1)		1.4 (0.9-2.0)
Combined[d]				840 (560,1220)	32.4 (16.7-62.9)	5000 (2000, 10,300)	
Hyperhomocysteinemia							2.5
Antiphospholipid Ab							2.5

VTE = venous thromboembolism; CI = confidence interval; Ab = antibody.

[a] per 100,000 person-years.

[b] Heterozygous carriers.

[c] Homozygous carriers' relative risk = 80.

[d] Combined factor V Leiden and prothrombin 20,210.

Reproduced with permission from Heit J. Thrombophilia: Clinical and laboratory assessment and management. In: C. Kitchens, B. Alving, C. Kessler, eds. Consultative Hemostasis and Thrombosis. Philadelphia, PA: Saunders; 2007:213-244. Copyright 2007, Elsevier.

Antithrombin (previously known as antithrombin III) deficiency is an autosomal-dominant disorder, and the prevalence of the heterozygous condition is 0.02% in the general population (homozygous antithrombin deficiency is generally not compatible with life). Antithrombin deficiency is associated with a risk for VTE of approximately 1% per year. Type 1 deficiency is a deficiency of the protein, whereas type II deficiency is characterized by a defective protein. Protein C and protein S are vitamin K–dependent proteins. Protein C requires activation by thrombomodulin-thrombin on the endothelial surface to neutralize factors VIIIa and Va, whereas protein S is a cofactor in this reaction. Protein C deficiency is inherited as an autosomal-recessive trait, with 1 in 200 to 300 individuals affected, many of whom are asymptomatic. Protein C has a half-life of approximately 6 hours, decreases to low levels soon after initiation of warfarin therapy, and is the cause of warfarin-induced skin necrosis in some patients. Concomitant treatment with heparin can prevent such an adverse event. Protein S deficiency is inherited as an autosomal-dominant trait. Its frequency is less than that of protein C deficiency. It circulates bound to C4b-binding protein, 40% of which is free and active. Deficiencies of protein C, S, and antithrombin all lead to an increased risk for VTE (see Table 18). Arterial thrombotic events are rare.

Acquired Causes of Thrombophilia

Antithrombin or protein C or S deficiency may occur rarely in patients with nephrotic syndrome due to loss of these proteins in the urine. The antiphospholipid syndrome is the most common acquired thrombophilia. The antiphospholipid antibody is actually an antibody to a protein bound to phospholipid identified as β_2-glycoprotein 1. Other proteins, such as prothrombin or protein C, may function as the epitope for binding. The antiphospholipid antibody sometimes interferes with the coagulation cascade as measured by the activated partial thromboplastin time (aPTT) or the prothrombin time (PT), causing a prolongation that is not corrected with a corresponding mix including normal plasma (that is, a lupus inhibitor). These antibodies, although they prolong in vitro coagulation tests, are associated with an increased risk for venous (approximately two thirds) and arterial thromboembolism. There is also a strong correlation between this syndrome and pregnancy loss, presumably due to placental insufficiency in affected patients secondary to thrombosis.

Criteria for the diagnosis of the antiphospholipid syndrome are listed in **Table 19**.

For individuals with antiphospholipid syndrome and a thromboembolic event, long-term oral anticoagulant therapy is indicated.

Laboratory Testing

Laboratory testing for thrombophilia is fraught with great confusion and misunderstanding concerning the use of assays. Expert opinion suggests that tests should be performed in patients with unusual or idiopathic events or for those whose events occurred at a young age. Tests that are not biologic assays, such as genetic testing, can be done if necessary. Testing should not be done in the setting of an acute thrombotic event but rather weeks or months after it has occurred and when anticoagulant therapy has been discontinued, because active thrombosis may alter the level of some proteins.

Screening for thrombophilia is based on whether patients are determined to be strongly or weakly thrombophilic; the former should undergo screening, whereas screening may not be cost-effective in the latter group. Patients who are considered strongly thrombophilic will often have had their first idiopathic venous thrombosis before 50 years of age, may have a history of recurrent thrombotic episodes, and may have first-degree relative(s) in whom a documented thromboembolism has occurred before the age of 50 years. Weakly thrombophilic patients with a venous thromboembolism have none, or perhaps one, of these characteristics.

Patients who are strongly thrombophilic should undergo testing for activated protein C resistance, factor V Leiden, the prothrombin gene mutation, antiphospholipid antibodies, a lupus inhibitor, antithrombin deficiency, protein C deficiency,

---

TABLE 19 Criteria for Diagnosis of Antiphospholipid Syndrome[a]

Clinical Criteria

1. Vascular thromboses:

 One or more episodes of a vascular thrombotic event.

2. Pregnancy morbidity:

 One or more unexplained deaths of a morphologically normal fetus beyond the 10th week of gestation.

 One or more premature births of a morphologically normal neonate before the 34th week of gestation because of eclampsia or severe preeclampsia or recognized features of placental insufficiency.

 Three or more unexplained consecutive spontaneous abortions before the 10th week of gestation.

Laboratory Criteria

1. Presence of lupus anticoagulant on two or more occasions at least 12 weeks apart.

2. Anticardiolipin antibody of IgG and or IgM isotype in medium or high titer on two or more occasions at least 12 weeks apart.

3. Presence of anti-β_2-glycoprotein 1 antibody of IgG and or IgM isotype present on two or more occasions at least 12 weeks apart.

[a]The diagnosis requires at least one clinical and one laboratory criterion.

Adapted with permission from Miyakis S, Lockshin MD, Atsumi T, et al. International consensus statement on an update of the classification criteria for definite antiphospholipid syndrome. J Thromb Haemost. 2006;4(2):295-306. [PMID: 16420554] Copyright 2006, The International Society on Thrombosis and Haemostasis.

and protein S deficiency. Those who are weakly thrombophilic should undergo either no special testing or testing for activated protein C resistance, factor V Leiden, the prothrombin gene mutation, antiphospholipid antibodies, and a lupus inhibitor. Testing for antithrombin deficiency, protein C deficiency, and protein S deficiency is not indicated in weakly thrombophilic patients.

Antithrombotic Agents

Three major classes of antithrombotic drugs are currently in use: anticoagulants, antiplatelet agents, and thrombolytic or fibrinolytic agents. Thrombolytic agents have a direct effect on thrombi by hastening their dissolution, whereas anticoagulants and antiplatelet agents are always prophylactic because they prevent de novo initiation of thrombosis (primary prophylaxis) or extension or recurrence of established thrombi (secondary prophylaxis).

Unfractionated Heparin

Unfractionated heparin, a glycosaminoglycan with a molecular weight ranging from 5000 to 30,000 daltons and derived primarily from porcine intestinal mucosa, binds to antithrombin through a unique pentasaccharide in the heparin molecule, enabling antithrombin to bind rapidly and neutralize the serine protease coagulation factors (IIa, IXa, Xa, XIa, and XIIa) (**Figure 24**). To neutralize thrombin, unfractionated heparin must also bind to thrombin, which requires a minimal chain length of 18 monosaccharides in the unfractionated heparin molecule. This is not required for Factor Xa inactivation. Unfractionated heparin has a half-life of approximately 1 hour after intravenous bolus administration and is metabolized in part by the liver and is partially excreted by the kidneys.

The frequent failure of heparin to achieve a therapeutic level of anticoagulation remains a challenge and is principally the result of inadequate dosing. Dosing nomograms help to standardize and improve therapy and facilitate achievement and maintenance of more rapid therapeutic levels of heparin. **Table 20** outlines a popular dosing nomogram.

The aPTT, used to measure the heparin response, is highly dependent on the reagent used in the test. Every laboratory is obligated to perform an in vitro or ex vivo heparin titration curve with the reagent currently in use and establish the reagent-specific therapeutic range (equivalent to 0.2–0.7 U/mL of heparin, depending on the type of titration curve used).

Low-Molecular-Weight Heparin

Low-molecular-weight heparin (LMWH) is a fragment of unfractionated heparin produced by chemical or enzymatic depolymerization of unfractionated heparin. The average molecular weight of LMWH agents ranges from 4000 to 6500 daltons and contains the pentasaccharide for antithrombin binding. Because LMWH lacks many of the larger monosaccharide chains (≥18) required for binding to thrombin, it has a greater relative ability to neutralize factor Xa than does

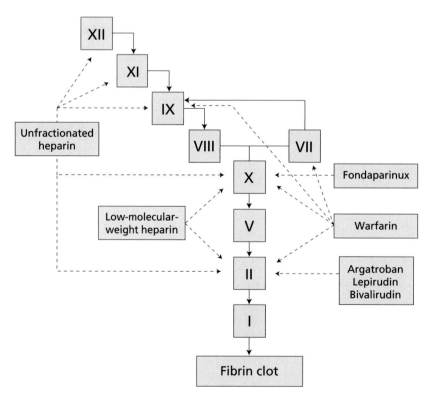

FIGURE 24.
The coagulation cascade illustrating the anticoagulants commonly used today and their specific targets.

TABLE 20 Heparin Dosing Nomogram	
Heparin Dosing and Monitoring Activities	
Check baseline aPTT, INR, CBC/platelet count	
Give heparin bolus, 80 U/kg, IV	
Begin IV heparin infusion, 18 U/kg/h	
Target aPTT for institution-specific therapeutic range[a]	
aPTT-based Dosing Adjustments	
aPTT	**Dosing Adjustment**
<35 sec[a]	80 U/kg bolus; increase drip by 4 U/kg/h
35–50 sec[a]	40 U/kg bolus; increase drip by 2 U/kg/h
51–70 sec[a]	No change
71–90 sec[a]	Reduce drip by 2 U/kg/h
>90 sec[a]	Hold heparin for 1 h; reduce drip by 3 U/kg/h

aPTT = activated partial thromboplastin time; IV = intravenous; CBC = complete blood count; INR = International Normalized Ratio.

[a]Each laboratory must perform its own in vitro heparin titration curve to establish the therapeutic range for the specific aPTT reagent in use, which is equivalent to a heparin concentration of 0.3-0.7 anti Xa U/mL (by anti Xa assay) or 0.2-0.4 U/mL (by protamine titration assay). The therapeutic range varies depending on the aPTT reagent in use.

Adapted with permission from Raschke RA, Reilly BM, Guidry JR, et al. The weight-based heparin dosing nomogram compared with a standard care nomogram. Ann Intern Med. 1993;119(9):874-881. [PMID: 8214998] Copyright 1993, American College of Physicians.

thrombin. LMWH agents have a significantly reduced ability to bind to plasma proteins, facilitating increased availability for binding to antithrombin, producing an anticoagulant effect, and requiring no laboratory monitoring, except, perhaps, during pregnancy. They are also more uniformly absorbed from subcutaneous depots and have a longer plasma half-life (range, 3 to 5 h). LMWH agents are excreted predominantly from the kidney. Alteration of dosing is required in patients with renal failure for whom it is recommended that full-dose therapy be instituted only with the aid of anti-Xa–factor assay monitoring capability. Monitoring may also be helpful in morbidly obese patients.

The indications for LMWH depend on the commercial preparation used and include VTE prophylaxis and treatment and prophylaxis of ischemic complications in the setting of acute coronary syndromes and ST-elevation myocardial infarction.

Fondaparinux

Fondaparinux is a further refinement on the mechanism of action of unfractionated heparin. It contains the pentasaccharide that binds to and activates antithrombin, and it is synthetically synthesized. It is a specific indirect inhibitor of factor Xa and has no antithrombin effect because it lacks the longer saccharide chains necessary for thrombin binding. Fondaparinux has essentially no protein binding, has a predictable antithrombotic effect, and requires no coagulation monitoring. This agent has good absorption from subcutaneous depots, reaches peak concentrations in 1 to 3 hours, and has an effective half-life of approximately 17 hours, allowing for once-daily dosing. Although fondaparinux may induce heparin/platelet factor-4 antibodies, these antibodies rarely cause heparin-induced thrombocytopenia (HIT) (see HIT). It is excreted entirely by the kidneys and is not recommended in patients with renal impairment (creatinine clearance <30 mL/min).

Fondaparinux is approved for prophylaxis of VTE in patients undergoing hip or knee replacement surgery or hip fracture surgery and in other medical or surgical conditions. It is also approved for the treatment of acute DVT or pulmonary embolism.

Fondaparinux, when initiated 4 to 8 hours after surgery, has been found to be superior to LMWH in preventing VTE after total hip replacement, total knee replacement, and hip fracture surgery. It has also been reported to be non-inferior to dalteparin in preventing postoperative VTE in patients who undergo high-risk abdominal surgery.

Vitamin K Antagonists (Warfarin)

Warfarin, the major vitamin K antagonist used in North America, interferes with the reduction and recycling of oxidized vitamin K (**Figure 25**). As a result, poorly functional coagulation precursors are secreted, leading to defective coagulation. Factor VII has the shortest half-life (approximately 6 h), and its concentration falls the most rapidly. Factor II has a half-life of approximately 60 hours; thus, several days of therapy are required to achieve a decrease in concentration, explaining why heparin and warfarin therapy must overlap for a minimum of 3 to 5 days to result in a reduction of all vitamin K–dependent coagulation factors.

Warfarin is indicated for the prevention or treatment of VTE; for prevention of systemic embolism in patients with prosthetic heart valves or atrial fibrillation; for the primary prevention of acute myocardial infarction in high-risk men; and for the prevention of stroke, recurrent infarction, or death in patients with acute myocardial infarction.

Warfarin has a narrow therapeutic window, exhibits considerable variability in dose response among patients, is subject to interactions with drugs and diet, requires laboratory control that can be difficult to standardize, and requires complex dosing regimens that can lead to compliance and communications errors. Warfarin therapy therefore must be managed carefully to avoid adverse events. Management by specialized anticoagulation clinics has been shown to yield improved outcomes (safety and efficacy) compared with care provided by individual physicians who do not employ a systematic approach to anticoagulation management. Patient-specific characteristics, such as heart, liver, and kidney disorders; cancer; anemia; and history of stroke are risk factors for adverse events in patients who receive warfarin.

The initial average maintenance dose of warfarin is 5 mg/d or lower in patients who are elderly or malnourished, or who have liver disease, heart failure, or are recently postoperative.

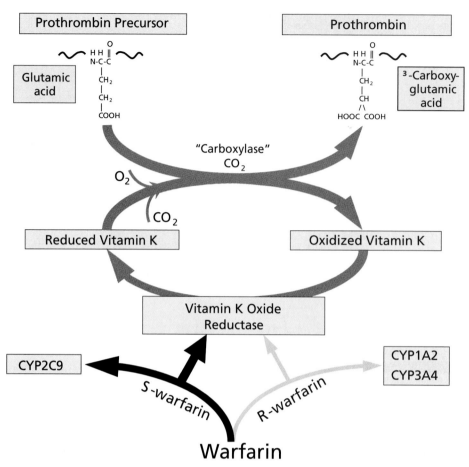

FIGURE 25.
The mechanism of action of warfarin.

Warfarin should overlap with heparin therapy for a period of 3 to 5 days, although it can be commenced out of hospital in some patients without initial heparin (for example, in patients with chronic stable atrial fibrillation).

Estimation of the maintenance dose is based on observations of the INR response. An individual who rapidly achieves a high therapeutic PT (INR >2.0) after two doses of warfarin is likely to require a low maintenance dose. Conversely, patients in whom little elevation of the PT (INR <1.5) is observed after two doses are likely to require a higher maintenance dose.

Pharmacogenetic-based dosing may play an important role in the pharmacokinetic and pharmacodynamic behavior of warfarin. Single nucleotide polymorphisms in the gene coding for CYP2C9 (see Figure 25), the principal enzyme responsible for metabolizing the S enantiomer of warfarin, alter the rate of metabolism (that is, half-life) of warfarin, affecting the rapidity of initial effect and the dose required to maintain a therapeutic INR. Similarly, various mutations in the gene coding for the VKORC1 enzyme, the target of warfarin, lead to a protein that is either sensitive or resistant to warfarin inhibition, and, consequently, also affect the initial dose and the maintenance dose required to achieve a therapeutic INR.

Retrospective analyses have shown that single nucleotide polymorphisms coding for these proteins may account for up to 50% of the variation in the dose required to achieve a therapeutic INR, and algorithms have been developed to help in the initial warfarin dosing. These mutations have also been shown to correlate with adverse events. Whether dosing algorithms based on pharmacogenetics add value to the conscientious monitoring of the INR and dose management remains to be determined. Pilot trials of genetic-based dosing have yielded mixed results, but a recent randomized prospective trial showed that dosing based on real-time pharmacogenetic information achieved a therapeutic range faster and maintained the therapeutic range longer than dosing based on INR response alone.

An elevated INR is managed by discontinuing warfarin, administering vitamin K, or infusing the patient with fresh frozen plasma, prothrombin concentrate, or recombinant factor VIIa. The choice of therapy is based on the severity of the clinical situation. Vitamin K should be administered orally or intravenously in urgent situations.

Perioperative management of patients who are taking warfarin when an invasive procedure is needed requires an assessment of the risk for surgical bleeding if anticoagulation is continued versus the risk for thrombosis if anticoagulation is discontinued. LMWH is currently recommended over unfractionated heparin as an alternative agent in this setting because it is a less-complex treatment modality, requires no monitoring, and can be administered at home. A recent review of LMWH versus unfractionated heparin in the perioperative setting summarizes the options and outcomes for a range of procedures. **Table 21** summarizes the 2008 American College of Chest Physicians Chest Consensus Conference recommendations for management.

TABLE 21 Pre- and Postoperative Bridging Guidelines for Patients Receiving Warfarin

Guideline	Grade of Recommendation[a]
Stop warfarin therapy ~5 days preoperatively	1B
Resume warfarin therapy ~12-24 h postoperatively if hemostasis is secure	1C
If INR >1.5 the day before procedure, can administer oral vitamin K, 1-2 mg	1C
For patients with MHV, AF, or VTE at high risk of TE, bridging with full-dose SC LMWH or IV UFH is recommended	1C
For patients with MHV, AF, or VTE at moderate risk of TE, bridging with full-dose SC LMWH, IV UFH, or low-dose SC LMWH is recommended	2C
For patients with MHV, AF, or VTE at low risk of TE, bridging with low-dose SC LMWH or no bridging is recommended	2C
When possible, outpatient SC LMWH over inpatient IV UFH is recommended from a cost-saving perspective	1C
Administer last dose of full-dose SC LMWH 24 h preoperatively at half the calculated dose	1C
If receiving IV UFH, stop infusion at ~4 h preoperatively	1C
Resume full-dose SC LMWH for minor procedures ~24 h postoperatively if hemostasis is secured	1C
Resume full-dose SC LMWH/UFH for major procedures or high bleeding-risk procedures ~48–72 h postoperatively if hemostasis is secured, or low-dose SC LMWH/UFH when hemostasis is secured	1C

MHV = mechanical heart valve; AF = atrial fibrillation; VTE = venous thromboembolism; TE = thromboembolism; SC LMWH = subcutaneous low-molecular-weight heparin; IV UFH = intravenous unfractionated heparin; INR = International Normalized Ratio.

[a] Grade 1 recommendations are considered strong and indicate that the benefits do (or do not) outweigh risks, burdens, and costs, whereas grade 2 recommendations are referred to as suggestions and imply that individual patient values may lead to different management choices.

Adapted with permission from Douketis JD, Berger P, Dunn AS, et al; American College of Chest Physicians. The perioperative management of antithrombotic therapy: American College of Chest Physicians Evidence-based Clinical Practice Guidelines (8th Edition). Chest. 2008;133(6 Suppl):299S-339S. [PMID: 18574269] Copyright 2008, American College of Chest Physicians.

Direct Thrombin Inhibitors

There are three direct thrombin inhibitors in clinical use: lepirudin, the recombinant form of the leech enzyme, hirudin; bivalirudin, an engineered form of hirudin that alters its thrombin-binding capacity and half-life; and argatroban, a small molecule that binds irreversibly to the active site of thrombin. Each of these is a parenterally administered drug with limited Food and Drug Administration–approved indications, and all require therapeutic monitoring. Lepirudin and argatroban are principally used as alternative anticoagulants for patients with HIT. Lepirudin is excreted in the urine and argatroban metabolized by the liver, attributes that often determine which of the two is to be used based on the patient's comorbidities. Bivalirudin is used in percutaneous coronary interventions as an alternative to unfractionated heparin. It is also approved for HIT in this setting.

KEY POINTS

- Factor V Leiden and PT^{20210} gene mutations are responsible for two of the most common inherited types of thrombophilia.
- Thrombophilia testing is best done after the acute thrombotic event has occurred and at least 2 weeks after completion of anticoagulation therapy in these patients.
- Thrombophilia screening is appropriate for selected patients who experience unusual thromboses or who were young when the event occurred.
- Fondaparinux, when initiated 4 to 8 hours after surgery, has been found to be superior to low-molecular-weight heparin in preventing venous thromboembolism after total hip replacement, total knee replacement, and hip fracture surgery.
- Patient-specific characteristics, such as heart, liver, and kidney disorders; cancer; anemia; and history of stroke are risk factors for adverse events in patients who receive warfarin.

Management of Venous Thromboembolism

The clinical features of DVT, such as pain, redness, warmth, and swelling, are nonspecific and may reflect other conditions (for example, cellulitis, heart failure, or ruptured Baker cyst). A definitive diagnosis of DVT can be made only with objective testing. Thus, even a moderate or strong suspicion of VTE must be confirmed by objective testing. Currently, compression ultrasonography is the most commonly used confirmatory diagnostic tool in patients with suspected DVT. In patients with DVT, compression ultrasonography will detect a noncompressible venous lumen, inside which echogenic material is visible. Contrast venography, the gold standard, is seldom used because of its invasiveness, cost, and associated morbidity.

Clinical rules have been developed and verified to help establish the diagnosis of DVT or pulmonary embolism to formalize clinical thinking and optimize clinical testing. The best-known predictive model is that of Wells et al. According to these criteria, each of the following characteristics earns 1 point: active cancer; paralysis or recent plaster cast; recent immobilization or major surgery; tenderness along the deep veins; swelling of the whole leg; greater than a 3-cm difference in calf circumference compared with other leg; pitting edema; and collateral superficial veins. Patients in whom an alternative diagnosis is likely earn -2 points. A high probability for DVT exists in patients with a score of greater than 3; a moderate probability exists in those with a score of 1 to 2; and low pretest probability exists in those with a score of 0 or less.

Immunologic D-dimer assays are particularly sensitive for detecting the presence of intravascular thrombosis, but they have a low specificity for predicting DVT. Therefore, a negative assay may be helpful in excluding an acute thrombotic process, but a positive assay is not helpful. Sensitive enzyme-linked immunosorbent assays (ELISAs) have been studied for their negative predictive value in excluding the presence of a DVT, and D-dimer assays have been included as part of diagnostic algorithms to aid in the diagnosis of DVT and minimize invasive testing. In the setting of low clinical probability and negative D-dimer assay results, a DVT can be excluded without the need for an objective test.

DVT and pulmonary embolism require initial treatment with an immediate-acting anticoagulant, usually unfractionated heparin, LMWH, or fondaparinux. Inadequate initial therapy with unfractionated heparin has been shown to result in a high recurrence rate. Warfarin is initiated simultaneously with heparin, and both therapies are overlapped for a minimum of 4 to 5 days and until the INR has reached the therapeutic range for two measurements taken 24 hours apart. In selected cases of severe iliofemoral thrombosis, catheter-directed thrombolysis has been used to restore patency with apparent effectiveness, but randomized controlled trials comparing this procedure with standard anticoagulant therapy are lacking; therefore, its routine use is not recommended.

The duration of therapy is determined by whether a DVT is associated with reversible or irreversible inciting factors or is idiopathic (**Table 22**).

DVT associated with transient reversible factors is associated with a low risk for recurrence after 3 to 6 months of anticoagulant therapy. DVT that is idiopathic or associated with certain congenital thrombophilic conditions has a rate of recurrence as high as 8% to 10% per year after 6 to 12 months of therapy; therefore, longer-term therapy is recommended for patients in these settings, and in some situations, lifelong therapy is appropriate. To reduce the risk for bleeding and the need for INR testing, the PREVENT investigators showed that administering a lower-intensity anticoagulation regimen (INR, 1.5–2.0) after the initial 3 to 6 months of therapy in patients with a high risk for DVT recurrence resulted in a significant reduction in recurrence risk and no increased major bleeding risk compared with placebo. The ELATE investigators, however, found that administering continued anticoagulation to achieve a target INR of 2.0 to 3.0 was more effective than reduced-intensity anticoagulation, without evidence of increased bleeding. The patient-specific estimated risk of bleeding should determine which of these two strategies to use.

Recently, results of D-dimer assay performed after 6 months of anticoagulation therapy have been shown to be predictive of thrombotic recurrence. An elevated high-sensitivity D-dimer assay result predicts an increased risk for recurrence by at least fourfold compared with a normal result. Thus, a positive assay provides further impetus to continue long-term anticoagulation, whereas a normal assay might lead to cessation of therapy because of an altered risk/benefit ratio for continued anticoagulation. The assay must be done 3 to 4 weeks after warfarin therapy is stopped.

In patients with VTE and cancer, several studies, including the CLOT study, have shown the potential benefit of LMWH over warfarin. Lee et al. found a significant difference in recurrent DVT between those randomized to receive 3 months of dalteparin (27/336; 8%) versus dalteparin followed by warfarin (53/336; 16%) (NNT = 13) in patients with VTE and cancer. There was no significant difference in major bleeding or death between these two groups.

There is a 20% to 40% incidence of postphlebitic syndrome after an episode of DVT manifested by intermittent discomfort, swelling, varicosities, and skin changes. A very small percentage of patients will develop severe symptoms including skin ulcerations.

KEY POINTS

- Compression ultrasonography is used as a confirmatory diagnostic test for patients in whom there is a strong or moderate clinical suspicion of venous thromboembolism.

- The Wells clinical prediction rules help to establish the likelihood of the presence of venous thromboembolism.

- The D-dimer assay is helpful in excluding venous thromboembolism in patients in whom the clinical suspicion for this condition is low.

- D-dimer assays may be helpful in predicting the risk for recurrent venous thromboembolism once anticoagulants are stopped.

- Venous thromboembolism in the setting of cancer is best treated with prolonged low-molecular-weight heparin (3 to 6 months) with subsequent transition to warfarin if necessary.

TABLE 22 Duration of Treatment and Management of Patients with Venous Thromboembolism[a]

Type of VTE	Duration of Therapy	Management
Associated with a transient reversible risk factor	3-6 months of anticoagulation with warfarin	Target INR of 2.5
Associated with a major continuing risk factor; associated with a major thrombophilic defect (APS, AT, or PC deficiency); recurrent; idiopathic	A minimum of 6-12 months of anticoagulation with warfarin, with consideration of long-term, indefinite anticoagulation	Target INR of 2.5 for the first 6 months. Depending on estimated risk of recurrence and risk for bleeding, target INR of 1.8 after 6 months is acceptable (an ongoing target of 2.5 is more effective, but could confer a higher risk for an adverse event)
Associated with cancer	3-6 months of anticoagulation with LMWH followed by warfarin if anticoagulation still required	Dalteparin, 200 U/kg/d × 1 month, followed by 150 U/kg/d × 5 months followed by warfarin, target INR of 2.5, if required

VTE = venous thromboembolism; INR = international normalized ratio; APS = antiphospholipid syndrome; AT = antithrombin; PC = protein C; LMWH = low-molecular-weight heparin.

[a]Patients must be assessed regularly for indefinite or long-term anticoagulation, and the duration is determined by assessing the risk of bleeding while receiving warfarin versus the risk for recurrent VTE after cessation of warfarin.

Bibliography

Agnelli G, Becattini C. Treatment of DVT: How long is long enough and how do you predict recurrence. J Thromb Thrombolysis. 2008:25(1):37-44. [PMID: 17906973]

Agnelli G; Bergqvist D; Cohen AT; Gallus AS; Gent M; PEGASUS investigators. Randomized clinical trial of postoperative fondaparinux versus perioperative dalteparin for prevention of venous thromboembolism in high-risk abdominal surgery. Br J Surg. 2005;92(10):1212-1220. [PMID: 16175516]

Ansell, J, Hirsh J, Hylek E, Jacobson A, Crowther M, Palareti G; American College of Chest Physicians. Pharmacology and management of the vitamin K antagonists: American College of Chest Physicians Evidence-Based Clinical Practice Guidelines (8th Edition). Chest. 2008;133:160S-198S. [PMID: 18574265]

Bauer KA. The thrombophilias: Well-defined risk factors with uncertain therapeutic implications. Ann Intern Med. 2001;135(5):367-373. [PMID: 11529700]

Caraco Y, Blotnick S, Muszkat M. CYP2C9 genotype-guided warfarin prescribing enhances the efficacy and safety of anticoagulation: a prospective randomized controlled study. Clin Pharmacol Ther. 2008;83(3):460-70. [PMID: 17851566]

Douketis JD, Berger PB, Dunn AS, et al; American College of Chest Physicians. The perioperative management of antithrombotic therapy: American College of Chest Physicians Evidence-Based Clinical Practice Guidelines (8th Edition). Chest. 2008;133(6 Suppl):299S-339S. [PMID: 18574269]

Gage BF, Eby C, Milligan PE, Banet GA, Duncan JR, McLeod HL. Use of pharmacogenetics and clinical factors to predict the maintenance dose of warfarin. Thromb Haemost 2004;91(1):87-94. [PMID: 14691573]

Kearon C, Ginsberg JS, Kovacs MJ, et al; Extended Low-Intensity Anticoagulation for Thrombo-Embolism Investigators. Comparison of low-intensity warfarin therapy with conventional-intensity warfarin therapy for long-term prevention of recurrent venous thromboembolism. N Engl J Med. 2003;349(7):631-639. [PMID: 12917299]

Lee AYY, Levine MN, Baker RI, et al; Randomized Comparison of Low-Molecular-Weight Heparin versus Oral Anticoagulant Therapy for the Prevention of Recurrent Venous Thromboembolism in Patients with Cancer (CLOT) Investigators. Low molecular weight heparin versus a coumarin for the prevention of recurrent venous thromboembolism in patients with cancer. N Engl J Med. 2003;349(2):146-153. [PMID: 12853587]

Lim W, Crowther MA, Eikelboom JW. Management of antiphospholipid antibody syndrome: A systematic review. JAMA. 2006;295(7):1050-1057. [PMID: 16507806]

Palareti G, Cosmi B, Legnani C, et al; PROLONG investigators. D-dimer testing to determine the duration of anticoagulation therapy [erratum in N Engl J Med. 2006;355(26):2797]. N Engl J Med. 2006;355(17):1780-1789. [PMID: 17065639]

Ridker PM, Goldhaber SZ, Danielson E, et al; PREVENT investorgatos. Long-term, low-intensity warfarin therapy for the prevention of recurrent venous thromboembolism. N Engl J Med. 2003;348(15):1425-1434. [PMID: 12601075]

Turpie AG, Bauer KA, Eriksson BI, Lassen MR. Fondaparinux vs enoxaparin for the prevention of venous thromboembolism in major orthopedic surgery: a meta-analysis of 4 randomized double-blind studies. Arch Intern Med. 2002;162(16):1833-1840. [PMID: 12196081]

Wells PS, Hirsh J, Anderson DR, et al. Accuracy of clinical assessment of deep vein thrombosis [erratum in Lancet 1995;346(8973):516]. Lancet. 1995;345(8961):1326-1330. [PMID:7752753]

Hematologic Issues in Pregnancy

Gestational Anemia

Normal pregnancy is associated with a mild anemia despite increases in erythropoietin and erythrocyte production and erythrocyte mass. The anemia is due to a dramatic increase in plasma volume as a consequence of an increased uterine vascular bed in addition to poorly defined hormonal mechanisms. The relatively greater increase in plasma volume compared with the increase in erythrocyte mass leads to a low-viscosity erythrocytosis that promotes oxygen delivery to the developing fetus.

Anemia usually becomes apparent in the eighth week of pregnancy and progresses throughout most of the third trimester. Several weeks before delivery, anemia stabilizes and then rapidly improves before delivery. Gestational anemia is defined as hemoglobin levels greater than 11.0 g/dL (110 g/L) in the first and third trimesters and greater than 10.5 g/dL (105 g/L) in the second trimester. Healthy pregnant women have normochromic, normocytic erythrocyte indices, and gestational anemia usually does not require further investigation. Additional studies are needed for pregnant women with marked normocytic anemia, which could indicate red cell aplasia, a rare cause of anemia in pregnancy. Prompt evaluation is also required for pregnant women with erythrocytes of abnormal size, an elevated reticulocyte count, or an abnormal leukocyte or platelet count.

Iron Deficiency

Iron deficiency is present in up to 40% of pregnant women worldwide. It occurs when dietary iron supplementation and iron storage provide less iron than that needed for both the developing fetus and the increased erythrocyte mass associated with pregnancy. As with iron deficiency in nonpregnant patients, iron deficiency in pregnant women is diagnosed by low serum iron and ferritin levels and elevated serum total iron-binding capacity in the setting of microcytic, hypochromic erythrocytes. Iron deficiency in pregnant women who do not have an obvious cause for blood loss is usually the result of the pregnancy. In these women, iron deficiency does not require further investigation and can be remedied with oral replacement of iron salts.

Although iron deficiency is associated with increased complications during pregnancy, including preterm delivery and low-birth-weight newborns, data from randomized trials do not provide clear support for routine iron prophylaxis for pregnant women who are not anemic. However, even in the absence of supporting data, iron supplements are routinely given to almost all pregnant women in the United States. Occasional pregnant patients will be unable to absorb oral iron adequately or will have such high iron requirements that parenteral iron therapy is indicated. Parenteral iron dextran is associated with significant side effects, including anaphylaxis, and is therefore a pregnancy class C drug (safety uncertain). Newer parenteral iron preparations, including iron sucrose and ferric gluconate, are better tolerated. These are pregnancy class B drugs (presumed safe) that may be effective for pregnant patients who require parenteral iron therapy. However, large, high-quality trials that assess clinical outcomes are needed to establish the efficacy and safety of these newer parenteral iron preparations during pregnancy.

Folate Deficiency

Pregnant women have approximately twice the folate requirements as nonpregnant women because of folate needs of the developing fetus. Folate deficiency is associated with neural tube defects. In order to prevent this birth defect, mandatory folate supplementation of grains and cereal products is required

in the United States. Additionally, pregnant women are routinely prescribed multivitamins with folate. Folate deficiency is therefore very rare in pregnant women in this country.

KEY POINTS

- Mild anemia (hemoglobin level greater than 10.5 to 11.0 g/dL [105 g/L to 110 g/L]) occurs during pregnancy and generally does not require evaluation or treatment.
- Evaluation is required for pregnant women with marked normocytic anemia, erythrocytes of abnormal size, an elevated reticulocyte count, or an abnormal leukocyte or platelet count.
- Iron deficiency is common during pregnancy and generally does not require extensive evaluation.
- Iron deficiency in pregnant women can usually be treated with oral iron supplementation.

Sickle Cell Disease in Pregnancy

Women who are homozygous for hemoglobin S (SS) have later menarche, later first pregnancies, and more spontaneous abortions than matched normal controls. Newborns of mothers with SS anemia have lower birth weights and lower gestational ages. The pregnancy-related mortality rate in affected women is between 0.5% and 2%. Because of the increased fetal morbidity and maternal mortality, pregnancy in these women should be managed by a team of medical personnel, including an obstetrician, primary care physician, and hematologist. If possible, patients should consult their physicians before planning a pregnancy. Despite earlier reports suggesting an increased risk of hypertension and eclampsia in patients with SS anemia, more recent studies showed no difference in these complications. In contrast to women who are homozygous for hemoglobin S or women with SC disease or S/β-thalassemia, women with sickle cell trait are not anemic and do not have an increased incidence of obstetric complications.

Based on results of randomized studies, prophylactic blood transfusions are generally not needed for pregnant women with SS anemia. However, transfusions may be indicated for certain patients, including those with severe uncompensated anemia evidenced by signs of heart failure (see Transfusion Medicine).

Pain crises may increase during pregnancy, and typical opiate analgesics can generally be used. However, meperidine is contraindicated in patients with sickle cell disease because of its tendency to induce seizures owing to accumulation of normeperidine. Hydroxyurea is contraindicated during pregnancy and should ideally be discontinued at least 3 months before conception. Although case reports of successful pregnancies in women taking hydroxyurea have been published, there are currently no guidelines concerning the management of patients who become pregnant while taking this drug. Discontinuing hydroxyurea immediately upon recognition of pregnancy therefore seems advisable.

Thrombocytopenia in Pregnancy

Gestational Thrombocytopenia

Gestational (mild) thrombocytopenia is the most common cause of pregnancy-associated thrombocytopenia. Although platelet concentrations tend to decrease progressively during pregnancy because of a corresponding progressive increase in plasma volume, levels generally do not reach the thrombocytopenic range. Most pregnant women who do have a mild thrombocytopenia, called gestational or incidental thrombocytopenia, have platelet counts ranging between 70,000/μL $(70 \times 10^9/L)$ and 150,000/μL $(150 \times 10^9/L)$. This occurs in approximately 5% of pregnancies and appears in late gestation. The cause of gestational thrombocytopenia is unknown; although it is not believed to have an immune basis. Specific therapy is not required. However, when the platelet count decreases to less than 100,000/μL $(100 \times 10^9/L)$, more serious causes should be excluded.

Immune Thrombocytopenic Purpura

Immune (idiopathic) thrombocytopenic purpura (ITP) accounts for approximately 10% of cases of thrombocytopenia in pregnant women. No diagnostic studies are available to differentiate ITP from gestational thrombocytopenia. One clue to distinguishing these disorders is that ITP is often present before pregnancy or is detected early in the pregnancy, whereas gestational thrombocytopenia usually develops later during gestation near term.

ITP is a diagnosis of exclusion in both pregnant and nonpregnant patients. Other diagnoses to consider are preeclampsia during the latter months of pregnancy, HELLP syndrome (hemolysis, elevated liver enzymes, low platelet count), HIV-related thrombocytopenia, thrombotic thrombocytopenic purpura, and, possibly, disseminated intravascular coagulation. The peripheral blood smear in patients with ITP may show large platelets, a finding consistent with increased platelet turnover. Bone marrow aspirate or biopsy is usually not indicated.

Pregnant patients with ITP require careful monitoring but no specific therapy if the platelet count remains above 50,000/μL $(50 \times 10^9/L)$. Platelet counts only slightly below 50,000/μL $(50 \times 10^9/L)$ can generally be tolerated early in pregnancy but become more dangerous later in the second trimester and during the third trimester. If therapy must be started, prednisone, 1 mg/kg daily, is used initially. Patients must be monitored for the development of gestational diabetes, which can be exacerbated by corticosteroids. If prednisone is not effective, intravenous immune globulin is administered and must be given approximately every 3 weeks to maintain an adequate platelet count. Splenectomy may rarely be needed and is best done during the mid-second trimester. When deciding whether to perform splenectomy, the risks of surgery must be balanced against potential harm from the underlying thrombocytopenia to the fetus and mother.

Approximately 10% of newborns of mothers with ITP will have thrombocytopenia. Neither the severity of maternal thrombocytopenia nor whether the mother received treatment for ITP correlates with the occurrence of thrombocytopenia in the newborn. Because of a poor correlation with maternal thrombocytopenia as well as potential artifacts in measurement and a small percentage of morbidity and mortality from the procedure, prenatal sampling of fetal blood from a scalp vein or the umbilical cord is generally not recommended.

Preeclampsia and the HELLP Syndrome

Approximately 20% of thrombocytopenia in pregnant patients is due to preeclampsia (formerly called pregnancy-induced hypertension). Preeclampsia most commonly occurs during the later stages of gestation, and the platelet count may be as low as 20,000/μL $(20 \times 10^9/L)$.

About 10% of patients with preeclampsia develop the HELLP syndrome (hemolysis, elevated liver enzymes, low platelet count). The cause is unknown but probably represents endothelial injury, platelet activation, and subsequent platelet destruction. The HELLP syndrome is associated with a wide range of systemic symptoms, and abnormal laboratory findings may be difficult to differentiate from those caused by thrombotic thrombocytopenic purpura, hemolytic uremic syndrome, and, occasionally, disseminated intravascular coagulation. Suggested criteria for diagnosis include microangiopathic hemolytic anemia, a platelet count less than 100,000/μL $(100 \times 10^9/L)$, a serum total bilirubin level greater than 1.2 mg/dL (20.52 μmol), a serum aspartate aminotransferase level greater than 70 U/L, and a serum lactate dehydrogenase level greater than 600 U/L. The HELLP syndrome is associated with significant postpartum maternal morbidity and a maternal mortality rate of 1% to 3%. Newborns may also be affected but usually less severely than their mothers. Although both preeclampsia and the HELLP syndrome usually resolve soon after delivery, the latter may be exacerbated during the postpartum period. Intensive monitoring of the mother should therefore be continued. In some patients, corticosteroids have been shown to hasten resolution of the HELLP syndrome in the postpartum period.

Thrombotic Thrombocytopenic Purpura

Thrombotic thrombocytopenic purpura (TTP) may also occur during pregnancy. The clinical and laboratory manifestations of TTP are the same in pregnant and nonpregnant patients. Treatment of TTP is also the same for both groups of patients and involves plasmapheresis.

KEY POINTS

- Gestational (mild) thrombocytopenia is the most common cause of pregnancy-associated thrombocytopenia.
- Gestational thrombocytopenia does not require specific treatment.
- No diagnostic studies are available to differentiate gestational thrombocytopenia from immune thrombocytopenic purpura, but the latter is often present before pregnancy or is detected early in the pregnancy, whereas gestational thrombocytopenia usually develops in the third trimester or at term.
- Initial therapy for immune thrombocytopenic purpura is prednisone; if prednisone is ineffective, intravenous immune globulin is administered.
- The HELLP syndrome is characterized by microangiopathic hemolytic anemia, elevated liver enzymes (greater than 70 U/L), and a low platelet count (less than 100,000/μL [100 × 10⁹/L]).

Thrombophilia, Venous Thromboembolism, and Pregnancy

Venous thromboembolism occurs in 0.1% of pregnancies, and an inherited thrombophilic defect is found in 30% to 50% of pregnant women who develop a venous thromboembolism. Some thrombophilic defects, such as the antiphospholipid antibody syndrome, have a strong association with recurrent fetal loss, fetal growth retardation, and abruptio placentae, whereas others, such as the factor V Leiden mutation, are less strongly associated with these abnormalities, or the association is controversial. The pathophysiology of these thrombophilic defects is thought to be due to placental ischemia caused by microvascular thrombi. Whether eclampsia and preeclampsia are also associated with these defects is less clear, and many studies show no association. **Table 23** summarizes the frequency of thrombophilic disorders during pregnancy based on several studies.

Pregnant patients with a history of venous thromboembolism, a family history of thrombophilia, or a history of recurrent fetal loss should be evaluated for a thrombophilic disorder, especially if establishing the diagnosis will alter the management of the pregnancy. Routine screening is otherwise not indicated.

Prophylaxis with low-dose unfractionated heparin or low-molecular-weight heparin (LMWH) is indicated for pregnant patients with selected thrombophilic defects (deficiency of antithrombin, protein C, or protein S; compound heterozygotes for prothrombin G20210A or factor V Leiden mutation). Prophylaxis with both low-dose aspirin and low- or moderate-dose unfractionated heparin or LMWH is indicated for women with recurrent fetal loss and the antiphospholipid antibody syndrome. Anticoagulant therapy for up to 6 weeks postpartum is recommended. Other defects require only close monitoring.

Unfractionated heparin and LMWH are safe to use during pregnancy because neither crosses the placental barrier and neither has been shown to have a teratogenic effect on the fetus. However, use of either agent may be associated with mild bone loss in the mother when administered for many months. If full-dose LMWH is used, periodic monitoring

TABLE 23 Prevalence of Thrombophilia and Risk for Venous Thromboembolism in Pregnant Women

Thrombophilic Disorder	Prevalence in the General Population	Prevalence in Women with VTE in Pregnancy (%)	Risk of VTE (Odds Ratio)
None	<50	4-10	
Factor V Leiden (heterozygote)	3-7 (of white women)	20-46	5-16
Factor V Leiden (homozygote)		9-17	10-41
PT gene mutation (heterozygote)		6-26	3-15
PT gene mutation (homozygote)		NA	NA
Compound heterozygote		7-9	9-107
Antithrombin deficiency	0.02-0.17	7-12	7-64
Protein C deficiency	0.14-0.5	0.1	4-7
Protein S deficiency	0.14-0.5	0.08	2-3

VTE = venous thromboembolism.

may be helpful because requirements for LMWH increase as pregnancy progresses. The target serum anti-Xa level should be between 0.5 and 1.0 U/mL measured approximately 5 to 6 hours after the last dose of LMWH is administered. Warfarin is contraindicated during the first trimester because of the potential for warfarin-induced embryopathy. In addition, warfarin is rarely used in the United States during the second and third trimesters generally because of the fear of liability if any fetal maloccurrence should develop, whether or not it is warfarin related.

Women with a history of idiopathic deep venous thrombosis or deep venous thrombosis associated with a thrombophilic defect should receive anticoagulation prophylaxis during pregnancy and the postpartum period. Women with a history of deep venous thrombosis due to a reversible risk factor may only need close surveillance without prophylaxis during pregnancy but should receive an anticoagulant after delivery. **Figure 26** summarizes recent recommendations for the use of prophylactic or treatment-dose anticoagulants in at-risk pregnant women.

Pregnant women without known thrombophilic defects have an increased risk of developing deep venous thrombosis. This is possibly due to an increasing thrombophilic profile during pregnancy and progressive venous obstruction from

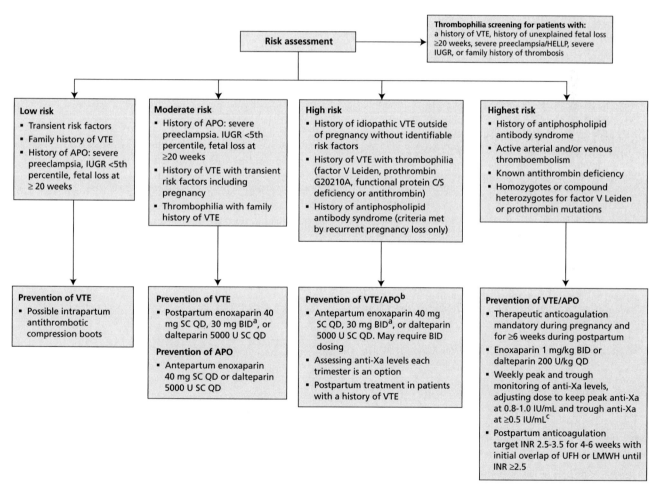

FIGURE 26.
Figure risk assessment and prevention of venous thromboembolism (VTE) and adverse pregnancy outcomes (APOs) in pregnant patients.

IUGR = intrauterine growth retardation; VTE = venous thromboembolism; APO = adverse pregnancy outcome; SC = subcutaneously; QD = daily; BID = twice daily; UFH = unfractionated heparin; LMWH = low-molecular-weight heparin.

[a]The choice of enoxaparin dose should be tailored according to the individual patient as these doses have not been compared in this setting.

[b]Aspirin and heparin are recommended in patients with antiphospholipid antibodies.

[c]The dose of enoxaparin may be increased to maintain peak level at the top end of the desired range.

Reprinted from Duhl AJ, Paidas MJ, Ural SH, et al; Pregnancy and Thrombosis Working Group. Antithrombotic therapy and pregnancy: consensus report and recommendations for prevention and treatment of venous thromboembolism and adverse pregnancy outcomes. Am J Obstet Gynecol. 2007;197:457.e1-457.e21. [PMID: 17980177] Copyright 2007, with permission from Elsevier.

the enlarging uterus. Most thrombotic events occur on the left side because of compression of the left iliac vein by the right iliac artery. If a venous thrombosis does develop, therapy with full-dose unfractionated heparin or, more conveniently, full-dose LMWH should be initiated, even though the latter is not approved by the U.S. Food and Drug Administration for this indication.

KEY POINTS

- Pregnant patients with a history of venous thromboembolism, a family history of thrombophilia, or a history of recurrent fetal loss should be evaluated for a thrombophilic disorder.

- Pregnant patients with known or at high risk for thrombophilic defects require anticoagulation prophylaxis; those at low risk need only close monitoring.

- Unfractionated heparin and low-molecular-weight heparin are the anticoagulants of choice for use during pregnancy.

- Warfarin is contraindicated during the first trimester of pregnancy.

Bibliography

Bates SM, Greer IA, Pabinger I, Sofaer S, Hirsh J; American College of Chest Physicians. Venous thromboembolism, thrombophilia, antithrombotic therapy, and pregnancy. Chest. 2008;133(6 Suppl): 844S-886S. [PMID: 18574280]

Deruelle P, Coudoux E, Ego A, Houfflin-Debarge V, Codaccioni X, Subtil D. Risk factors for post-partum complications occurring after preeclampsia and HELLP syndrome: A study in 453 consecutive pregnancies. Eur J Obstet Gynecol. 2006;125(1):59-65. [PMID: 16118033]

Duhl AJ, Paidas MJ, Ural SH, et al; Pregnancy and Thrombosis Working Group. Antithrombotic therapy and pregnancy: consensus report and recommendations for prevention and treatment of venous thromboembolism and adverse pregnancy outcomes. Am J Obstet Gynecol. 2007;197(5):457.e1-e21. [PMID: 17980177]

Karin R, Sacher RA. Thrombocytopenia in pregnancy. Current Hematol Reports. 2004;3(2):128-133. [PMID: 14965489]

Kher A, Bauersachs R, Nielsen JD. The management of thrombosis in pregnancy: role of low molecular weight heparin. Thromb Haemost. 2007;97(4):505-513. [PMID: 17393011]

Krivak TC, Zorn KK. Venous thromboembolism in obstetrics and gynecology. Obstet Gynecol. 2007;109(3):761-777. [PMID: 17329532]

Kwon JY, Shin JC, Lee JW, Lee JK, Kim SP, Rha JG. Predictors of idiopathic thrombocytopenic purpura in pregnant women presenting with thrombocytopenia. Int J Gynecol Obstet. 2007;96(2):85-88. [PMID: 17239378]

Lim W, Eikelboom JW, Ginsberg JS. Inherited Thrombophilia and pregnancy associated venous thromboembolism. BMJ. 2007;334(7607): 1318-21. [PMID: 17585161]

Parnas M, Sheiner E, Shoham-Vardi, et al. Moderate to severe thrombocytopenia during pregnancy. Eur J Obstet Gynecol Reprod Biol. 2006;128(1-2):163-168. [PMID: 16533554]

Pena-Rosas JP, Viteri FE. Effects of routine oral iron supplementation with or without folic acid for women during pregnancy. Cochrane Database Syst Rev. 2006;3:CD004736. [PMID: 16856058]

Current Issues in Cancer Treatment

The past several years have seen great advancements in the treatment of many solid tumors and lymphoma. With a better understanding of carcinogenesis, tumor progression, and metastasis, several key molecular targets have been identified and exploited to develop therapeutic agents designed to interfere with these cellular pathways.

Monoclonal antibodies such as trastuzumab, which binds to the *HER2* receptor in breast cancer cells, have now been shown to improve survival of patients with *HER2*-positive, early-stage disease. Additional antibodies targeting other members of the epidermal growth factor receptor family (cetuximab and panitumumab) have been approved for use in metastatic disease and are now being studied in clinical trials in the adjuvant setting.

Following the success of imatinib in the treatment of chronic myeloid leukemia, newer specific or multi-targeted oral tyrosine kinase inhibitors such as erlotinib and sorafenib are now available and are generally well tolerated, showing clinical efficacy in previously treatment-resistant diseases such as gastrointestinal stromal tumors and renal cell carcinoma.

Tumor dependency on angiogenesis has been better defined. Novel antiangiogenic agents such as bevacizumab, a monoclonal antibody against the vascular endothelial growth factor that targets the tumor microenvironment, have been shown to have broad-spectrum activity against solid tumors.

We are ushering in an unprecedented era of successful drug development for the treatment of cancer.

Cancer Risk

Environmental Risk Factors

Tobacco use is a strong and common cancer risk factor and the leading cause of preventable death. Smoking and other tobacco use cause about 30% of all cancer-related deaths in the United States. Almost 90% of lung cancer is caused by tobacco, and the risk for lung cancer is 10 to 20 times higher in smokers than it is in never-smokers. Smoking also causes cancers of the upper respiratory tract, genitourinary tract, gastrointestinal tract, and pancreas, whereas the use of chewing tobacco and snuff causes primarily upper respiratory tract cancers. Second-hand smoke modestly increases the risk for lung cancer and appears to account for about 5000 cancer-related deaths in the United States annually.

Alcohol, although not a carcinogen, is associated with development of cancer in the upper respiratory passages and esophagus, apparently by increasing the permeability of the mucosa to active carcinogens, especially in smokers. Alcoholic cirrhosis predisposes patients to hepatocellular carcinoma.

Sun exposure dramatically increases the risk for squamous or basal cell carcinoma of the skin, and intermittent intense sun exposure, especially in childhood or adolescence, increases the risk for melanoma. The carcinogenic effects of sun exposure are the result of direct DNA damage to skin cells. Melanomas appear to be the result of genetic and environmental factors in addition to ultraviolet light exposure.

Ionizing radiation is a well-established etiologic factor in the development of leukemia in populations exposed to the atomic bomb and in radiologists before the advent of safety measures. The cancer risk in individuals exposed to radiation appears to be higher when the same dose is accumulated for a short period rather than for long periods. Thyroid cancer risk is increased in individuals who were exposed to radiation during adolescence. Patients who have received radiation therapy (for example, survivors of Hodgkin lymphoma) have a lifelong increased risk for tumors originating in the irradiated field.

Asbestos-related cancers of the lung, pleura, and abdominal peritoneum cause several thousand deaths every year. Most cases of mesothelioma occur in patients who were exposed to asbestos. Smoking in association with asbestos exposure increases the risk for lung cancer and mesothelioma.

It is estimated that 17% of all new cases of cancer worldwide are due to infections. Viruses may increase cancer risk through cellular transformation, disruption of cell-cycle control, increased cell turnover rates, and immune suppression. Multiple links between infectious agents and cancer have been established, including human papillomavirus (HPV) with cervical and other anogenital cancers and oropharyngeal cancer; hepatitis B and C virus with hepatocellular carcinoma; human T-cell lymphotropic virus (HTLV-1) with adult T-cell leukemia; human immunodeficiency virus (HIV-I) with Kaposi sarcoma and non-Hodgkin lymphoma; human herpesvirus 8 (HHV-8) with Kaposi sarcoma and primary effusion lymphoma; and Epstein-Barr virus (EBV) with Burkitt lymphoma, Hodgkin lymphoma, posttransplantation lymphoma, and oro- and nasopharyngeal carcinomas. In addition, Robin Warren and Barry Marshall were awarded the Nobel Prize for Medicine or Physiology in 2005 for their discovery of an association between *Helicobacter pylori* and peptic ulcer disease and gastritis as well as gastric cancer.

Most of these infectious agents are spread through contact with infected blood or body fluids, thus offering opportunities for prevention. Successful methods of prevention that have been widely implemented include vaccines for HPV and hepatitis B. Mucosa-associated lymphoid tissue non-Hodgkin lymphoma (NHL) often is eradicated with antibiotic-based therapy.

KEY POINTS

- Smoking and other tobacco use cause about 30% of all cancer-related deaths in the United States.
- Patients who have received radiation therapy have a lifelong increased risk for tumors originating in the irradiated field.
- Smoking in association with asbestos exposure increases the risk for lung cancer and mesothelioma.
- Alcohol, although not a carcinogen, is associated with development of cancer in the upper respiratory passages.
- The most common infectious agents implicated in cancer include human papillomavirus in cervical, anogenital, and oropharyngeal cancer; hepatitis B and C in hepatocellular carcinoma; *Helicobacter pylori* in gastric adenocarcinoma and mucosa-associated lymphoid tissue non-Hodgkin lymphoma; and Epstein-Barr virus in Hodgkin lymphoma.

Genetic Susceptibility Risk Factors

Individuals with certain germline heritable traits have a substantially increased susceptibility for cancer. These familial syndromes are relatively rare, accounting for less than 5% of all detected cancers. Individuals born with a critical tumor suppressor gene mutation have a "head start" in developing cancer. They are more susceptible to environmental carcinogens than are individuals without such genetic mutations.

Penetrance, or the frequency of genotypic expression, is incomplete in individuals with tumor suppressor gene mutations, and cancer incidence in such individuals ranges from 30% to 85% depending on the type of genetic mutation. Penetrance is likely related to the specific mutation identified in a family as well as other genetic or environmental factors that affect disease expression.

Breast Cancer

About 5% of breast cancer cases are attributable to rare, high-penetrance mutations in a few specific genes (for example, *BRCA1*, *BRCA2*, *ATM*, *PTEN*, and *TP53*); mutations in *BRCA1* and *BRCA2* account for up to 50% of cases of hereditary and familial breast cancer. This proportion is higher in patients with breast cancer at a younger age of onset and in families with multiple breast or ovarian cancer cases. Each gene shows some differences in the familial pattern of the cancer: *BRCA1* is more strongly associated with ovarian cancer, *BRCA2* with male breast cancer, *ATM* with radiosensitivity, *PTEN* with Cowden syndrome (including hamartomas of the skin and other organs), and *p53* with Li-Fraumeni syndrome (which includes cancer of the brain, lung, and soft tissue).

Hereditary Colorectal Cancer Syndromes

There are four primary hereditary colorectal cancer syndromes: familial adenomatous polyposis (FAP), hereditary nonpolyposis colorectal cancer (HNPCC), Peutz-Jeghers syndrome, and juvenile polyposis. Although less than 10% of colorectal cancer cases occur in individuals with high-penetrance genetic abnormalities, a mutation in the germline *APC* gene is a risk factor for FAP, and a mutation in the germline *MSH2*, *PMS1*, and *PMS2* genes is a risk factor for HNPCC. Although HNPCC may be associated with frequent polypoid precursors of cancer, polyps occur much less commonly in HNPCC than in FAP. In addition to colorectal cancer, ovarian and endometrial cancer may be more common in individuals with HNPCC.

KEY POINTS

- Individuals born with a critical tumor suppressor gene mutation are more susceptible to environmental carcinogens than are individuals without such genetic mutations.

- About 5% of breast cancer is attributable to rare, high-penetrance mutations in a small number of specific genes, with *BRCA1* and *BRCA2* mutations accounting for up to 50% of cases of hereditary and familial breast cancer.

- Polyps occur much less commonly in hereditary nonpolyposis colorectal cancer than in familial adenomatous polyposis.

- In addition to colorectal cancer, ovarian and endometrial cancer may be more common in individuals with hereditary nonpolyposis colorectal cancer.

Risk Assessment and Genetic Counseling

A cancer risk assessment should consist of questions about family history and lifestyle and a physical examination. Genetic counseling relies on education, risk assessment, and risk management to help individuals and their families cope with a disorder or the heightened risk for a disorder. The specific goals of the counseling process are to: (1) provide accurate information on the genetic, biologic, and environmental factors related to the individual's risk of disease; (2) provide a sufficient understanding of the genetic basis of cancer to assist in decisions regarding genetic testing; (3) formulate appropriate options and recommendations for prevention and screening; (4) offer psychologic support to facilitate adjustment to an altered risk perception and to promote adherence to the recommended actions; and 5) avoid discrimination in regard to employment and insurance coverage if one is at increased risk for developing cancer.

KEY POINT

- Cancer risk assessment consists of a history to determine family and lifestyle risks and a physical examination to identify signs consistent with genetic cancer syndromes.

Bibliography

Alberg AJ, Ford JG, Samet JM; American College of Chest Physicians. Epidemiology of lung cancer: ACCP evidence-based clinical practice guidelines (2nd edition).Chest. 2007 Sep;132(3 Suppl):29S-55S. [PMID: 17873159]

Croce CM. Oncogenes and cancer. N Engl J Med. 2008;358(5):502-11. [PMID: 18234754]

Dong LM, Potter JD, White E, Ulrich CM, Cardon LR, Peters U. Genetic susceptibility to cancer: the role of polymorphisms in candidate genes. JAMA. 2008;299(20):2423-2436. [PMID: 18505952]

Kushi LH, Byers T, Doyle C, et al; American Cancer Society 2006 Nutrition and Physical Activity Guidelines Advisory Committee. American Cancer Society Guidelines on Nutrition and Physical Activity for Cancer Prevention : Reducing the Risk of Cancer with Healthy Food Choices and Physical Activity [erratum in CA Cancer J Clin. 2007;57(1):66]. CA Cancer J Clin. 2006;56(5):254-281. [PMID: 17005596]

Markowitz LE, Dunne EF, Saraiya M, Lawson HW, Chesson H, Unger ER; Centers for Disease Control and Prevention (CDC); Advisory Committee on Immunization Practices (ACIP). Quadrivalent Human Papillomavirus Vaccine: Recommendations of the Advisory Committee on Immunization Practices (ACIP). MMWR Recomm Rep. 2007;56(RR-2):1-24. [PMID: 17380109]

Robson M, Offit K. Clinical practice. Management of an inherited predisposition to breast cancer. N Engl J Med. 2007;357(2):154-62. [PMID: 17625127]

Breast Cancer

Introduction

Breast cancer is the most common non–skin cancer malignancy diagnosed in women. In 2008, an estimated 184,000 cases of breast cancer were diagnosed and 41,000 patients died of the disease in the United States.

Epidemiology and Risk Factors

The risk factors for breast cancer in the general population are older age, family history of breast cancer, specific benign breast biopsy conditions (atypical ductal hyperplasia, lobular carcinoma in situ), early menarche, nulliparity/late first birth, late menopause, radiation exposure (for example, Hodgkin lymphoma survivors), and alcohol.

The Women's Health Initiative (WHI) indicates that limiting exogenous estrogen combined with progestin is the best documented method for reducing breast cancer risk. The effect of estrogen therapy alone (without progestin) on breast cancer risk is less clear. Data from the National Cancer Institute's Surveillance, Epidemiology, and End Results (SEER) registries showed a sharp decrease (6.7%) in the incidence of breast cancer in the United States in 2003, which has been attributed to a decrease in the use of hormone-replacement therapy. Data from 2004 showed little additional decrease in incidence compared with 2003.

BRCA1 and *BRCA2* mutations lead to a significantly increased breast and ovarian cancer risk; however, this risk applies to less than 1% of the population excluding Ashkenazi Jewish women and members of high-risk populations, and less than 5% of all cases of breast cancer are attributed to germline abnormalities in these genes.

Testing for *BRCA1* and *BRCA2* gene mutations should be done if (1) the individual has personal or family history of features suggestive of genetic cancer; and (2) the test results will help to establish the diagnosis or influence the management of the patient or family members at risk. According to the United States Preventive Services Task Force, family history patterns of increased risk for *BRCA1/BRCA2*-associated breast cancer in non-Ashkenazi Jewish women include the following:

- two first-degree relatives with breast cancer, in one of whom the diagnosis was established at age 50 years or younger;
- a combination of three or more first- or second-degree relatives with breast cancer regardless of age at diagnosis;
- a combination of breast and ovarian cancer among first- and second-degree relatives;
- a first-degree relative with bilateral breast cancer;
- a combination of two or more first- or second-degree relatives with ovarian cancer regardless of age at diagnosis;
- a first- or second-degree relative with both breast and ovarian cancer at any age; or
- a history of breast cancer in a male relative.

A family history associated with an increased breast cancer risk in women of Ashkenazi Jewish descent includes any first-degree relative (or two second-degree relatives on the same side of the family) with breast or ovarian cancer.

Such women and their families should be referred to a qualified genetic counseling program before and after testing.

KEY POINTS

- Older age, a family history of breast cancer, benign breast biopsy history, early menarche, nulliparity/late first birth, late menopause, radiation exposure, and alcohol are breast cancer risk factors in the general population.
- Limiting exogenous estrogen in combination with progestin is the best documented method for reducing breast cancer risk.
- Testing for *BRCA1* and *BRCA2* gene mutations should be done in women with personal or family history features suggestive of genetic breast or ovarian cancer and if the findings will help to establish the diagnosis or influence management.
- Women and their family members who may be at risk for *BRCA1* and *BRCA2* gene mutations should be referred to genetic counseling before and after genetic testing.

Risk-Reduction Strategies

The two most highly effective breast cancer risk-reduction strategies are surgical removal of breast tissue (prophylactic mastectomy) and endocrinologic manipulation using selective estrogen receptor modulators (SERMs).

Among *BRCA* carriers, the largest risk reduction results from prophylactic mastectomy. Although this option is not acceptable to many women because of its resulting morbidity, bilateral prophylactic mastectomy as a prevention strategy is much more acceptable to *BRCA* mutation carriers who have an extraordinarily high lifetime risk of developing breast cancer. Premature cessation of ovarian function (through early menopause or oophorectomy) reduces breast cancer risk. In *BRCA* mutation carriers, oophorectomy is done to reduce the risk of ovarian cancer, and if done premenopausally, reduces breast cancer risk.

The SERMs tamoxifen and raloxifene reduce the risk for new breast cancer by as much as 50%. For premenopausal women, tamoxifen is the only Food and Drug Administration–approved SERM for breast cancer prevention. For postmenopausal women, both tamoxifen and raloxifene are Food and Drug Administration–approved therapies. Use of these agents is approved for women with Gail model scores of greater than 1.7% for the risk of breast cancer over the next 5 years (go to www.cancer.gov/bcrisktool/ for additional information on the Gail model).

Raloxifene is as effective as tamoxifen in reducing the risk for invasive breast cancer but is slightly less effective at reducing the risk for noninvasive breast cancer; however, compared with tamoxifen, raloxifene is associated with less risk for thromboembolic events and cataracts; fewer hysterectomies from gynecologic problems such as bleeding; and fewer cases of endometrial cancer. Patient-reported outcomes show that those treated with raloxifene experienced more musculoskeletal symptoms, weight gain, and dyspareunia compared with those who received tamoxifen, whereas patients treated with tamoxifen reported more vasomotor symptoms, leg cramps, and bladder and gynecologic problems.

The decision as to whether to choose tamoxifen or raloxifene in the prevention of invasive breast cancer in postmenopausal women should be made jointly between the physician and patient and should include a frank discussion of the benefits and side-effect profiles of these two agents.

KEY POINTS

- Among *BRCA* carriers, the largest breast cancer risk reduction results from prophylactic mastectomy.
- The selective estrogen receptor modulators tamoxifen and raloxifene reduce the risk for new breast cancer by as much as 50%.
- In postmenopausal women, raloxifene is as effective as tamoxifen in reducing the risk for invasive breast cancer but is slightly less effective at reducing the risk for noninvasive breast cancer.

Primary Therapy for Newly Diagnosed Invasive Breast Cancer

Breast-conserving therapy consists of excision of the primary tumor followed by radiation to the remaining ipsilateral breast tissue. Randomized clinical trials have shown that the survival rate for women undergoing breast-conserving therapy is equivalent to that of those who undergo mastectomy, with breast-conserving therapy resulting in improved cosmetic outcomes and less morbidity than mastectomy.

Although whole-breast radiation is considered a standard component of breast-conserving therapy, it may not be necessary for selected patients, such as elderly women with small, estrogen receptor (ER)–positive, lymph node–negative tumors, who are treated with endocrine therapy. Radiation therapy may cause both immediate and late side effects.

Approximately 25% of women with breast cancer are not appropriate candidates for breast-conserving therapy because complete excision cannot be achieved unless mastectomy is performed or because radiation is contraindicated (**Table 24**).

By decreasing tumor size, preoperative (neoadjuvant) chemotherapy allows a few patients with larger tumors to undergo postchemotherapeutic breast-conserving therapy, although this strategy has not resulted in improved survival compared with postoperative or adjuvant chemotherapy.

Sentinel lymph node biopsy has replaced full axillary lymph node dissection for the staging of disease in many women with early-stage, clinically lymph node–negative breast cancer. The first draining (or sentinel) lymph node is identified by injecting blue dye and radioactive colloid into the tumor site. If the sentinel lymph node does not contain

TABLE 24 Summary of Breast-Conserving Therapy Consensus Standards of Care

Patient Selection Criteria	Comments
History and physical examination findings	History of prior therapeutic radiation, collagen vascular disease, presence of breast implants, date of last menstrual period (i.e., pregnant). Physical examination findings of tumor size and location, fixation to skin, ratio of breast to tumor size, evidence of multiple primary tumors, enlarged supraclavicular lymph nodes, evidence of locally advanced cancer (e.g. skin ulceration, peau d'orange, inflammatory carcinoma, fixed axillary lymph nodes, lymphedema of ipsilateral arm)
Breast imaging results	Multicentricity, evidence of diffuse microcalcifications
Histologic assessment of the resected breast specimen	Margins of resection, extensive DCIS
Assessment of needs and expectations	Patient preference
Absolute Contraindications to Breast-Conserving Therapy	**Comments**
Two or more primary tumors in separate breast quadrants	None
Pregnancy (except in some cases in the third trimester, with radiotherapy deferred until after delivery)	None
Mammogram showing diffuse malignant-appearing microcalcifications	This often represents extensive DCIS within the breast
History of breast-region radiotherapy resulting in an unacceptably high cumulative radiation dose to the chest wall when combined with proposed treatment	Women treated for Hodgkin lymphoma with mantle radiation have a high incidence of breast cancer later in life
Repeated positive resection margins after reasonable re-excision attempts	Microscopic resection margins on the lumpectomy specimen are the major selection criteria for breast-conservation therapy
Relative Contraindications to Breast-Conserving Therapy	**Comments**
Collagen vascular disease history	Scleroderma is the major concern
Large tumor size in a small breast	Concern about significant cosmetic alteration
Breast size	Large pendulous breasts may lead to technical problems in reproducibility of patient set-up for radiation

DCIS = Ductal carcinoma in situ.

Information from Morrow M, Harris JR; American College of Radiology. Practice Guideline For Breast Conservation Therapy In The Management Of Invasive Breast Carcinoma. www.acr.org/SecondaryMainMenuCategories/quality_safety/guidelines/breast/invasive_breast_carcinoma.aspx. Revised 2006. Accessed January 22, 2008.

metastases, it is unlikely that more distal axillary lymph nodes will contain metastases; consequently, no further surgery is indicated in this setting, and the toxicity from a full axillary lymph node dissection is avoided. However, if the sentinel lymph node shows metastatic involvement, then axillary lymph node dissection is performed to determine the number of involved lymph nodes (which has prognostic value) and, possibly, to reduce the odds for recurrence.

Most patients undergoing mastectomy do not require radiation to complete local therapy. However, radiation therapy to the chest wall and surrounding lymph nodes may be indicated after mastectomy, particularly for patients with large tumors (greater than 5 cm) or with four or more positive axillary lymph nodes. Postmastectomy radiation therapy for patients with one to three positive lymph nodes is controversial.

The incidence of ductal carcinoma in situ (DCIS) has increased as a result of widespread screening interventions. Local therapy for patients with DCIS consists of breast-conserving therapy with lumpectomy plus radiation therapy or mastectomy. Chemotherapy is not indicated for patients with pure DCIS; however, tamoxifen is indicated for women with DCIS after lumpectomy and radiation therapy to reduce the incidence of local recurrences and second primary breast cancer.

KEY POINTS

- Survival of patients who undergo breast-conserving therapy is equal to that of mastectomy, with improved cosmetic outcomes and less morbidity.
- Sentinel lymph node biopsy has replaced full axillary lymph node dissection for the staging of many women with early-stage, clinically lymph node–negative breast cancer.
- Local therapy for patients with ductal carcinoma in situ consists of breast-conserving therapy with lumpectomy plus radiation therapy or mastectomy, but not chemotherapy.
- Tamoxifen is indicated for patients with ductal carcinoma in situ after lumpectomy and radiation therapy to reduce the risk for local recurrences and second primary breast cancer.

Systemic Breast Cancer Therapy

Adjuvant Systemic Therapy

Adjuvant systemic therapy is indicated for patients with early-stage breast cancer who are at significant risk for recurrence in a distant metastatic site. The purpose of adjuvant systemic therapy is to reduce the burden of clinically undetectable, distant micrometastatic disease. Estimating an individual patient's risk of harboring clinically silent metastatic deposits based on established prognostic factors is essential.

A prognostic factor is any measurement that correlates with disease-free or overall survival in the absence of therapy and therefore correlates with the natural history of the disease. Conversely, a predictive factor is any measurement that predicts response to a given therapy. Examples of prognostic factors include lymph node status and tumor size, whereas an example of a predictive factor is the presence or absence of hormone receptors (such as in predicting the benefit of endocrine therapy) or *HER2/neu* overexpression (such as in predicting the benefit of trastuzumab). Factors such as *HER2/neu* expression may be prognostic and predictive.

The most important prognostic factors used to determine the need for adjuvant therapy in patients with breast cancer are lymph node involvement and tumor size. The use of genomic profiling, which evaluates individual gene expression at a molecular level in a patient's tumor to determine the prognosis and benefits in patients who undergo adjuvant chemotherapy—particularly those with lymph node–negative, ER-positive cancer—is increasing.

Endocrine therapy is beneficial only in patients with ER-positive or progesterone receptor (PR)–positive tumors. In premenopausal women with ER-positive and PR-positive tumors, 5 years of tamoxifen is the standard adjuvant endocrine therapeutic regimen; treatment longer than 5 years with this drug is not recommended. Several large, prospective, randomized trials have shown that the aromatase inhibitors, such as anastrozole, letrozole, or exemestane, appear to be more effective in reducing risk for recurrence than is tamoxifen in postmenopausal women with ER-positive breast cancer. Although the aromatase inhibitors do not increase the risk for thromboembolic disease or endometrial cancer, they are associated with postmenopausal symptoms such as hot flushes, musculoskeletal symptoms such as arthralgia, and an increased risk for osteoporosis. The American Society of Clinical Oncology has suggested that "adjuvant therapy for postmenopausal women with hormone receptor–positive breast cancer should include an aromatase inhibitor to lower the risk of tumor recurrence"; however, the optimal strategy (primary therapy with an aromatase inhibitor vs. sequential therapy with tamoxifen followed by an aromatase inhibitor) is currently unclear. Aromatase inhibitors are contraindicated in premenopausal women because reduced feedback of estrogen to the hypothalamus and pituitary gland leads to an increase in gonadotropin secretion with potential adverse effects.

Adjuvant chemotherapy generally consists of 2 to 6 months of treatment with two or more agents, administered concurrently or sequentially. Therapy is generally individualized based on prognostic factors such as lymph node status. Commonly used agents include cyclophosphamide, doxorubicin or epirubicin, methotrexate, 5-fluorouracil, and one of the taxanes (docetaxel or paclitaxel). But what the optimal regimen is remains controversial.

Common chemotherapeutic side effects include nausea, vomiting, alopecia, and peripheral neuropathies. Rare (<1%) life-threatening toxicities include neutropenia with associated infection, thrombocytopenia with associated hemorrhage, anthracycline-induced cardiomyopathy, and secondary malignancies, especially leukemia and myelodysplastic syndromes (see Oncologic Urgencies and Emergencies).

HER2 is a member of the epidermal growth factor receptor family of tyrosine kinases and is amplified or overexpressed in 20% to 30% of breast cancers. Trastuzumab is a humanized monoclonal antibody to the *HER2* receptor. Several large, randomized trials have demonstrated that 52 weeks of adjuvant trastuzumab therapy reduces the risk for breast cancer recurrence by approximately 50% and may even reduce mortality by as much as 30%. Trastuzumab has been associated with induction of heart failure, particularly when used concurrently with an anthracycline. Patients should undergo monitoring of left ventricular function before trastuzumab treatment, and frequently during and after trastuzumab treatment.

Depending on their prognosis, patients with ER-positive tumors may receive endocrine treatment alone or chemotherapy and endocrine treatment. In general, adjuvant chemotherapy is considered for patients with tumors of 1 cm or greater in size. Computerized programs are now available to assist in decision-making for adjuvant therapy (www.adjuvantonline .com/index1.html).

KEY POINTS

- Lymph node involvement and tumor size are the most important prognosticators used to determine the need for adjuvant therapy in patients with early-stage breast cancer.
- Gene expression profiling is beginning to supplant the use of clinical prognostic factors in patients with breast cancer.
- Endocrine therapy is beneficial only in patients with estrogen receptor– or progesterone receptor–positive tumors.
- In premenopausal women with estrogen receptor-positive tumors, 5 years of tamoxifen is the standard adjuvant endocrine therapeutic regimen.
- Aromatase inhibitors appear to be more effective in reducing recurrence risk than tamoxifen in postmenopausal women with estrogen receptor–positive breast cancer.
- Trastuzumab may reduce the risk for breast cancer recurrence by 50% and mortality by possibly as much as 30%.

Metastatic Breast Cancer

Metastatic breast cancer is generally incurable with currently available therapies, although systemic therapy may improve the survival of some patients and palliate symptoms for many

more. Minimizing toxicity and maintaining a good quality of life are extremely important issues in these patients. Patients with ER–positive tumors are usually managed, at least initially, with serial endocrine therapies, including tamoxifen, aromatase inhibitors, fulvestrant (an ER down-regulator), and megestrol acetate. Patients whose tumors are ER-negative or are refractory to endocrine treatment are eligible to receive chemotherapy in the form of sequential single agents or as combination therapy.

Trastuzumab is active alone and in combination with chemotherapy for patients with *HER2*-positive metastatic breast cancer, resulting in tumor shrinkage and prolonged survival. Patients who receive trastuzumab should undergo careful evaluation for signs of cardiotoxicity (see Adjuvant Systemic Therapy). Trastuzumab should not be given concurrently with anthracycline agents.

For patients with metastatic bone disease, routine administration of an intravenous bisphosphonate, either pamidronate or zoledronic acid, reduces the incidence of morbidity (including bone pain), analgesic use, and fracture. Although the most common toxicities of these drugs are musculoskeletal symptoms and low-grade fever, rarely, renal dysfunction can occur. Osteonecrosis of the jaw (**Figure 27**) is also an emerging bisphosphonate-induced toxicity in the setting of metastatic bone disease, but its incidence is currently unclear. The benefits of bisphosphonates in the adjuvant setting to reduce recurrences and prevent osteoporosis are currently being studied.

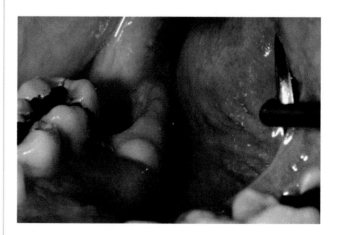

FIGURE 27.
Osteonecrosis of the jaw, a complication related to bisphosphonate therapy.

Reprinted with permission from Woo SB, Hellstein JW, Kalmar JR. Systematic Review: Bisphosphonates and Osteonecrosis of the Jaws. Ann Intern Med. 2006;144(10):753-761. [PMID: 16702591] Copyright 2006, American College of Physicians.

- Routine bisphosphonate administration (pamidronate or zoledronic acid) reduces the incidence of morbidity, analgesic use, and fracture in patients with metastatic breast cancer.
- Bisphosphonates may cause musculoskeletal symptoms, low-grade fever, and renal dysfunction (rarely), and have also been associated with osteonecrosis of the jaw in the setting of metastatic bone disease.

Follow-up Monitoring

In the absence of suspicious symptoms, intensive laboratory and radiologic follow-up testing to detect metastases in patients with early-stage breast cancer after systemic therapy has not demonstrated a survival or quality-of-life benefit. Therefore, the standard posttherapy follow-up monitoring of these patients should address long-term complications of therapy, quality-of-life issues, and routine medical care (See Care of Cancer Survivors). The American Society of Clinical Oncology recommends monthly breast self-examination, annual mammography of the preserved and contralateral breast, and a careful history and physical examination every 3 to 6 months for 3 years, then every 6 to 12 months for 2 years, and then annually. The role of MRI breast imaging in patients at high risk for breast cancer, particularly those with a personal history of breast cancer, is controversial and continues to be studied.

- In the absence of suspicious symptoms, intensive laboratory and radiologic follow-up testing in survivors of early-stage breast cancer does not improve survival or quality of life.

Quality of Life in Breast Cancer Survivors

Nearly 80% of women with early-stage breast cancer achieve long-term disease-free and overall survival after local and systemic therapy; however, many women experience therapy-related bodily changes, including chemotherapy-induced menopause, endocrine-induced menopause-like symptoms, and weight gain. Recent studies have focused on the effects of systemic therapy, particularly chemotherapy, on cognitive function.

For women with a history of breast cancer, estrogen-replacement therapy should be avoided because of the increased risk for inducing a breast cancer recurrence or a second primary breast cancer. Selective serotonin reuptake inhibitors are useful in reducing the incidence of hot flushes in breast cancer survivors; however, some of these drugs can lead to a pharmacologic drug interaction resulting in reduced efficacy of tamoxifen and should therefore be avoided in patients taking this agent. Because selective serotonin reuptake inhibitors inhibit CYP2D6 enzymes, which are responsible for conversion of tamoxifen to endoxifen, reduced levels of endoxifen have been reported in patients who take tamoxifen concurrently. Vaginal estrogen preparations may be used for the treatment of vaginal dryness, although systemic absorption of these agents is a concern. Over-the-counter, nonhormonal, vaginal lubricants administered at the time of intercourse are also helpful for many women with these symptoms.

Osteoporosis is a major concern for women who have undergone natural or therapy-induced menopause, and the aromatase inhibitors can further increase this risk. Periodic screening for osteoporosis with dual-energy X-ray absorptiometry scanning is therefore recommended in this setting. Healthy lifestyle habits, including weight-bearing exercise, tobacco avoidance, and calcium/vitamin D supplementation, are routinely recommended for all patients with breast cancer who are at risk for osteoporosis. If evidence of progressive bone loss persists despite these strategies, the use of oral bisphosphonates is recommended. Raloxifene is specifically approved for the treatment of osteoporosis; however, there are no data regarding its efficacy as adjuvant therapy for breast cancer, and it therefore should not be substituted for tamoxifen in this setting. Raloxifene and tamoxifen or an aromatase inhibitor should not be given concomitantly, and raloxifene should not be used after 5 years of tamoxifen use.

- For women with a history of breast cancer, estrogen-replacement therapy should be avoided.
- Selective serotonin reuptake inhibitors may reduce the incidence of hot flushes in breast cancer survivors; however, caution is indicated in women taking tamoxifen.
- Vaginal estrogen preparations may be helpful for women with vaginal dryness caused by breast cancer therapy, although systemic absorption of these agents is a concern.
- Aromatase inhibitors can further increase the risk for osteoporosis in postmenopausal women with breast cancer.
- Weight-bearing exercise, tobacco avoidance, and calcium/vitamin D supplementation are recommended osteoporosis risk-reduction measures.
- Oral bisphosphonates are appropriate for postmenopausal women with a history of breast cancer who have evidence of progressive bone loss.

Bibliography

Anderson GL, Limacher M, Assaf AR, et al; The Women's Health Initiative Steering Committee. Effects of conjugated equine estrogen in postmenopausal women with hysterectomy: the women's health initiative randomized controlled trial. JAMA 2004; 291(14): 1701-1712. [PMID: 15082697]

Fisher B, Anderson S, Bryant J, et al. Twenty-year follow-up of a randomized trial comparing total mastectomy, lumpectomy and lumpectomy plus irradiation for the treatment of invasive breast cancer. N Engl J Med. 2002; 347(16):1233-1241. [PMID: 12393820]

Fisher B, Dignam J, Wolmark N, et al. Tamoxifen in treatment of intraductal breast cancer: National Surgical Adjuvant Breast and Bowel Project B-24 randomized controlled trial. Lancet. 1999;353 (9169):1993-2000. [PMID: 10376613]

Heemskerk-Gerritsen BA, Brekelmans CT, Menke-Pluymers MB, et al. Prophylactic mastectomy in BRCA1/2 mutation carriers and women at risk of hereditary breast cancer: long-term experiences at the Rotterdam Family Cancer Clinic. Ann Surg Oncol.2007; 14(12):3335-3344. [PMID: 17541692]

Howell A, Cuzick J, Baum M, et al. Results of the ATAC (Arimidex, Tamoxifen, Alone or in Combination) trial after completion of 5 years' adjuvant treatment for breast cancer. Lancet. 2005; 365(9453):60-62. [PMID: 15639680]

Morrow M, Harris JR, eds; American College of Radiology. Practice Guideline For Breast Conservation Therapy In The Management Of Invasive Breast Carcinoma. Revised 2006. Accessed at www.acr.org/ SecondaryMainMenuCategories/quality_safety/guidelines/breast/i nvasive_breast_carcinoma.aspx on January 22, 2008.

Paik S, Shak S, Tang G, et al. A multigene assay to predict recurrence of tamoxifen-treated, node-negative breast cancer. N Engl J Med. 2004;351(27):2817-2826. [PMID: 15591335]

Paik S, Tang G, Shak S, et al. Gene expression and benefit of chemotherapy in women with node-negative, estrogen-receptor-positive breast cancer. J Clin Oncol. 2006;24(23):3726-3734. [PMID: 16720680]

Piccart-Gebhardt MJ, Procter M, Leyland-Jones B, et al. Trastuzumab after adjuvant chemotherapy in HER2 positive breast cancer. N Engl J Med. 2005; 353(16):1659-1672. [PMID: 16236737]

Ravdin PM, Cronin KA, Howlader N, et al. The decrease in breast-cancer incidence in 2003 in the United States. N Engl J Med. 2007;356(16):1670-1674. [PMID: 17442911]

Romond EH, Perez, EA, Bryant J, et al. Trastuzumab plus adjuvant chemotherapy for operable HER2-positive breast cancer. N Engl J Med. 2005;353(16):1673-1684. [PMID: 16236738]

Rossouw JE, Anderson GL, Prentice RL, et al; Writing Group for the Women's Health Initiative Investigators. Risks and benefits of estrogen plus progestin in healthy postmenopausal women. Principal results from the women's health initiative randomized controlled trial. JAMA. 2002;288(3):321-33. [PMID: 12117397]

Thurlimann B, Keshaviah A, Coates AS, et al. A comparison of letrozole and tamoxifen in postmenopausal women with early breast cancer. N Engl J Med. 2005;353(26):2747-57. [PMID: 16382061]

Vogel VG, Costantino JP, Wickerham DL, et al. Effects of tamoxifen vs raloxifene on the risk of developing invasive breast cancer and other disease outcomes. The NSABP study of tamoxifen and raloxifene (STAR) P-2 trial [erratum in JAMA. 2006;296(24):2926][erratum in JAMA. 2007;298(9):973]. JAMA 2006; 295(23): 2727-2741. [PMID: 16754727]

Winer EP, Hudis C, Burstein HJ, et al. American Society of Clinical Oncology technology assessment on the use of aromatase inhibitors as adjuvant therapy for postmenopausal women with hormone receptor positive breast cancer: status report 2004. J Clin Oncol. 2005;23(3):619-629. [PMID: 15545664]

Ovarian Cancer

Introduction

Ovarian cancer is the fifth leading cause of cancer-related death among women after lung, breast, colorectal, and pancreatic cancer. It is a disease of older women, with a median age at onset of 61 years. This disease occurs rarely in women younger than 40 years except for cases with a hereditary disposition.

Tumors of low malignant potential represent about 15% of cases of ovarian cancer and usually occur in younger women (median age, 49 years). Histologically, these tumors, also called "borderline tumors," are characterized by atypical epithelial proliferation without stromal invasion.

Risk Factors

Hereditary-based ovarian cancer represents approximately 5% to 10% of cases, most commonly due to *BRCA1* and *BRCA2* gene mutations, and also is occasionally part of the phenotype of hereditary nonpolyposis colorectal cancer syndrome (see Breast Cancer section).

Some risk factors for ovarian cancer may be environmental (for example, a high-fat diet), although these risk factors are not well defined (**Table 25**). Parity is associated with a 30% to 45% reduction in ovarian cancer risk compared with nulliparity, and each additional birth decreases the risk by another 10% to 15%. Oral contraceptive use decreases ovarian cancer risk by 30% to 60% depending on duration of use. In women who took oral contraceptives for at least 5 years, the protective effect may last up to 20 years after last use. Sharply rising pituitary gonadotropin levels and decreasing estrogen contribute to increased ovarian cancer incidence beginning at menopause.

Ovarian cancer screening is not recommended for the general population because no tests or series of tests are sufficiently sensitive or specific enough to establish a diagnosis, and no data have shown a survival benefit resulting from earlier diagnosis and therapy. Women who are at high risk for this disease because of hereditary factors should undergo pelvic examinations, CA-125 measurement, and transvaginal ultrasonography every 6 to 12 months, usually beginning at age 35 years or 5 to 10 years earlier than the earliest age at diagnosis of ovarian cancer in a family member according to a National Institutes of Health Consensus Conference panel of experts. Currently, no data conclusively show that this screening strategy affects survival.

Prophylactic bilateral salpingo-oophorectomy prior to age 40 is strongly recommended for women with a family history of ovarian cancer, particularly for *BRCA1* or *BRCA2* carriers who want to diminish their risk for developing this disease. This procedure is the only known reliable strategy for

TABLE 25 Putative Ovarian Cancer Risk Factors

Nulliparity

Hormones
  Endogenous (increased gonadotropin)
  Exogenous (mixed findings)

Environmental
  Diet (high fat)
  Talc
  Asbestos

Chronic Inflammation
  Endometriosis
  Pelvic inflammatory disease

Hereditary (only truly established risk factor)

risk reduction, reducing risk by approximately 90%. A small (2%) risk for developing primary peritoneal carcinomatosis after bilateral salpingo-oophorectomy remains, suggesting that the genetic defect may involve the entire epithelial lining of the abdominal cavity. An additional benefit of prophylactic oophorectomy is the 50% decrease in breast cancer risk it confers in this high-risk population. It is not clear whether women with a high genetic risk of ovarian cancer should be treated with oral contraceptives.

KEY POINTS

- Parity and oral contraceptive use are associated with a decreased risk for ovarian cancer.

- Ovarian cancer screening is not recommended for the general population.

- The ovarian cancer risk reduction achieved by prophylactic salpingo-oophorectomy is approximately 90%.

- Oral contraceptives may reduce the risk for ovarian cancer by 30% to 60%.

Diagnosis and Staging

Patients with ovarian cancer have vague symptoms that often are not apparent until late in the disease owing to the free-floating position of the ovaries within the peritoneal cavity; consequently, more than 70% of women with ovarian cancer have metastatic disease beyond the pelvis at presentation. Ovarian cancer symptoms include changes in urinary patterns, abdominal and/or pelvic pain, bloating, early satiety, increasing abdominal girth, difficulty breathing owing to ascites formation, and changes in bowel function, including a complete or partial obstruction.

On physical examination of patients with ovarian cancer, abdominal distention and a fluid wave may be detected. Chest examination may disclose dullness to percussion resulting from pleural effusion(s). Because the normal postmenopausal ovary is not palpable, any palpable adnexal mass found during the pelvic examination of postmenopausal women should be considered suspicious, requiring a workup and, often, removal. Such a finding in a premenopausal woman may represent a functional cyst, and such patients may be observed for a menstrual cycle or two after additional evaluation, such as pelvic or transvaginal ultrasonography, is performed. Additionally, the finding of nodularity in the cul-de-sac, ascites, and an abdominal mass should be evaluated for the possibility of ovarian cancer in any woman. Vaginal discharge is uncommon in patients with ovarian cancer.

A markedly elevated CA-125 concentration in a postmenopausal woman with an adnexal mass strengthens the presumptive diagnosis of ovarian cancer; however, abnormal levels of CA-125 are not specific for cancer, and this test alone is not used to establish the diagnosis. CA-125 can be elevated in nonmalignant conditions, such as uterine leiomyomata, endometriosis, pregnancy, liver disease, and inflammation or irritation of the peritoneal lining.

Pelvic ultrasonography is often the first imaging study performed for purposes of documenting a mass in patients with ovarian cancer because many gynecologists can perform this test in their offices. CT of the abdomen and pelvis may be helpful in evaluating the remainder of the peritoneal cavity. Usually, MRI does not provide additional information in the evaluation of patients with ovarian cancer. Positron emission tomographic scanning in ovarian cancer is fraught with a high rate of false-positive and false-negative results.

Staging is performed at the time of initial surgery concurrently with tumor debulking (also termed "surgical cytoreduction"). Detailed tissue sampling is mandatory during surgery because up to 30% of patients with disease grossly confined to the ovary will have metastatic disease (**Table 26**). Studies have shown that the best results are obtained when this procedure is performed by a trained gynecologic oncologist. Patients with true stage I disease with well-differentiated tumors have a greater than 90% survival rate, even without adjuvant chemotherapy (**Table 27**).

TABLE 26 Components of Laparotomy for Ovarian Cancer

En bloc resection of primary tumor, ovaries, and uterus

Partial infracolic omentectomy

Selective lymphadenopathy

Bowel resection (as indicated)

Sampling of undersides of diaphragms

Selective lymphadenectomy (pelvic and para-aortic)

Removal of all other resectable tumor

Appendectomy

In the rare patients in whom full staging and debulking surgery cannot be performed because of poor prognosis, neoadjuvant therapy (chemotherapy administered prior to debulking surgery) may facilitate cytoreduction after therapy.

KEY POINTS

- A markedly elevated CA-125 concentration in a postmenopausal woman with an adnexal mass strengthens the presumptive diagnosis of ovarian carcinoma, but elevated CA-125 is not specific for or diagnostic of cancer.

- More than 70% of women with ovarian cancer have metastatic disease beyond the pelvis at diagnosis.

- The first and most important step in treatment of ovarian cancer is maximal surgical cytoreduction performed by a trained gynecologic oncologist with comprehensive staging at laparotomy.

- Detailed tissue sampling is mandatory during cytoreduction surgery because up to 30% of patients with disease grossly confined to the ovary have micrometastatic disease.

Treatment

Surgical Cytoreduction

In most other solid tumors, anything short of complete surgical resection will have no impact on survival. However, ovarian cancer is unique in that maximal surgical cytoreduction of all tumor sites is associated with increased survival. The goal of such surgery is to achieve no visible residual disease. A large (>6000 patients) meta-analysis found that for each 10% increase in maximal cytoreduction, there was a 4.1% increase in median survival time. Optimal debulking, defined as no residual single lesion being greater than 1 cm, occurs in

approximately 82% of patients when performed by a gynecologic oncologist compared with 29% when performed by physicians from other surgical specialties. Maximal cytoreduction was one of the most powerful determinants of survival among patients with advanced-stage disease in a population uniformly treated with platinum-based chemotherapy.

KEY POINTS

- In patients with ovarian cancer, there is a 4.1% increase in median survival time for each 10% increase in maximal cytoreduction.

- Maximal cytoreduction preferably by a trained gynecologic oncologist is one of the most powerful determinants of survival in patients with advanced-stage ovarian cancer.

Chemotherapy

High-Risk, Early-Stage Disease

Well-staged patients with grade 1, stage I (A or B) disease require no postoperative chemotherapy. Whether patients with stage I, grade 2 disease require adjuvant chemotherapy remains controversial. Patients with high-risk, early-stage disease defined as stage IC or II disease, grade 3 tumor, or clear-cell histology should receive adjuvant chemotherapy because they have a 30% to 40% relapse rate. All patients with relapsed disease will go on to die of their disease.

Recently, two large randomized European trials were conducted comparing surgery alone with surgery followed by chemotherapy in patients with early-stage, high-risk (grade 3, clear-cell histology, and/or stage IC or II) ovarian cancer. Although there was no statistically significant difference in survival in one of those trials in which patients underwent more complete staging, there was an increment of 11% for

TABLE 27 Staging, Treatment, and Prognosis of Ovarian Cancer

Stage	Histologic Description	Typical Therapy	5-Year Survival (%)
I	Limited to the ovaries	Low risk[a] – surgery only High risk[b] – surgery followed by chemotherapy[c]	>90 75-80
II	Pelvic extension	Surgery followed by chemotherapy[c]	60-70
III	Peritoneal implants outside the pelvis and/or retroperitoneal or inguinal lymph nodes, or superficial liver metastases	Surgery followed by chemotherapy[c,d]	25-40
IV	Distant metastases	Surgery (dependent on distribution and resectability of disease) and chemotherapy[c]	10-15

[a]Low risk: grade 1.

[b]High risk: grade 3 or clear cell histology and/or stage IC or II.

[c]Chemotherapy usually consists of some form of a platinum/taxane doublet.

[d]Chemotherapy can be given either intravenously or intraperitoneally in patients who have been optimally debulked (no residual disease greater than 1 cm).

disease-free survival and 8% for overall survival in patients who received chemotherapy postoperatively when the studies were analyzed together. Another trial suggests that three cycles of chemotherapy seem as effective as six in patients with high-risk, early-stage disease.

Advanced-Stage Disease

Research supporting the modern era of chemotherapy for ovarian cancer began with the Gynecologic Oncology Group 111 trial, which compared patients who received combination cisplatin plus paclitaxel with a control group of patients receiving combination cisplatin plus cyclophosphamide. The cisplatin-paclitaxel–containing arm had a higher response rate, complete response rate, progression-free survival, and overall survival compared with the control group. As a result of this study and others, paclitaxel combined with either cisplatin or carboplatin has become the standard of care for the treatment of advanced-stage ovarian cancer.

Because ovarian cancer is primarily confined to the abdominal cavity, intraperitoneal chemotherapy has been added to systemic chemotherapy in patients with minimal residual disease. The Gynecologic Oncology Group 172 trial demonstrated a significant survival advantage of intraperitoneally plus intravenously delivered chemotherapy (IP arm) versus intravenously delivered chemotherapy only (66 months vs. 50 months; $P = 0.03$). However, toxicity was increased, and only 42% of patients assigned to the IP arm completed their assigned chemotherapy.

No clear consensus exists on the role of maintenance chemotherapy, which is not now the standard of care but is still being evaluated in ongoing randomized clinical trials.

KEY POINTS

- Standard therapy for patients with advanced-stage ovarian cancer consists of a platinum-based agent plus paclitaxel.
- Intraperitoneally plus intravenously delivered chemotherapy confers a significant survival advantage but greater toxicity compared with intravenously delivered chemotherapy in patients with ovarian cancer.

Second-Look Ovarian Cancer Surgery

Second-look surgery refers to the surgical re-exploration of patients with ovarian cancer after completion of chemotherapy to pathologically confirm the presence of a complete remission. This surgery has fallen from favor as part of standard practice because it has been shown to have no impact on survival. In addition, 50% of the patients who have no evidence of disease at the time of second-look surgery will still relapse.

KEY POINT

- Second-look ovarian cancer surgery is no longer in favor because it does not affect survival.

Management of Recurrent Ovarian Cancer

Surgery

Retrospective studies suggest that patients with ovarian cancer who undergo surgery for relapsed disease (an approach also termed "secondary cytoreduction") may experience enhanced survival if they can be completely cytoreduced again. Surgery should be considered for patients with a solitary focus of recurrence at a site amenable to resection, a long disease-free interval (>12 months) before recurrence, good performance status, and few comorbidities, although there are no randomized trials supporting these criteria. National Comprehensive Cancer Network guidelines recommend resection of recurrent disease if it is a focal recurrence of low volume after a disease-free interval of at least 6 months.

KEY POINT

- Patients with relapsed ovarian cancer who are being considered for surgery may experience enhanced survival if they undergo comprehensive secondary cytoreduction.

Chemotherapy

The goals of therapy in the recurrent setting are to control disease, maintain quality of life, and extend survival. The platinum-free interval is the time from the completion of primary platinum-based treatment to the time of recurrence. This characteristic is the major determinant for choosing the subsequent antineoplastic drugs or agents in the treatment of ovarian cancer, because platinum compounds remain the preferred drugs for patients deemed to have platinum-sensitive disease. Patients who relapse longer than 6 months after the completion of primary chemotherapy are considered to be platinum-sensitive, with response rates increasing with lengthening platinum-free intervals based on several retrospective studies. Response rates to platinum compounds exceed all other agents once the platinum-free interval is longer than 12 months. In recent years, platinum-containing doublets have been shown to be superior to platinum alone in large, randomized trials. In a trial of 800 patients with relapsed disease, a statistically significant improvement in progression-free survival and overall survival was reported in women who received combined carboplatin plus paclitaxel compared with carboplatin alone. Administration of the combination regimen was complicated mostly by worsening neuropathy.

There are multiple nonplatinum agents for treating patients with recurrent ovarian cancer who are no longer responsive to platinum-based therapy. Choosing the appropriate agent for these patients should be based on which drugs have already been used, residual toxicities from prior regimens, current gastrointestinal tract status, convenience, and the toxicities of remaining drug options. Multiple new molecularly targeted agents are being evaluated initially in the setting of relapse. The most promising of these agents has been bevacizumab, a humanized monoclonal antibody against vascular endothelial growth factor.

KEY POINTS

- Platinum-based doublets are the treatment of choice for patients with ovarian cancer who relapse 6 months or more after completion of front-line therapy unless contraindicated.
- Which drugs have already been used, residual toxicities from the prior regimens, current status of the gastrointestinal tract, convenience, and the toxicities of remaining options should be considered when choosing drugs for patients with relapsed ovarian cancer who are no longer platinum-responsive.

Monitoring and Follow-up

The National Comprehensive Cancer Network recommends that once a woman with ovarian cancer achieves a complete response, she should undergo physical examination and be asked to provide an interim history every 2 to 4 months for 2 years, then every 6 months for 3 years, and then annually. Serologic CA-125 concentration should be measured at each visit if initially elevated. Complete blood count and other serum chemistries should be evaluated as clinically indicated. There are no specific recommendations regarding imaging studies, such as abdominal CT, MRI, or PET, other than to perform them as clinically warranted.

KEY POINT

- In the follow-up management of patients with ovarian cancer, laboratory and imaging studies should be performed only when clinically indicated.

Supportive Care

Supportive care of patients with ovarian cancer most frequently involves patients receiving chemotherapy and includes monitoring and support of blood counts, proper mouth care, and, when appropriate, catheter maintenance. Patients with refractory ascites present a more unique problem; they feel bloated, are unable to eat, and often experience dyspnea because they cannot fully expand their lungs because of limited excursion of the diaphragm. This condition often develops late in the disease when the cancer no longer is

responsive to chemotherapy. Weekly or twice-weekly paracentesis is often required in these patients to provide comfort. Patients with ovarian cancer also experience large protein losses due to drainage procedures in addition to poor nutrition, which contributes to worsening third-space fluid.

Another relatively common complication of ovarian cancer requiring special supportive care is bowel obstruction caused by mass effect of carcinomatosis. These patients often have end-stage disease and are given the option of draining gastrostomy tube placement before they enter hospice care. For a single-focus bowel obstruction, surgery may be indicated, especially in settings in which postoperative chemotherapy is still likely to be active.

KEY POINTS

- Weekly or twice-weekly paracentesis is often required in patients with ovarian cancer–induced ascites to provide comfort.
- Patients with end-stage ovarian cancer who have a bowel obstruction are given the option of draining gastrostomy tube placement before entering hospice care.
- For a single-focus bowel obstruction in patients with ovarian cancer, surgery may be indicated, especially in settings in which postoperative chemotherapy is still likely to be active.

Bibliography

Armstong DK, Bundy B, Wenzel L, et al. Intraperitoneal cisplatin and paclitaxel in ovarian cancer. N Engl J Med. 2006;354(1):34-43. [PMID: 16394300]

Bandera CA. Advances in the understanding of risk factors for ovarian cancer. J Reprod Med 2005;50(6):399-406. [PMID: 16050564]

Bell J, Brady MF, Young RC, et al; Gynecologic Oncology Group. Randomized phase III trial of three versus six cycles of adjuvant carboplatin and paclitaxel in early stage epithelial ovarian carcinoma: a Gynecologic Oncology Group study. Gynecol Oncol. 2006;102(3):432-439. [PMID: 16860852]

Bristow RE, Tomacruz RS, Armstrong DK, Trimble EL, Montz FJ. Survival effect of maximal cytoreductive surgery for advanced ovarian carcinoma during the platinum era: A meta-analysis. J Clin Oncol. 2002;20(5):1248-1259. [PMID: 11870167]

Bukowski RM, Ozols RF, Markman M. The management of recurrent ovarian cancer. Semin Oncol. 2007;34(2 Suppl 2):S1-15. [PMID: 17512352]

Goff BA, Mandel LS, Drescher CW, et al. Development of an ovarian cancer symptom index. Possibilities for earlier detection. Cancer. 2007;109(2):221-227. [PMID: 17154394]

McGuire WP, Hoskins WJ, Brady MF, et al. Cyclophosphamide and cisplatin compared with paclitaxel and cisplatin in patients with stage III and stage IC ovarian cancer. N Engl J Med. 1996;334(1):1-6. [PMID: 7494563]

Morgan RJ, Alvarez RD, Armstrong DK, et al. Ovarian cancer. Clinical practice guidelines in oncology. N Natl Compr Canc Netw. 2006;4(9):912-939. [PMID: 17020669]

Ozols RF, Bundy BN, Greer BE, et al; Gynecologic Oncology Group. Phase III trial of carboplatin and paclitaxel compared with cisplatin and paclitaxel in patients with optimally resected stage III ovarian cancer: a Gynecologic Oncology Group study. J Clin Oncol. 2003; 21(17):3194-3200. [PMID: 12860964]

Trimbos JB, Vergote I, Bolis G, et al; EORTC-ACTION collaborators. European Organisation for Research and Treatment of Cancer-Adjuvant ChemoTherapy in Ovarian Neoplasm. Impact of adjuvant chemotherapy and surgical staging in early-stage ovarian carcinoma: European Organisation for Research and Treatment of Cancer-Adjuvant ChemoTherapy in Ovarian Neoplasm trial. J Natl Cancer Inst. 2003;95(2):113-125. [PMID: 12529344]

Gastrointestinal Malignancies

Colorectal Cancer

In 2008, there were approximately 149,000 new cases of colorectal cancer in the United States, making it the fourth most common malignancy behind lung, prostate, and breast cancer. Approximately 50,000 patients died of colorectal cancer, making it the second leading cause of cancer-related death in the United States behind lung cancer. The incidence of colorectal cancer in the United States appears to be declining, although there is a shift toward more proximally located tumors. Identification and removal of premalignant polyps as a result of screening sigmoidoscopy and colonoscopy may explain the declining incidence.

There are various hereditary cancer syndromes that predispose affected persons to colorectal cancer (see Cancer Risk section). Inflammatory bowel disease (Crohn disease and ulcerative colitis) also predisposes patients to colorectal cancer. However, most colorectal cancers are sporadic. A personal history of adenomatous polyps or polyps with villous or tubulovillous histology or a history of such polyps in a first-degree relative increases the relative risk for colorectal cancer. Other risk factors include diabetes mellitus, obesity, and the use of tobacco and alcohol. Although some studies have shown that a diet high in red meat is a risk factor for colorectal cancer, the overall evidence about dietary factors remains inconclusive. However, diets high in fiber, including fruits and vegetables, may be protective. The lifetime risk for colorectal cancer is 1 in 18, and the risk increases with age.

Signs and symptoms of colorectal cancer include anemia as a result of occult blood loss, melena, hematochezia, abdominal pain, and a change in bowel habits. Patients with metastatic disease often have right upper quadrant pain, abdominal bloating, early satiety, and weight loss. Surgical resection is the primary curative therapy, but 40% to 60% of patients who undergo surgical resection for cure relapse, usually within the first 3 years and peaking in the second year after resection.

Staging

The four-stage American Joint Committee on Cancer (AJCC) TNM (tumor, node, metastasis) staging system has replaced the Dukes classification and staging system for colorectal cancer (**Table 28** and **Table 29**). Pathologic staging is performed on the surgical specimens and is important for defining prognosis and for identifying patients who may benefit from adjuvant chemotherapy. The survival rate increases with the number of lymph nodes analyzed, whether or not the lymph nodes are positive for metastatic disease; therefore, at least 12 lymph nodes should be examined for accurate staging. Additional features associated with risk of recurrence include obstruction or perforation at presentation, tumor adherence to other organs, positive radial margins, poorly differentiated histology, and the presence of lymphovascular or perineural invasion.

Adjuvant Therapy of Colon Cancer

The goal of postoperative adjuvant therapy is to eradicate micrometastases and thereby to improve the postresection survival rate. Patients with lymph node–positive disease (stage III) benefit from adjuvant chemotherapy. Adjuvant therapy for patients with stage II colon cancer is controversial. However, there are patients with high-risk disease (T4 lesions, poorly differentiated histology, or inadequately sampled lymph nodes) who may benefit from adjuvant therapy. There are ongoing studies using molecular genetic factors to identify which patients with stage II disease are at higher risk for recurrence and more likely to benefit from adjuvant chemotherapy.

The most active chemotherapeutic agent in colon cancer is 5-fluorouracil (5-FU), which inhibits thymidylate synthase, the rate-limiting enzyme in pyrimidine nucleotide synthesis. 5-FU is usually administered with leucovorin, a reduced folate that stabilizes the binding of 5-FU to thymidylate synthase, thereby enhancing the inhibition of DNA synthesis. There is now available an oral fluoropyrimidine, capecitabine, a prodrug of 5-FU, which is converted to 5'-deoxyfluorocytidine in the liver and is in turn converted to 5'-deoxyfluorouridine in tissues. The final conversion to active 5-FU is by thymidine phosphorylase, an enzyme expressed in high levels within the tumor microenvironment.

TABLE 28 The AJCC TNM Staging and Dukes Staging for Colorectal Cancer

Stage	AJCC TNM	Dukes	5-Year Survival Rate (%)
I	T1-2, N0, M0	A	93
IIA	T3, N0, M0	B	84.7
IIB	T4, N0, M0	B	72.2
IIIA	T1-2, N1, M0	C	83.4
IIIB	T3-4, N1, M0	C	64.1
IIIC	T any, N2, M0	C	44.3
IV	T any, N any, M1	–	8.1

AJCC = American Joint Committee on Cancer; TNM = tumor, node, metastasis.

TABLE 29 The AJCC TNM Definitions for Colorectal Cancer
Primary Tumor (T)
TX: Primary tumor cannot be assessed
T0: No evidence of primary tumor
Tis: Carcinoma in situ: intraepithelial or invasion of the lamina propria
T1: Tumor invades submucosa
T2: Tumor invades muscularis propria
T3: Tumor invades through the muscularis propria into the subserosa or into nonperitonealized pericolic or perirectal tissues
T4: Tumor directly invades other organs or structures and/or perforates visceral peritoneum
Regional Lymph Nodes (N)
NX: Regional nodes cannot be assessed
N0: No regional lymph node metastasis
N1: Metastasis in one to three regional lymph nodes
N2: Metastasis in four or more regional lymph nodes
Distant Metastasis (M)
MX: Distant metastasis cannot be assessed
M0: No distant metastasis
M1: Distant metastasis
AJCC = American Joint Committee on Cancer; TNM = tumor, node, metastasis.

The chemotherapy choices in the adjuvant setting include 5-fluorouracil (5-FU), often given by continuous infusion and with leucovorin to enhance its activity. Oral capecitabine, a prodrug of 5-FU, is replacing prolonged infusional 5-FU in many chemotherapy regimens. The newest agent used in the adjuvant setting in colon cancer is oxaliplatin, a diaminocyclohexane platinum derivative that impairs DNA synthesis. A multicenter international study of oxaliplatin, 5-FU, and leucovorin (FOLFOX) for adjuvant treatment of patients with stage II and stage III colon cancer showed an improvement in disease-free survival at 4 years for patients with stage II disease (85% versus 81%) and stage III disease (70% versus 61%). The benefits of adding oxaliplatin to 5-FU and leucovorin were confirmed in a subsequent study. The FOLFOX regimen has therefore been approved for adjuvant chemotherapy in patients with stage II and III colon cancer.

Rectal Cancer

There were an estimated 41,420 new cases of rectal cancer and 8500 deaths from rectal cancer in the United States in 2008. Approximately 30% of all colorectal cancers are located in part or entirely below the peritoneal reflection. Endoscopic ultrasound is more accurate than CT scan or MRI for determining T stage and as accurate as these modalities for determining nodal involvement. Surgery is the mainstay of therapy for both colon and rectal cancer, but because the rectum is a retroperitoneal organ without a serosa, obtaining wide margins at resection is technically difficult; there is, therefore, a higher incidence of local recurrence.

Because 75% of patients with rectal cancer die with both local and distant recurrence and only 25% with solely distant recurrences, the goal of adjuvant therapy for rectal cancer is to decrease the risk for both. Radiation therapy is often used in patients with rectal cancer either preoperatively (that is, in the neoadjuvant setting) or postoperatively for better local control. Randomized trials have clearly shown the benefit of treating patients with stage II and stage III rectal cancer either adjuvantly or neoadjuvantly with combinations of concurrent 5-FU/radiation therapy and systemic FOLFOX. Clinical trials are evaluating the role of the newer monoclonal antibodies in the adjuvant treatment of resected colorectal tumors.

Management of Patients with Metastatic Disease

Newer targeted therapies have resulted in marked improvements in response rates, 1-year overall survival, and 2-year overall survival in patients with metastatic colorectal cancer. However, the 5-year overall survival rate for patients with unresectable disease is still 10% or less. Aggressive surgical approaches in patients with limited and surgically resectable metastases can result in cure in about 25% of cases. In addition to oxaliplatin and 5-FU, irinotecan, a topoisomerase inhibitor that did not show benefit in adjuvant studies, is used in patients with metastatic disease as a single agent or in combination with 5-FU. As first-line therapy, irinotecan combinations have a response rate of about 40% and improved time-to-progression and overall survival over 5-FU therapy alone. Uridine diphosphoglucuronosyltransferase (UGT1A1) is an enzyme involved in the metabolism of irinotecan, and patients who are homozygous for the *UGT1A1*28* allele may develop neutropenia from this agent; patients are now routinely genotyped before receiving irinotecan. Oxaliplatin therapy can cause neurotoxicity and hepatotoxicity. Therefore, first-line therapy with irinotecan or oxaliplatin is largely based on physician and/or patient preference and on preexisting toxicities such as neuropathy or hepatic dysfunction, or the presence of *UGT1A1* polymorphisms.

Monoclonal antibody therapies are generally well-tolerated and do not share overlapping toxicities with standard cytotoxic agents. Bevacizumab, an antiangiogenic agent that targets the vascular endothelial growth factor that is overexpressed in many solid tumors, is approved for use in combination with chemotherapy. Bevacizumab has been shown to improve survival when used with irinotecan and oxaliplatin-based treatment. Typical toxic effects include proteinuria and hypertension. Another approved monoclonal antibody cetuximab targets the epidermal growth factor receptor. Many patients treated with this agent develop a potentially dose-limiting acneiform rash over the face, neck, chest, and back. Cetuximab given with irinotecan-based therapy improved progression-free survival, but only if the tumor has no K-*ras* mutations. The next generation EGFR monoclonal antibody, panitumumab, is a fully human anti-EGFR monoclonal antibody that results in fewer allergic reactions and has been shown to improve progression-free survival over best supportive care. There are ongoing studies to determine the role of combinations of these antibodies with and without cytotoxic therapy.

Postresection Colorectal Cancer Surveillance

Guidelines for follow-up surveillance of patients who have undergone resection for colorectal cancer have been produced by the National Comprehensive Cancer Network (NCCN) (www.nccn.org) and the American Society of Clinical Oncology (ASCO) (www.ASCO.org). The NCCN recommends a history and physical examination with digital rectal examination and measurement of serum carcinoembryonic antigen (CEA) every 3 to 6 months for the first 2 years after resection and then every 6 months for the subsequent 3 years, along with a colonoscopy at 1 year with a repeat in 1 year if abnormal or in 3 years if negative for polyps and then every 5 years. Based on results from three meta-analyses of randomized controlled clinical trials, CT scan of the chest, abdomen, and pelvis is now recommended annually for 3 years for patients with perineural invasion or poorly differentiated tumors. The benefit to CT imaging of the liver is that it can identify limited metastases that can be treated with liver resection, with a 25% lower mortality rate for successfully resected patients.

KEY POINTS

- Administering monoclonal antibodies such as bevacizumab and cetuximab with standard chemotherapy has improved overall survival in patients with metastatic colorectal cancer.
- Oxaliplatin, a cytotoxic agent with proven effectiveness in the metastatic setting, has been shown to be beneficial in adjuvant therapy for colon cancer.
- Stage for stage, rectal cancer has a poorer prognosis than colon cancer because the retroperitoneal location of the rectum and its lack of a serosa result in a high local recurrence rate.
- Postresection surveillance of patients with colorectal cancer is important because up to 25% of patients with limited distant recurrence can undergo surgery with curative intent.
- The survival rate in colorectal cancer increases with the number of lymph nodes analyzed, whether or not the lymph nodes are positive for metastatic disease; therefore, at least 12 lymph nodes should be examined for accurate staging.

Gastric Cancer

In 2008, there were approximately 21,500 new cases of gastric cancer and approximately 10,800 deaths from the disease. Gastric cancer is more common in black Americans than whites, and there is a 2:1 male-to-female predominance. Risk factors for gastric cancer include *Helicobacter pylori* infection, male sex, advanced age, a history of smoking, a family history of gastric cancer, and familial adenomatous polyposis. The relative risk for gastric cancer is twofold greater after partial gastrectomy for peptic ulcer disease.

Affected patients typically present with anemia as a result of occult blood loss, melena, abdominal pain, nausea and vomiting, and weight loss. Such patients should be referred for upper endoscopy and endoscopic ultrasound. After the diagnosis is made, staging workup includes chest radiograph and CT scan of the abdomen with optional PET scan. For patients with localized and resectable disease, the 5-year overall survival rate is approximately 58%. The 5-year survival rate for patients with metastatic disease is about 23%.

The AJCC TNM system is used to stage gastric cancer (**Table 30** and **Table 31**). Most patients present with advanced and unresectable metastatic disease, and their disease is considered incurable. For patients with localized tumors, surgery with curative intent is undertaken. However, up to 50% of these patients has microscopic or macroscopic disease at the surgical margins or peritoneal involvement, distant metastases, or invasion of major blood vessels.

In one study, 556 patients with lymph node–negative resected gastric cancer or cancer of the gastroesophageal

TABLE 30 AJCC TNM Classification for Gastric Cancer
AJCC Stage Groupings
Stage 0
Tis, N0, M0
Stage IA
T1, N0, M0
Stage IB
T1, N1, M0
T2a, N0, M0
T2b, N0, M0
Stage II
T1, N2, M0
T2a, N1, M0
T2b, N1, M0
T3, N0, M0
Stage IIIA
T2a, N2, M0
T2b, N2, M0
T3, N1, M0
T4, N0, M0
Stage IIIB
T3, N2, M0
Stage IV
T4, N1, M0
T4, N2, M0
T4, N3, M0
T1, N3, M0
T2, N3, M0
T3, N3, M0
Any T, any N, M1

AJCC = American Joint Committee on Cancer; TNM = tumor, node, metastasis.

TABLE 31 AJCC Gastric Cancer TNM Definitions	
T0	No evidence of primary tumor
Tis	Carcinoma in situ: intraepithelial tumor without invasion of the lamina propria
T1	Tumor invades lamina propria or submucosa
T2	Tumor invades muscularis propria or subserosa
T2a	Tumor invades muscularis propria
T2b	Tumor invades subserosa
T3	Tumor penetrates serosa (visceral peritoneum) without invasion of adjacent structures
T4	Tumor invades adjacent structures
N0	No regional lymph node metastasis
N1	Metastasis in 1 to 6 regional lymph nodes
N2	Metastasis in 7 to 15 regional lymph nodes
N3	Metastasis in more than 15 regional lymph nodes
M0	No distant metastasis
M1	Distant metastasis

AJCC = American Joint Committee on Cancer; TNM = tumor, node, metastasis.

junction were randomized to receive chemotherapy and radiation therapy or observation. The chemotherapy consisted of 5-FU/leucovorin followed by concurrent 5-FU/radiation therapy followed by additional 5-FU/leucovorin. Patients who received adjuvant therapy had a median overall survival of 36 versus 27 months for the patients who were observed only, a median relapse-free survival of 30 versus 19 months, and a 3-year disease-free survival rate of 48% versus 31%. Therefore, combination adjuvant chemotherapy and radiation therapy is considered the standard of care. Of the patients who relapsed, 65% were regional lymph node relapses, 19% local relapses, and 33% distant relapses.

Another study randomized patients to receive neoadjuvant chemotherapy with epirubicin, cisplatin, and 5-FU, followed by resection, followed by adjuvant epirubicin, cisplatin, and 5-FU versus surgery and observation. Patients who received neoadjuvant and adjuvant therapy had an improvement in median progression-free survival as well as 5-year overall survival rate (36% versus 23%). Other recent studies have suggested that a pathologic response to neoadjuvant therapy with chemotherapy and radiation therapy may result in potentially better outcomes. Therefore, standard adjuvant therapy for gastric cancer is concurrent chemotherapy and radiation therapy. For patients fit enough to receive aggressive therapy, neoadjuvant therapy with epirubicin, cisplatin, and 5-FU followed by postoperative adjuvant therapy is a reasonable treatment option.

Posttreatment surveillance includes a physical examination every 3 to 4 months for 3 years and then annually. For patients who have undergone a proximal or total gastrectomy, monitoring of bone density and concentrations of serum vitamin B_{12}, iron, folate, and calcium are warranted.

For patients with metastatic or recurrent disease, there is no standard of care. Active single agents for metastatic gastric cancer include oxaliplatin, capecitabine, epirubicin, and docetaxel; combination regimens include epirubicin, cisplatin, and 5-FU or docetaxel, cisplatin, and 5-FU. Patients should be encouraged to enroll in clinical trials.

KEY POINTS

- Neoadjuvant and adjuvant chemotherapy and radiation therapy improve overall survival in patients with resectable gastric cancer; however, relapse remains high.
- Serum vitamin B_{12} concentration should be monitored in patients who have undergone proximal or total gastrectomy.

Esophageal Cancer

Esophageal cancer represents only 6% of all gastrointestinal cancers in the United States. In 2008, there were approximately 16,500 new cases of esophageal carcinoma and 14,300 deaths from the disease. Esophageal carcinoma is more common in black Americans than whites, and there is a 3:1 male-to-female predominance. Esophageal carcinomas are squamous cell or adenocarcinoma, with the less common squamous cell tumors accounting for approximately 30%. The incidence of esophageal adenocarcinoma is increasing.

Risk factors for esophageal cancer include smoking, alcohol consumption, advanced age, male sex, Barrett esophagus, gastroesophageal reflux disease, and achalasia. Barrett esophagus, a metaplastic condition in which columnar or glandular epithelium replaces normal squamous epithelium in the distal esophagus, is the most important risk factor and confers a 40-fold increased risk for esophageal adenocarcinoma compared with the unaffected population. Although endoscopic surveillance can detect early cancers in asymptomatic patients, no study has shown that routine surveillance improves survival, and it therefore remains controversial.

Patients with esophageal carcinoma typically present with dysphagia, initially for solid foods and then liquids, accompanied by weight loss in 90% of cases. Other symptoms may include odynophagia, retrosternal pain, cough, and hoarseness. Workup includes barium swallow and/or upper esophagogastroduodenoscopy with biopsy. For patients with localized disease, the overall 5-year survival rate is 31%, whereas in patients with unresectable metastatic disease, the 5-year survival rate is only approximately 15%.

The AJCC TNM system is used to stage esophageal carcinoma. Imaging with endoscopic ultrasound and PET/CT has become increasingly useful in accurately predicting the surgical stage and identifying patients with distant metastases at presentation.

Increasingly, trimodality therapy consisting of chemotherapy, radiation therapy, and surgery is used to manage locally advanced esophageal cancer. In fit patients who can undergo surgical resection, patient management should include an experienced thoracic surgeon, a radiation therapist, and a medical oncologist. Esophagectomy is recommended in patients with T1 lymph node–negative disease. Patients who are not candidates for resection typically undergo definitive chemoradiation followed by observation. Patients who are candidates for resection undergo preoperative chemoradiation and, if they remain able to undergo surgery, esophagectomy.

Six randomized trials have compared radiation therapy alone with combined chemotherapy and radiation therapy. One such trial, RTOG 85-01, showed the superiority of concurrent chemotherapy with 5-FU/cisplatin and radiation therapy over radiation therapy alone, with a median survival of 14 versus 9 months and a 5-year overall survival rate of 27% versus 0%. Despite excellent responses with chemotherapy and radiation therapy, up to 40% of patients with no detectable disease on posttreatment biopsies had residual tumor at surgery, suggesting that disease is not eradicated with chemotherapy and radiation therapy alone. This study supports the recommendation for posttreatment resection in otherwise healthy patients.

There have been several studies comparing preoperative chemotherapy and radiation therapy followed by surgery versus surgery alone; the results of these studies have been equivocal. The patients who received preoperative chemotherapy and radiation therapy had 3-year overall survival rates ranging from 30% to 45%, which in two of the studies were significantly better than surgery alone, with 3-year survival rates ranging from 6% to 16%. The CALGB 97-81 study consisted of patients with stage I, II, and III esophageal cancer who received 5-FU/cisplatin with concurrent radiation therapy followed by surgery or surgery alone. The 5-year overall survival rate was 39% in patients given combination therapy versus 16% in patients who underwent surgery alone. The median survival in patients treated with the trimodality approach was 6.8 years versus 4.5 years for surgery alone. Therefore, chemoradiation therapy followed by surgery is superior to surgery alone. Furthermore, pathologic complete response rates have been shown to correlate with higher cure rate.

There is no standard regimen for metastatic esophageal cancer. Several agents have been shown to be active, including 5-FU, cisplatin, and the taxanes, but it is recommended that affected patients be enrolled in clinical trials when possible.

KEY POINTS

- Smoking and alcohol use are risk factors for squamous cell carcinoma of the esophagus.

- Gastroesophageal reflux disease and Barrett esophagus are risk factors for adenocarcinoma of the esophagus.

- Chemoradiation therapy followed by surgery is superior to surgery alone in the treatment of esophageal cancer.

Pancreatic Cancer

Patients with pancreatic cancer have a dismal prognosis: in 2008 in the United States, there were approximately 37,600 new cases and 34,200 deaths from the disease, making it the fourth leading cause of cancer-related death. Less than 5% of all patients with pancreatic cancer lives for 5 years after diagnosis. Even in patients who undergo resection with curative intent, the median overall survival is 15 months, and the 5-year survival rate is only approximately 20%. In patients with unresectable but locally advanced pancreatic cancer, median survival is 8 to 10 months, and in patients with metastatic disease the median overall survival is 6 months. About 25% of patients present with resectable disease, another 25% with locally advanced unresectable disease, and 50% with metastatic disease. Risk factors for pancreatic cancer include cigarette smoking, which confers a 2.5 relative risk. There is weaker evidence that diabetes mellitus, obesity, and chronic pancreatitis predispose patients to pancreatic cancer. The exception is hereditary pancreatitis, which confers a very increased risk for pancreatic cancer; however, cases of hereditary pancreatitis constitute only 1% of cases of chronic pancreatitis.

Patients often present with nonspecific abdominal pain (or pain radiating through to the back), bloating, nausea, anorexia, and weight loss. The diagnosis is more readily suspect in patients who present with jaundice, either with or without pain.

The evaluation of patients with suspected pancreatic cancer consists of high-resolution, dynamic-phase helical or spiral CT scan of the abdomen and liver chemistry tests. Endoscopic ultrasound is being increasingly used; the procedure better delineates smaller tumors than CT and gives more accurate guidance for fine-needle aspiration to confirm the pathology and provide a better assessment of the extent of the tumor, including whether nodal disease is present. In addition, endoscopic ultrasound–guided biopsy carries a much lower risk for peritoneal seeding of tumor than CT-guided biopsy. Endoscopic retrograde cholangiopancreatography may be indicated, particularly for the endoscopic placement of a biliary stent in patients who present with obstructive jaundice.

The AJCC system is used to stage pancreatic cancer. The presence of distant metastases, encasement of the superior mesenteric artery or celiac artery, and occlusion of the superior mesenteric vein or portal vein preclude resection. Patients with potentially resectable disease may undergo a Whipple procedure (cholecystectomy, partial gastrectomy, removal of the proximal jejunum and a portion of the pancreas followed by gastrojejunostomy) in the hands of an experienced surgeon. Neoadjuvant chemotherapy with or without radiation therapy is typically used for locally advanced but potentially resectable or locally advanced unresectable disease. Palliative systemic chemotherapy is recommended for patients with incurable metastatic disease.

The two chemotherapeutic agents most commonly used for pancreatic cancer are gemcitabine and 5-FU; however, the optimal regimen for adjuvant therapy is unsettled. In a recent study, patients who received chemotherapy had a better outcome than patients who did not, with a median survival of 20.1 versus 15.5 months and a 5-year survival of 21% versus 8%. Patients who received chemotherapy and radiation therapy had a worse prognosis than patients who did not, with a median survival of 15.9 versus 17.9 months and a 5-year overall survival of 10% versus 20%. Therefore, the role of radiation therapy postoperatively is uncertain. No standard postoperative regimen has emerged as superior, and there are ongoing adjuvant studies to determine optimal treatment

after resection, incorporating newer monoclonal antibodies such as cetuximab or bevacizumab.

In patients with metastatic disease, gemcitabine is the standard therapy. Gemcitabine received Food and Drug Administration approval for use in pancreatic cancer based on a study showing clinical benefit response of 24% for gemcitabine versus 5% for 5-FU. The antitumor response rate was only 5% in the gemcitabine arm and 0% in 5-FU, with a median survival of 5.7 versus 4.4 months. Multiple chemotherapy regimens, including capecitabine and oxiliplatin, have failed to show an improvement in survival over gemcitabine alone.

Despite the success of newer targeted therapies in other solid tumors, there has been little advancement in the treatment of pancreatic cancer. A recent randomized trial of gemcitabine with or without erlotinib, an oral tyrosine kinase inhibitor of the epidermal growth factor receptor, showed a very modest improvement in overall survival from 5.91 months to 6.24 months and an improvement in 1-year overall survival rate from 17% to 23%. Erlotinib received Food and Drug Administration approval for this indication, but whether this improvement is clinically meaningful is unclear. Two other randomized phase III studies evaluating the additional benefit of either bevacizumab or cetuximab to single-agent gemcitabine failed to show any statistically significant benefit in overall survival.

KEY POINTS

- Neoadjuvant chemotherapy with or without radiation therapy is typically used for locally advanced but potentially resectable or locally advanced unresectable pancreatic cancer.

- Pancreatic cancer has an extremely poor prognosis; newer targeted therapies have failed to add any substantial benefit to standard gemcitabine.

Bibliography

Ajani, JA, Mansfield, PF, Crane, CH, et al. Paclitaxel-based chemoradiotherapy in localized gastric carcinoma: degree of pathologic response and not clinical parameters dictated patient outcome. J Clin Oncol, 2005;23(6):1237-1244. [PMID: 15718321]

Ajani JA, Winter K, Okawara GS. Phase II trial of preoperative chemoradiation in patients with localized gastric adenocarcinoma (RTOG 9904): quality of combined modality therapy and pathologic response. J Clin Oncol. 2006;24(24)3953-3958. [PMID: 16921048]

Andre T, Boni C, Mounedji-Boudiaf L, et al; Multicenter International Study of Oxaliplatin/5-Fluorouracil/Leucovorin in the Adjuvant Treatment of Colon Cancer (MOSAIC) Investigators. Oxaliplatin, fluorouracil, and leucovorin as adjuvant treatment for colon cancer. N Engl J Med. 2004;350(23):2343-2351. [PMID: 15175436]

Benson AB 3rd, Schrag D, Somerfield MR, et al. American Society of Clinical Oncology recommendations on adjuvant chemotherapy for stage II colon cancer. J Clin Oncol. 2004;22(16):3408-3419. [PMID: 15199089]

Chang GJ, Rodriguez-Bigas MA, Skibber JM, Moyer VA. Lymph node evaluation and survival after curative resection of colon cancer:

systematic review. J Natl Cancer Inst. 2007;99(6):433-441. [PMID: 17374833]

Cunningham D, Allum WH, Stenning SP, et al; MAGIC trial participants. Perioperative chemotherapy versus surgery alone for resectable gastroesophageal cancer. N Engl J Med. 2006;355(1):11-20. [PMID: 16822992]

Desch CE, Benson AB 3rd, Somerfield MR, et al; American Society of Clinical Oncology. Colorectal cancer surveillance: 2005 update of an American Society of Clinical Oncology practice guideline. J Clin Oncol. 2005;23(33):8512-8519. [PMID: 16260687]

Karapetis CS, Khambata-Ford C, Jonker DJ, et al. K-ras Mutations and Benefit from Cetuximab in Advanced Colorectal Cancer. N Engl J Med. 2008;359(17):1757-1765. [PMID: 18946061]

Kelsen DP, Ginsberg R, Pajak TF, et al. Chemotherapy followed by surgery compared with surgery alone for localized esophageal cancer. N Engl J Med. 1998;339(27):1979-1984. [PMID: 9869669]

Kuebler JP, Wieand HS, O'Connell MJ, et al. Oxaliplatin combined with weekly bolus fluorouracil and leucovorin as surgical adjuvant chemotherapy for stage II and III colon cancer: results from NSABP C-07. J Clin Oncol. 2007;25(16):2198-2204. [PMID: 17470851]

Moore MJ, Goldstein D, Hamm J, et al; National Cancer Institute of Canada Clinical Trials Group. Erlotinib plus gemcitabine compared with gemcitabine alone in patients with advanced pancreatic cancer: a phase III trial of the National Cancer Institute of Canada Clinical Trials Group. J Clin Oncol. 2007;25(15):1960-1966. [PMID: 17452677]

Oettle H, Post S, Neuhaus P, et al. Adjuvant chemotherapy with gemcitabine vs observation in patients undergoing curative-intent resection of pancreatic cancer: a randomized controlled trial. JAMA. 2007;297(3):267-77. [PMID: 17227978]

Lung Cancer

Introduction

Lung cancer is the leading cause of cancer death in the United States, accounting for approximately 29% of all cancer deaths. During 2008, approximately 213,380 new cases of lung cancer were diagnosed (114,760 among men and 98,620 among women). Nearly 70% of patients with lung cancer are older than 65 years, and fewer than 3% are younger than 45 years. Despite the poor prognosis of lung cancer, some people are cured, and there are currently about 330,000 long-term survivors of this disease.

Clinical Presentation

Cough is a common manifestation in patients with lung cancer and occurs in most patients. Because many patients with lung cancer are current or former smokers and may have chronic cough from irritation caused by cigarette smoke or underlying chronic bronchitis, a cough with increasing frequency or severity requires investigation. Increasing dyspnea, hemoptysis, chest pain, or clinical features suggesting pneumonia are other symptoms of lung cancer. Patients with pleural or pericardial effusions may have dyspnea, cough, and chest pain. Patients with apical tumors that infiltrate surrounding structures may have Pancoast syndrome (**Figure 28**), which is characterized by shoulder pain, lower brachial plexopathy,

and Horner syndrome (ptosis, miosis, and ipsilateral anhidrosis) (**Figure 29**). See **Table 32** for a listing of manifestations of lung cancer.

Hoarseness may be caused by vocal cord paresis or paralysis when tumors or lymph node metastases compress or invade the recurrent laryngeal nerve. This symptom more commonly occurs in left-sided tumors in which the recurrent laryngeal nerve passes under the aortic arch but also occasionally occurs in patients with high, right-sided, mediastinal lesions.

Lung cancer can metastasize to multiple sites, most commonly to bone and the liver, brain, and adrenal glands. Bone metastases often cause pain, may predispose to pathologic fracture, and may cause hypercalcemia-induced symptoms. Patients with brain metastases may experience headaches, neurologic symptoms, or decreased mental acuity. In addition, metastatic lung cancer may also cause spinal cord compression, resulting in a characteristic sequence of symptoms including pain followed by motor weakness.

Lung cancer is commonly associated with systemic manifestations, including weight loss, anorexia, fatigue, and generalized weakness. Small cell lung cancer (SCLC) characteristically produces peptide hormones, which can cause endocrine syndromes, such as hyponatremia from the syndrome of inappropriate antidiuretic hormone secretion (SIADH) and hypercortisolism through secretion of adrenocorticotropic hormone (ACTH), in a subset of patients. Patients with SIADH may be asymptomatic, or they may have symptoms such as headache, decreased mental acuity, and even seizures. Neurologic symptoms, such as the Lambert-Eaton syndrome, cortical cerebellar degeneration, limbic

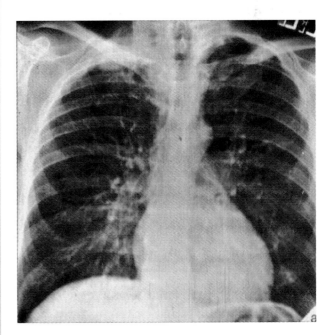

FIGURE 28.
Radiographic findings of a tumor infiltrating the apical area, indicative of Pancoast syndrome.

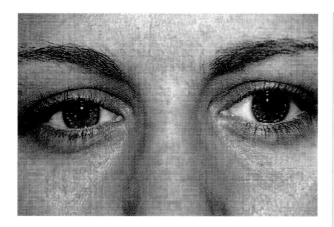

FIGURE 29.
A patient with Horner syndrome, as depicted by smaller right pupil and ptosis of the right eye.

Reproduced with permission from Bradford CA, Basic Ophthalmology, 8th Edition, American Academy of Ophthalmology, Copyright 2004.

encephalitis, and peripheral neuropathy, may also occur in patients with lung cancer, but they are relatively rare and all more commonly occur in patients with SCLC. A few patients with lung cancer may have symptomatic hypertrophic osteoarthropathy (**Figure 30**), a syndrome in which periosteal inflammation causes pain in affected areas, most commonly in the knees and ankles. Clubbing, a form of hypertrophic osteoarthropathy that consists of enlargement of the distal, compared with the proximal, digits, may also occur, and early recognition of this finding could hasten the diagnosis of lung cancer (**Figure 31**).

KEY POINTS

- A cough with increasing frequency or severity requires investigation for possible lung cancer.
- Patients with apical tumors infiltrating surrounding structures may have Pancoast syndrome, characterized by shoulder pain, lower brachial plexopathy, and Horner syndrome.
- Bone metastases in lung cancer often cause pain, may predispose to pathologic fracture, and may cause hypercalcemia-induced symptoms.
- Brain metastases are characterized by headaches, neurologic symptoms, or decreased mental acuity.
- Spinal cord compression in lung cancer typically consists of pain followed by motor weakness.
- Early recognition of clubbing (enlargement of the distal, compared with the proximal, digits) could hasten the diagnosis of lung cancer.

Non–Small Cell Lung Cancer

Non–small cell lung cancer (NSCLC) accounts for approximately 85% to 90% of cases of lung cancer. Although

TABLE 32 Common Lung Cancer Manifestations
Primary (Localized) Tumor
Postobstructive pneumonia
Cough
Hemoptysis
Wheezing
Dyspnea
Incidentally found lung mass
Intrathoracic Spread
Hoarseness (laryngeal nerve)
Ptosis, miosis, anhidrosis (Horner syndrome)
Shoulder pain, shoulder and arm weakness (brachial plexopathy)
Facial edema and venous distention in the neck and chest wall (superior vena cava syndrome)
Paralyzed hemidiaphragm (phrenic nerve)
Pleural effusion
Metastatic Spread
Bone pain and fracture, isolated elevated alkaline phosphatase
Headache, focal neurological findings, seizures
Lymphadenopathy
Hepatomegaly
Anemia, leukopenia, thrombocytopenia, elevated serum lactate dehydrogenase concentration
Skin nodules
Remote Effects of Tumor and Paraneoplastic Syndromes
Anorexia, weight loss, nausea, vomiting
Confusion, rapidly progressive dementia, seizures (paraneoplastic encephalomyelitis)
Paresthesias, sensory ataxia, multimodal sensory loss (paraneoplastic sensory neuropathy)
Hyponatremia (SIADH secretion)
Hypercalcemia (parathyroid hormone-related protein)
Proximal upper and lower extremity weakness (Lambert-Eaton myasthenic syndrome)

SIADH = syndrome of inappropriate antidiuretic hormone secretion.

histologically distinct, three subtypes of NSCLC (adenocarcinoma, squamous cell carcinoma, and large cell carcinoma) are grouped together because of similarities in presentation, treatment, and natural history. Adenocarcinoma is the most common histologic type of lung cancer in the United States and is the most common type of lung cancer among never smokers; the incidence of adenocarcinoma among never smokers is increasing. Adenocarcinoma generally presents as a peripheral lesion. A subtype of adenocarcinoma termed bronchioloalveolar carcinoma, which is less strongly associated with tobacco use, has a propensity for intrapulmonary metastases and a more indolent course. Squamous cell carcinoma, which

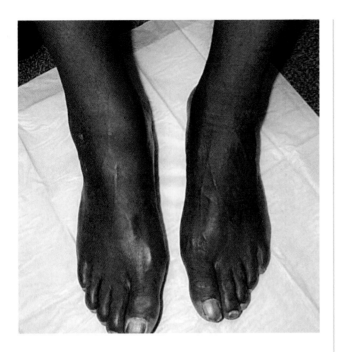

FIGURE 30.
Bilateral synovial effusions and soft-tissue edema in a patient with lung cancer–associated hypertrophic osteoarthropathy.

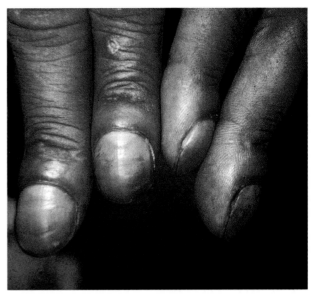

FIGURE 31.
Clubbing, which is caused by painless enlargement of the connective tissue in the terminal phalanges, producing a hyponychial angle of ≥190 degrees.

accounts for 25% to 30% of all lung cancers, tends to occur centrally, with endobronchial lesions. Large cell undifferentiated carcinoma accounts for only 10% of lung cancers.

Staging

The primary goals of staging are to identify patients who can receive treatment with curative intent as quickly and efficiently as possible, to minimize expense and invasive testing, and to identify patients with incurable disease to diminish the risks associated with surgery or combined-modality approaches. Clinical staging includes a thorough history and physical examination, radiologic imaging, and laboratory studies; pathologic studies may include lymph node biopsy, bronchoscopy, thoracentesis, or mediastinoscopy. The staging system for lung cancer has been recently revised with changes in the TNM descriptors for tumor size, ipsilateral and contralateral lung nodules, and pleural involvement. The current staging system is briefly summarized in **Table 33**.

Histologic confirmation of the presence or absence of tumor within the mediastinal lymph nodes is necessary whenever this information will change treatment recommendations. CT scans are routinely used to assess mediastinal lymphadenopathy. In a review of 20 studies assessing the value of CT scan to determine mediastinal involvement in patients with lung cancer, CT had a pooled sensitivity of 57%, a specificity of 82%, and a negative predictive value of 83%. Benign enlargement of mediastinal lymph nodes occurs more commonly in patients who have postobstructive infection. In patients who are considered surgical candidates, metastatic tumor is found in approximately 15% to 20% of mediastinal lymph nodes that are less than 1 cm in greatest diameter. A review of 18 studies of the usefulness of positron emission tomography with 18-fluorodeoxyglucose (PET-FDG) to assess disease involvement within the mediastinal lymph nodes demonstrated a pooled sensitivity of 84% and a specificity of 89%, with a positive predictive value of 79% and a negative predictive value of 93%. The combined positive predictive value and negative predictive value of CT scanning and PET-FDG were 83% to 93% and 88% to 95%, respectively. Thus, PET-FDG is superior to CT scanning in the staging of disease in patients with mediastinal lymph node involvement. An estimated 15% to 20% of patients with a known or suspected diagnosis of early-stage lung cancer derive benefit from preoperative PET-FDG because previously unrecognized metastatic disease will be discovered with this diagnostic strategy and these patients will thus be spared unnecessary surgery.

KEY POINTS

- Disease staging in patients with non–small cell lung cancer includes a history and physical examination, radiologic imaging, and laboratory studies; lymph node biopsy, bronchoscopy, thoracentesis, or mediastinoscopy may also be appropriate.

- Positron emission tomography with 18-fluorodeoxyglucose is superior to CT scanning in evaluating the extent of mediastinal lymph node involvement in patients with lung cancer.

TABLE 33 Staging, Treatment, and Prognosis for Patients with Non–Small Cell Lung Cancer

Stage	Definition	Treatment	Prognosis
I	Tumor surrounded by lung or pleura, more than 2 cm from carina	Surgery and adjuvant chemotherapy, radiotherapy if not a surgical candidate; intent is cure	60% to 70% long-term disease-free survival
II	Locally advanced disease, without mediastinal involvement	Surgery and adjuvant chemotherapy, radiotherapy if not a surgical candidate; intent is cure	40% to 50% long-term disease-free survival
III	Mediastinal involvement	Combined modalities of chemotherapy, radiotherapy, and/or surgery	5% to 20% long-term disease-free survival

Treatment

Surgery is the treatment of choice for patients with stage I or II NSCLC (and selected stage III patients). Despite detection of early disease and complete resection, many patients with NSCLC experience recurrent metastatic disease. The use of adjuvant chemotherapy has been shown to consistently improve survival in patients with early-stage NSCLC (stage IB-III). Conversely, the use of adjuvant radiation therapy in patients with early-stage NSCLC has not been associated with a survival benefit and may actually be deleterious to overall survival.

Patients with stage III disease represent a heterogeneous group. Most have mediastinal lymphadenopathy, and survival rates depend on extent of mediastinal disease. For patients with minimal mediastinal lymphadenopathy and potentially resectable disease, chemotherapy is often administered before surgery. For patients with unresectable disease, multiple studies have proved that chemoradiation is superior to radiation alone, although the optimal sequence for administering these agents is not certain. Patients with superior sulcus, or Pancoast tumors, are also included among those with stage III NSCLC. Chemoradiation followed by surgery in these patients has yielded 5-year survival rates of 40% in phase II trials, which is an improvement compared with most patients with stage III lung cancer (defined by N2 lymph node positivity).

Patients with stage IIIB disease with malignant pleural or pericardial effusion do not benefit from radiation and should be treated with palliative-intent chemotherapy only. Also included among patients with stage IIIB disease are those with T4 lesions (characterized as a mass with a satellite lesion); these patients should receive initial treatment with surgery because they have potentially curable disease. Selected patients with disseminated (stage IV) disease have a solitary brain metastasis, and they may experience improved survival with surgical resection of the metastasis. However, surgical resection of a solitary metastasis located in sites other than the brain remains controversial.

Multiple phase III studies have determined the superiority of systemic chemotherapy over best supportive care in patients with stage IV, or metastatic, NSCLC, provided that those patients have a reasonable performance status. Chemotherapy improves overall survival by months compared with best supportive care in patients with NSCLC; it also relieves lung cancer–related symptoms, improves overall quality of life, and is cost-effective compared with best supportive care. There is no proof of benefit of chemotherapy in patients with NSCLC who are bed-bound. Palliative or hospice care may be indicated for such patients depending on their preferences.

Platinum-based chemotherapy has been widely accepted as the standard of care in patients with NSCLC. Generally, cisplatin or carboplatin is combined with one of several agents including paclitaxel, docetaxel, vinorelbine, gemcitabine, irinotecan, or pemetrexed. Because similar response and survival rates have been shown to result from the various regimens used to treat NSCLC, quality of life has become a critical issue to consider when choosing a particular regimen, in addition to ease of administration, side effects, and the personal preference and experience of the oncologist.

Although chemotherapy is an appropriate treatment for many patients with lung cancer, the use of traditional chemotherapeutic agents is believed to have reached a therapeutic plateau. Increased understanding of cancer biology has revealed numerous potential therapeutic strategies, including epidermal growth factor receptor and angiogenesis pathway targeting. The use of inhibitors of the epidermal growth factor receptor pathway with tyrosine kinase inhibitors such as erlotinib has caused consistent, although modest, improvements in survival and tumor reduction in many patients. Dramatic and rapid responses to erlotinib have been noted in patients who have an acquired mutation in the binding domain of the *EGFR* gene, which causes increased growth-factor signaling. Furthermore, the addition of the antivascular endothelial growth factor agent bevacizumab has been examined in patients with advanced-stage nonsquamous cell carcinoma. Patients who received bevacizumab combined with chemotherapy experienced a 2.3-month increase in median survival compared with patients who received chemotherapy alone.

Although many new active drugs are available for lung cancer, the reported response rates to second-line chemotherapy have generally been less than 10%. Patients who experience disease progression after initial first-line therapy may be treated with single agents such as docetaxel, erlotinib, or pemetrexed.

Patients who have undergone prior resection for early-stage lung cancer and go on to experience a recurrence in the form of a solitary pulmonary nodule generally have a second primary tumor. Resection of the new lesion with possible adjuvant chemotherapy may result in long-term survival.

Radiation can palliate lung cancer symptoms by decreasing bronchial compression, reducing hemoptysis, improving superior vena cava syndrome, and treating bony metastases. Monthly intravenous bisphosphonate therapy with pamidronate or zolendronate decreases skeletal-related events in patients with bony metastases. In those with central nervous system disease and airway obstruction, photodynamic therapy, endoscopic laser therapy, airway stenting, and cryotherapy may be used.

Many patients with NSCLC eventually develop brain metastases. The primary approach to the treatment of patients with brain metastases includes whole-brain radiation therapy; surgery; and stereotactic radiosurgery depending on number, size, and location of lesions and the status of systemic disease.

KEY POINTS

- Surgery is the treatment of choice for patients with stage I or II non–small cell lung cancer.
- Adjuvant chemotherapy has been shown to consistently improve survival in patients with early-stage non–small cell lung cancer, but adjuvant radiation therapy does not, and may actually be harmful.
- For patients with unresectable non–small cell lung cancer, chemotherapy plus radiation is superior to radiation alone.
- Patients with stage IIIB non–small cell lung cancer with malignant pleural or pericardial effusion do not benefit from radiation and should be treated with palliative-intent chemotherapy only.
- Treatment of patients with brain metastases includes whole-brain radiation therapy, surgery, and stereotactic radiosurgery depending on number, size, and location of lesions and the status of systemic disease.

Small Cell Lung Cancer

Small cell lung cancer (SCLC) accounts for less than 15% of all new lung cancer cases, more than 95% of which result from smoking. SCLC is an aggressive form of lung cancer that tends to disseminate early. Symptoms are related to bulky intrathoracic disease or to distant metastases. SCLC is usually centrally located, with hilar masses and hilar and mediastinal lymphadenopathy.

Staging

Patients with SCLC rarely present with disease that is sufficiently localized to allow for surgical resection, so the TNM system is generally not used in these patients. Instead, the Veterans Administration Lung Study Group staging system is typically used, which classifies disease as limited or extensive. The definition of limited-stage disease consists of disease limited to one hemithorax, with hilar and mediastinal lymphadenopathy that can be encompassed within one tolerable radiotherapy portal. Extensive-stage disease consists of any disease that exceeds those boundaries. Most patients (60% to 70%) with SCLC present with clinically extensive-stage disease. There are significant differences in median and 5-year survival among these patients depending on the presence of limited- or extensive-stage disease.

Given its prognostic and therapeutic implications, the main goal of staging is to identify disease sites outside of a potential radiation portal. Good prognostic factors include limited-stage disease, female sex, and good performance status.

CT of the chest facilitates assessment of the extent of intrathoracic involvement, including the presence of pleural effusion, lobar collapse, hilar and mediastinal lymphadenopathy, and contralateral parenchymal disease. Evaluation of the liver and adrenal glands should also be done simultaneous to CT scanning of the chest. Additional staging should include CT or MRI of the brain to identify central nervous system metastases and bone or PET scan to determine distant metastatic sites. Patient-specific symptoms or unexpected laboratory abnormalities may warrant additional imaging or bone scans. A bone marrow aspiration and biopsy should be done in patients with significant hematologic abnormalities because marrow infiltration in patients with SCLC has been reported. Once extensive-stage disease has been established, further staging does not guide treatment.

KEY POINTS

- Most patients with small cell lung cancer present with clinically extensive-stage disease.
- CT of the chest, with simultaneous liver and adrenal gland evaluation; CT or MRI of the brain; and bone or positron emission tomography scan may be appropriate in the staging of small cell lung cancer.

Treatment

Combination chemotherapy is the cornerstone of treatment for both limited-stage and extensive-stage SCLC. In general, the administration of etoposide and cisplatin plus chest radiotherapy for patients with good performance status and limited-stage disease should produce a complete response rate of 80% or higher, a median survival of 18 months, and 5-year cancer-free survival of 12% to 25%. Patients with extensive-stage disease who receive combination chemotherapy should have a complete response rate of more than 20% and a median survival of longer than 7 months. Notably, 2% of patients with extensive-stage SCLC are alive and cancer free at 5 years. The mortality rate from therapeutic complications is less than 3%.

For patients with limited-stage disease, etoposide and cisplatin are generally administered with chest radiation during the first cycles of chemotherapy. For patients with extensive-stage SCLC, combination chemotherapy remains the focus of treatment, with cisplatin or carboplatin plus etoposide the most widely used regimen. Routine use of chest radiotherapy in extensive-stage disease does not prolong survival. Radiotherapy in extensive-stage disease is reserved for the prevention or treatment of brain metastases; the treatment of symptomatic bone metastases; the treatment of spinal cord compression; or for palliative treatment of lobar collapse or superior vena cava syndrome in patients who have not responded to chemotherapy. Monthly intravenous bisphosphonate administration with pamidronate or zoledronate decreases skeletal-related events for patients with bony metastases.

Patients with limited-stage SCLC who have been successfully treated have a 50% to 60% risk of developing central nervous system metastases. Therefore, prophylactic cranial irradiation is used in patients who have had a complete response to chemotherapy. A meta-analysis of prophylactic cranial irradiation showed that this intervention reduces the risk of brain metastases by 45% and increases likelihood for survival by 5% compared with those who do not receive this therapy. Recently, a randomized trial of prophylactic cranial irradiation versus best supportive care after initial chemotherapy in patients with extensive-stage disease demonstrated a survival advantage in patients who received prophylactic cranial irradiation. Patients who undergo prophylactic cranial irradiation sometimes report a decline in neuropsychologic function; the degree to which prophylactic cranial irradiation contributes to this decline is controversial.

Because of the exquisite chemosensitivity of SCLC, patients with extensive-stage disease and poor performance status due to tumor burden should be offered chemotherapy because it can significantly improve symptoms and increase survival. However, chemotherapy is not appropriate for patients with advanced NSCLC and poor performance status.

Most patients with SCLC relapse within 1 year of initiation of treatment. Patients who are primarily resistant to therapy or have received many chemotherapeutic regimens rarely respond to more therapy, whereas those who respond to initial chemotherapy and experience a relapse more than 6 months after the conclusion of treatment are more likely to respond to additional chemotherapy.

Long-term survivors of SCLC usually have limited-stage disease at diagnosis. After 2 years, the risk of dying from the initial disease in these patients begins to decrease. The lung cancer mortality risk remains elevated in long-term survivors of SCLC, owing partly to the development of second primary tumors. The risk for developing a second primary tumor in patients with lung cancer is 2% to 10% per patient per year, a risk 10 times that of adult male smokers in whom a previous lung cancer has not developed. Any new lung masses in these patients should be promptly investigated, and biopsy should be performed because such findings may represent surgically resectable second primary tumors.

KEY POINTS

- Combination chemotherapy is the cornerstone of treatment for both limited-stage and extensive-stage small cell lung cancer.

- Routine use of chest radiotherapy in extensive-stage small cell lung cancer does not prolong survival.

- Monthly intravenous bisphosphonate administration with pamidronate or zoledronate decreases skeletal-related events for patients with bony metastases.

- Prophylactic cranial irradiation after initial chemotherapy in patients with limited- and extensive-stage small cell lung cancer improves survival rates.

- Patients with extensive-stage small cell lung cancer and poor performance status should be offered chemotherapy to improve symptoms and increase survival.

Bibliography

Arriagada R, Bergman B, Dunant A, Le Chevalier T, Pignon JP, Vansteenkiste J; International Adjuvant Lung Cancer Trial Collaborative Group. Cisplatin-based adjuvant chemotherapy in patients with completely resected non-small-cell lung cancer. N Engl J Med. 2004;350(4):351-360. [PMID: 14736927]

Auperin A, Arriagada R, Pignon JP, et al. Prophylactic cranial irradiation for patients with small-cell lung cancer in complete remission. Prophylactic Cranial Irradiation Overview Collaborative Group. N Engl J Med. 1999;341(7):476-484. [PMID: 10441603]

Douillard JY, Rosell R, De Lena M, et al. Adjuvant vinorelbine plus cisplatin versus observation in patients with completely resected stage IB-IIIA non-small-cell lung cancer (Adjuvant Navelbine International Trialist Association [ANITA]): a randomised controlled trial. Lancet Oncol. 2006;7(9):719-727. [PMID: 16945766]

Goldstraw P, Crowley J, Chansky K, et al; International Association for the Study of Lung Cancer International Staging Committee; Participating Institutions. The IASLC Lung Cancer Staging Project: Proposals for the Revision of the TNM Stage Groupings in the Forthcoming (Seventh) Edition of the TNM Classification of Malignant Tumors [erratum in J Thorac Oncol. 2007;2(10):985]. J Thorac Oncol. 2007;2(8):706-714. [PMID: 17762336]

Gould MK, Kuschner WG, Rydzak CE, et al. Test performance of positron emission tomography and computed tomography for mediastinal staging in patients with non-small-cell lung cancer: a meta-analysis. Ann Intern Med. 2003;139(11):879-892. [PMID: 14644890]

Pignon JP, Arriagada R, Ihde DC, et al. A meta-analysis of thoracic radiotherapy for small-cell lung cancer. N Engl J Med. 1992;327(23):1618-1624. [PMID: 1331787]

Rusch, VW, Giroux, DJ, Kraut, MJ, et al. Induction chemoradiation and surgical resection for superior sulcus non-small-cell lung carcinomas: long-term results of southwest oncology group trial 9416 (intergroup trial 0160). J Clin Oncol 2007; 25(3):313-318. [PMID: 17235046]

Sandler A, Gray R, Perry MC, et al. Paclitaxel-carboplatin alone or with bevacizumab for non-small cell lung cancer [erratum in N Engl J Med. 2007;356(3):318]. N Engl J Med. 2006; 355(24):2542-2540. [PMID: 17167137]

Schiller JH, Harrington D, Belani C, et al; Eastern Cooperative Oncology Group. Comparison of four chemotherapy regimens for advanced non-small cell lung cancer. N Engl J Med. 2002;346(2):92-98. [PMID: 11784875]

Shepherd FA, Rodrigues Pereira J, Ciuleanu T, et al; National Cancer Institute of Canada Clinical Trials Group. Erlotinib in previously treated non-small-cell lung cancer. N Engl J Med. 2005;353(2):123-132. [PMID: 16014882]

Slotman B, Faivre-Finn C, Kramer G, et al; EORTC Radiation Oncology Group and Lung Cancer Group. Prophylactic Cranial Irradiation in Extensive Small-Cell Lung Cancer. New Engl J Med. 2007; 357(7):664-672. [PMID: 17699816]

Winton, T, Livingston, R, Johnson, D, et al; National Cancer Institute of Canada Clinical Trials Group; National Cancer Institute of the United States Intergroup JBR.10 Trial Investigators. Vinorelbine plus cisplatin vs. observation in resected non-small-cell lung cancer. N Engl J Med. 2005;352(25):2589-2597. [PMID: 15972865]

Head and Neck Cancer

Squamous Cell Carcinoma

Head and neck cancer encompasses a diverse group of uncommon tumors that can be aggressive and can require complex multimodality treatment. In 2008, it was estimated that head and neck malignancies comprised 3% to 4% of all cancers in the United States and accounted for 1% to 2% of all cancer-related deaths. This disease occurs more commonly in men, and the incidence increases with age, especially after age 50 years (See Cancer Risk section for discussion of head and neck cancer risk factors).

Most head and neck cancers are local or regional squamous cell carcinomas; distant, metastatic cancer occurs in only about 10% of patients at diagnosis. In addition, there is a high frequency of secondary head and neck and lung cancers, suggesting that the entire respiratory mucosa may be predisposed to malignancy, the so-called field effect. No chemoprevention strategy to prevent these second cancers has been successful.

KEY POINT

- Because of a field cancerization effect, patients with head and neck cancer are at considerable risk for the development of a second primary tumor.

Physical Examination, Diagnosis, and Staging

Common symptoms and signs of head and neck cancer include the presence of a painless mass or mucosal ulcer; localized (often referred) pain of the mouth, teeth, throat, or ear; odynophagia or dysphagia; proptosis; diplopia or loss of vision; hearing loss; persistent unilateral sinusitis; and unilateral tonsillar enlargement in adults. Five to 10% of white plaques, often initially diagnosed as leukoplakia, contain carcinoma in situ. Examination of tissue should be done to differentiate leukoplakia (**Figure 32**) from *Candida* infection and lichen planus.

Physical examination is the best method for detecting upper aerodigestive tract lesions. Patients with such lesions should receive referral to a specialist experienced in head and neck cancers. Endoscopy is required to facilitate direct visualization of the nasopharynx, larynx, hypopharynx, cervical esophagus, and proximal trachea. This examination is not only useful for documenting the presence, site, and extent of tumors in the upper aerodigestive tract, but it can also identify other primary tumors.

Chest imaging should be performed to exclude occult lung metastases or second primary tumors. CT or MRI is useful for delineating tumor location and extent. Pathologic confirmation of carcinoma is done primarily by fine-needle aspiration. Open biopsy of a cervical lymph node is performed only when fine-needle aspiration of a primary tumor is non-diagnostic to avoid compromise of subsequent management in patients in whom tissue planes in the neck are disrupted by a diagnostic open biopsy.

The TNM system for the head and neck is widely used in the staging of this disease. Prognosis correlates strongly with stage at diagnosis. For many head and neck cancer sites, survival in patients with stage I disease exceeds 80%; however, most patients with head and neck cancer have stage III or IV disease at diagnosis with a long-term survival of less than 40%.

KEY POINTS

- Common symptoms and signs of head and neck cancer include the presence of a painless mass or mucosal ulcer; localized mouth, tooth, throat, or ear pain; odynophagia or dysphagia; proptosis; diplopia or loss of vision; hearing loss; persistent unilateral sinusitis; and unilateral tonsillar enlargement in adults.

- Examination of tissue should be done to differentiate leukoplakia from *Candida* infection and lichen planus in patients with oral lesions.

- Physical examination, endoscopy, and chest radiography are used in the diagnostic evaluation of patients with upper aerodigestive tract lesions.

- Pathologic confirmation of head and neck cancer is done primarily by fine-needle aspiration.

- For many head and neck cancer sites, survival in patients with stage I disease exceeds 80%.

- Most patients with head and neck cancer are diagnosed with stage III or IV tumors, and these patients have a long-term survival of less than 40%.

Treatment

Treatment for head and neck cancer is highly complex, not only because of the variety of tumor subsites involved in this disease, but also because of the anatomic constraints of the head and neck region and the importance of maintaining organ function during and after treatment. Radiation and surgery are the standard treatment modalities, reflecting the disease's locoregional predominance; however, chemotherapy is frequently added.

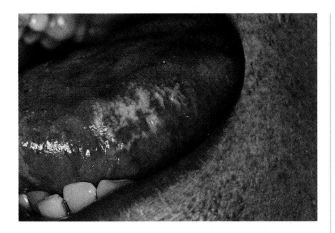

FIGURE 32.
Findings of leukoplakia, white patches that in some cases (5% to 10%) contain carcinoma in situ.
Tissue examination is required in patients with leukoplakia.

Patients with early-stage (stages I and II) head and neck cancer receive surgery or radiation with curative intent. Because both modalities result in similar rates of local control and survival, the therapeutic choice is usually based on an assessment of competing modalities, functional outcomes, and accessibility. For example, laryngeal cancer might best be treated with radiation therapy to preserve the voice, whereas oral cavity cancer is better managed with surgery, which eliminates the long-term radiation–associated side effects of xerostomia and loss of taste.

The treatment of patients with locoregionally advanced head and neck cancer (stages III and IVA and IVB disease without distant metastases) generally involves a combination of multiple treatment modalities, including radiation, chemotherapy, and surgery. Selection of therapy for this group of patients depends on careful assessment of prognosis as well as preservation of organ function. Integration of multiple modalities of treatment into the therapeutic regimen of patients with head and neck cancer has led to improvements in cure and local control rates, but multimodality therapy–associated toxicity is substantially increased compared with single-modality treatment.

For patients with distant metastatic or recurrent disease, chemotherapy provides major palliative benefits. The average survival of patients with advanced disease who receive chemotherapy is 6 to 8 months; survival is only slightly lower when supportive care alone is provided. Active drugs in treating metastatic head and neck cancer include platinum compounds, taxane agents, and 5-fluorouracil. A newer agent, cetuximab (a monoclonal antibody targeting the epidermal growth factor receptor [EGFR]), is combined with radiation therapy for the treatment of locally advanced head and neck cancer based on a randomized trial that showed a near doubling of median survival.

KEY POINTS

- Surgery or radiation therapy with curative intent is appropriate for patients with stages I and II head and neck cancer.

- The treatment of patients with stages III and IVA and IVB disease without distant metastases involves a combination of treatment modalities, including radiation, chemotherapy, and surgery.

- For patients with distant metastatic or recurrent disease, chemotherapy provides major palliative benefits but may or may not prolong survival.

Thyroid Cancer

Thyroid cancer is the most common endocrine cancer, occurring in an estimated 33,550 individuals in the United States and resulting in 1500 deaths per year. The incidence of thyroid nodules in the general population is 4% to 7% and is higher in women than men (2:1 ratio). The prevalence of thyroid cancer in patients with a solitary nodule or multinodular thyroid gland is 10% to 20%. Nodules occurring in the very young or the very old are more likely to be cancerous than those occurring in other populations.

Thyroid cancer is classified into four main types according to morphology and biologic behavior: papillary, follicular, medullary, and anaplastic. Differentiated (papillary and follicular) tumors account for more than 90% of thyroid malignancies. Gender- and age-adjusted survival rates for patients with papillary, follicular, and anaplastic carcinoma are 98%, 92%, and 13%, respectively. Medullary thyroid cancer represents 5% to 10% of all thyroid neoplasms. Approximately 80% of patients with medullary thyroid cancer have a sporadic form of the disease, whereas the remaining 20% have inherited disease. Anaplastic carcinoma represents less than 5% of all thyroid carcinomas.

KEY POINTS

- Gender- and age-adjusted survival rates for patients with papillary, follicular, and anaplastic thyroid carcinoma are 98%, 92%, and 13%, respectively.

- Patients with older age or more advanced disease stage may experience a worse prognosis regardless of thyroid cancer type.

Evaluation and Diagnosis

Most cases of thyroid cancer present as asymptomatic thyroid nodules. On examination, a hard or firm and fixed thyroid nodule may represent malignancy. See **Table 34** for clinical features suggestive of a malignancy in patients with thyroid nodules. Laboratory evaluation, including a thyroid-stimulating hormone test, can help differentiate a thyrotoxic nodule from an euthyroid nodule. In euthyroid patients with a nodule, fine-needle aspiration biopsy should be performed to

TABLE 34 Clinical Features Suggestive of Malignancy in Patients With Nodular Thyroid Disease

Category	Notes
Highest suspicion of malignancy	Rapid tumor growth, very firm nodule, fixation to adjacent structures, vocal cord paralysis, enlarged regional lymph nodes
Moderate suspicion of malignancy	Male: age <20 or >60 years; history of radiation; solitary nodule; diameter >4 cm
Low suspicion of malignancy	Female: age >20 years; no significant historical features; soft or rubbery nodule <4 cm

establish diagnosis, and radionuclide scanning should be reserved for patients with indeterminate cytology or thyrotoxicosis. The likelihood of obtaining insufficient specimens from fine-needle aspiration biopsy decreases when ultrasound guidance is used.

A characteristic feature of medullary thyroid carcinoma is the production of calcitonin. In addition, the C cells in medullary thyroid carcinoma originate from the embryonic neural crest; as a result, these tumors often have the clinical and histologic features of other neuroendocrine tumors such as carcinoid and islet-cell tumors. Thus, serum calcitonin levels can be used to monitor disease status. Although greater than 80% of cases are sporadic, medullary thyroid carcinoma may be associated with multiple endocrine neoplasia type 2A (MEN-2A), MEN-2B, or familial non-MEN.

The MEN-2A and MEN-2B syndromes are characterized by medullary thyroid cancer and pheochromocytoma. Therefore, it is imperative that 24-hour urine catecholamine levels are measured in patients with familial medullary thyroid cancer to rule out the presence of pheochromocytoma. Germline mutations in the *RET* proto-oncogene are responsible for familial non-MEN medullary thyroid carcinoma in addition to MEN-2A and MEN-2B. It is important to search for an inherited form of medullary thyroid cancer in patients with this disease unless inherited status has already been established. Approximately 95% of patients with the *RET* mutation eventually develop medullary thyroid cancer; consequently, prophylactic thyroidectomy is recommended in these patients.

KEY POINTS

- Patients found to have a euthyroid single thyroid nodule should undergo fine-needle aspiration biopsy to rule out malignancy.

- Most patients with the *RET* mutation eventually develop medullary thyroid cancer; therefore, prophylactic thyroidectomy is recommended in these patients.

- Twenty-four–hour urine catecholamine levels must be measured in patients with familial medullary thyroid cancer to rule out the presence of pheochromocytoma.

- Prophylactic thyroidectomy is recommended in patients with the *RET* mutation because of the high likelihood for thyroid cancer in this population.

Treatment

If cytologic results of the nodule show malignant or indeterminate cells, then thyroidectomy is generally performed. Surgery is the primary mode of therapy for patients with differentiated thyroid carcinoma and should be done by experienced surgeons to reduce the risk for hypoparathyroidism and recurrent laryngeal nerve injury. Total thyroidectomy is generally recommended if the primary tumor is at least 1 to 2 cm in diameter or if extrathyroidal extension or metastases are present. Unilateral lobectomy and isthmusectomy may be appropriate for patients with lower-risk tumors. Neck dissection is generally performed in patients with clinically involved lymph nodes, large tumors with poor features, and medullary carcinoma. After initial surgery, all patients should receive levothyroxine both to prevent hypothyroidism and to minimize potential thyroid-stimulating hormone (TSH) stimulation of tumor growth.

Radioactive iodine is then administered postoperatively to patients who have multiple tumors of the thyroid gland, large tumors, locally invasive tumors, or remote metastases. Iodine 131 (^{131}I) administered postoperatively to ablate remnants of thyroid tissue or residual disease may improve survival in patients with papillary and follicular tumors. This is important because relapsing disease develops in approximately 12% of patients who have no evidence of disease after primary therapy. Tumors that are not treatable with the combination of surgery, levothyroxine therapy, and repeat doses of ^{131}I are treated with external-beam radiation therapy or chemotherapy, but the response to these therapies is poor. Radioiodine is not taken up by C cells and is therefore not a treatment option for patients with medullary thyroid cancer.

Anaplastic carcinoma of the thyroid is an exceptionally aggressive disease. There is no effective therapy for advanced or metastatic anaplastic thyroid carcinoma, and the disease is uniformly fatal. The median survival from diagnosis ranges from 3 to 7 months. Death is usually attributable to upper-airway obstruction and suffocation (often despite tracheostomy) or to a combination of complications of local and distant disease.

Bibliography

Bonner JA, Harari PM, Giralt J, et al. Radiotherapy plus Cetuximab for Squamous-Cell Carcinoma of the Head and Neck. N Engl J Med. 2006;354(6):567-578. [PMID: 16467544]

Burtness B, Goldwasser MA, Flood W, et al; Eastern Cooperative Oncology Group. Phase III randomized trial of cisplatin plus cetuximab in metastatic/ recurrent head and neck cancer: An Eastern Cooperative Oncology Group study. J Clin Oncol. 2005;23(34): 8646-8654. [PMID: 16314626]

Cooper DS, Doherty GM, Haugen BR, et al; The American Thyroid Association Guidelines Taskforce. Management guidelines for patients with thyroid nodules and differentiated thyroid cancer. Thyroid. 2006;16(2):109-142. [PMID: 16420177]

Erkal HS, Mendenhall WM, Amdur RJ, Villaret DB, Stringer SP. Synchronous and metachronous squamous cell carcinomas of the head and neck mucosal sites. J Clin Oncol. 2001;19(5):1358-1362. [PMID: 11230479]

Hegedus L. Clinical practice. The thyroid nodule. N Engl J Med. 2004;351(17):1764-1771. [PMID: 15496625]

Jonklaas J, Sarlis NJ, Litofsky D, et al. Outcomes of patients with differentiated thyroid carcinoma following initial therapy. Thyroid. 2006;16(12):1229-42. [PMID: 17199433]

Kebebew E, Ituarte PH, Siperstein AE, Duh QY, Clark OH. Medullary thyroid carcinoma: clinical characteristics, treatment, prognostic factors, and a comparison of staging systems. Cancer. 2000;88(5):1139-1148. [PMID: 10699905]

Khuri FR, Lee JJ, Lippman SM, et al. Randomized phase III trial of low-dose isotretinoin for prevention of second primary tumors in stage I and II head and neck cancer patients. J Natl Cancer Inst. 2006;98(7):441-450. [PMID: 16595780]

Pfister DG, Laurie SA, Weinstein GS, et al; American Society of Clinical Oncology. American Society of Clinical Oncology clinical practice guideline for the use of larynx-preservation strategies in the treatment of laryngeal cancer. J Clin Oncol. 2006;24(22):3693-3704. [PMID: 16832122]

Soo KC, Tan EH, Wee J, et al. Surgery and adjuvant radiotherapy vs concurrent chemoradiotherapy in stage III/IV nonmetastatic squamous cell head and neck cancer: a randomised comparison. Br J Cancer. 2005;93(3):279-286. [PMID: 16012523]

Genitourinary Cancer

Prostate Cancer

Prostate cancer is the most common cancer in men and accounts for 29% of all malignancies in male patients. It is also the second most common cause of cancer-related deaths in men, after lung cancer. Approximately 218,900 new cases are diagnosed in the United States each year, and about 27,000 deaths related to prostate cancer occur annually. The lifetime risk of developing prostate cancer is 1 in 6 with a risk of death from this malignancy of 1 in 30. Risk factors include increasing age, race (highest in blacks, second highest in whites, and lowest in Asian Americans), and family history (twofold higher risk if a first-degree relative has prostate cancer). The role of modifiable risk factors is more controversial, although some studies suggest that a diet high in fats and low in vegetable content and selenium may increase the risk. Men with a history of prostatitis have a modestly increased risk. Vasectomy does not increase the risk of developing this malignancy.

Diagnosis and Staging

Prostate cancer is most often diagnosed following prostate-specific antigen (PSA) screening in asymptomatic men. Patients may also present with symptoms of prostatic hyperplasia, such as incomplete voiding, a decreased urinary stream, and frequent nocturia. The most common symptoms in patients with metastatic disease are bone pain and, less frequently, spinal cord compression and neurologic deficits.

The prostate may be normal or diffusely enlarged on digital rectal examination. The presence of palpable nodules or asymmetric areas of induration is more suggestive of malignant disease. If abnormalities are found on digital rectal examination, transrectal ultrasonography should be done to evaluate the anterior and medial portions of the prostate that are difficult to assess by physical examination. Transrectal biopsy of the prostate is the definitive diagnostic study and should be done in all patients with asymmetric induration or nodularity. Patients with an elevated or rising serum PSA level noted during routine screening should also undergo prostate biopsy, even if they are asymptomatic. Once a diagnosis of prostate cancer is made, additional studies such as a bone scan or CT scan of the abdomen and pelvis should be considered in patients with signs or symptoms suggestive of distant spread of the malignancy.

The risk of death from prostate cancer is determined by the stage of the disease, Gleason score, and serum PSA level. Staging is based on the TNM (tumor-node-metastasis) classification developed by the American Joint Committee on Cancer. The clinical tumor stage varies from T1 to T4 lesions. T1 tumors are clinically inapparent lesions that are not palpable on digital rectal examination or visible on diagnostic imaging studies. T2 tumors are confined to the prostate gland, T3 lesions extend through the prostate capsule, and T4 lesions are fixed tumors that invade adjacent tissue. Involvement of regional lymph nodes is classified as N1 disease, and metastasis to distant nonregional lymph nodes and other organs is considered M1 disease. Tumors may also be classified by pathologic stage (**Table 35**).

In addition to TNM staging, prostate cancer is graded histologically by determining the Gleason score. This method takes into account the heterogeneity in histologic patterns that is often found in prostate cancer specimens and has been shown to be of significant prognostic value. Criteria for patients at risk for metastasis and for failure of serum PSA levels to normalize after definitive therapy have also been identified and are based primarily on the clinical stage of the tumor, Gleason score, and serum PSA level at the time of diagnosis (**Table 36**).

Treatment

The National Comprehensive Cancer Network has developed guidelines for the initial treatment of men with prostate cancer based on their risk score and general life expectancy. As prostate cancer is more common in elderly men with comorbid disorders, the general life expectancy is critical to making informed decisions about treatment options (**Table 37**).

Surgery

Radical prostatectomy, with or without pelvic lymph node dissection, is generally considered for patients with disease limited to the prostate who have a life expectancy of 10 years or more. Prostatectomy can now be performed laparoscopically or with robotic assistance, preferably by surgeons experienced in these techniques. Advances in surgical techniques have decreased the long-term risks of erectile dysfunction and urinary incontinence. However, the risks associated with general anesthesia must always be considered because of the high incidence of comorbid disorders in this patient population.

TABLE 35 AJCC Stage Groupings for Prostate Cancer

Stage I
T1a, N0, M0, G1
Stage II
T1a, N0, M0, G2–4
T1b, N0, M0, any G
T1c, N0, M0, any G
T1, N0, M0, any G
T2, N0, M0, any G
Stage III
T3, N0, M0, any G
Stage IV
T4, N0, M0, any G
Any T, N1, M0, any G
Any T, any N, M1, any G

AJCC = American Joint Committee on Cancer.

TABLE 36 Prostate Cancer Recurrence Risk

Risk	Tumor (T) Stage	Gleason Score	PSA at Diagnosis (ng/mL)
Low	T1–T2a	2–6	<10
Intermediate	T2b–T2c	7	10–20
High	T3a	8–10	>20

PSA = prostate-specific antigen.

Radiation Therapy

Because of significantly improved techniques for external-beam radiation therapy for prostate cancer, patients who undergo either radiation therapy or surgery now have similar disease-free survival. Radiation therapy is less likely to cause

TABLE 37 Initial Treatment of Prostate Cancer

Risk	Life Expectancy	Treatment Options
Low	<10 years	Observation
	>10 but <20 years	Observation *or* Radiation therapy *or* Radical prostatectomy
	≥20 years	Radiation therapy *or* Radical prostatectomy
Intermediate	<10 years	Observation *or* Radiation therapy *or* Radical prostatectomy
	≥10 years	Radiation therapy *or* Radical prostatectomy
High	<5 years	Observation with hormonal therapy
	≥5 years	Radiation therapy with hormonal therapy *or* Radiation therapy alone *or* Radical prostatectomy

Information from NCCN Clinical Practice Guidelines in Oncology: Prostate Cancer. National Comprehensive Cancer Network. www.nccn.org/professionals/physician_gls/PDF/prostate.pdf. Accessed on December 21, 2008.

erectile dysfunction and urinary incontinence in the short term and avoids the risks associated with general anesthesia, perioperative bleeding, and infection. However, radiation treatment often must be given for 8 or more weeks and is associated with long-term toxic effects, including radiation proctitis and cystitis. In addition, the risk for erectile dysfunction may increase over time. Newer modalities such as intensity-modulated radiation therapy decrease these risks, as does brachytherapy (implantation of radioactive sources directly into the prostate), which attempts to avoid irradiating surrounding tissues, such as the bladder and rectum.

Androgen Deprivation Therapy

Patients with high-risk disease may benefit from short-term (4 to 6 months) androgen deprivation therapy (hormonal therapy) using a gonadotropin-releasing hormone (GnRH) agonist plus bicalutamide, with or without pelvic lymph node irradiation. Androgen-blocking agents given before, during, and after radiation therapy have been shown to improve survival in patients with high-risk localized or locally advanced disease. Androgen deprivation therapy is also used as first-line treatment for patients with a rising serum PSA level after initial definitive therapy for prostate cancer or for those with metastatic disease.

Use of GnRH agonists (chemical castration) is as effective as bilateral orchiectomy (surgical castration) in treating patients with metastatic disease. Chemical castration is often preferred psychologically and is reversible after discontinuation of therapy but requires repeated intramuscular or subcutaneous administration of hormonal agonists over long periods of time. GnRH agonists act by disrupting the pituitary–testes axis, thereby decreasing testosterone levels. Oral antiandrogens such as bicalutamide, flutamide, and nilutamide act by blocking the androgen receptors on cancer cells.

Typical adverse effects of androgen deprivation therapy include impotence, hot flushes, weight gain, fatigue, gynecomastia, osteopenia, diarrhea, hepatotoxicity, diabetes, and cardiovascular disease, and, possibly, decreased night vision. Men taking antiandrogens should add calcium and vitamin D supplements to their diet, and those with osteopenia should be treated with bisphosphonates.

Chemotherapy

Patients with metastatic prostate cancer are first treated with androgen deprivation therapy. Although prostate cancer initially is androgen dependent, over time, cancer cells become androgen independent, resulting in hormone-refractory disease in patients in whom metastatic disease progresses despite androgen deprivation therapy. Chemotherapy has recently been shown to prolong life expectancy in many of these patients. Several randomized trials have demonstrated a 3- to 6-month survival benefit for patients treated with docetaxel-based therapy compared with those treated with mitoxantrone plus prednisone. Patients who receive docetaxel now have a median survival of 16 to 18 months. Newer investigational agents, either alone or in combination with docetaxel and mitoxantrone, are currently undergoing clinical trials.

Bone is a common site of prostate cancer metastases, and supportive measures such as bone-directed therapies are often warranted. Bisphosphonates such as zoledronic acid or pamidronate reverse or prevent osteopenia, inhibit tumor-mediated bone resorption, decrease morbidity from bone fractures or bone pain, and may directly inhibit the growth of tumor cells. Other bone-directed radiopharmaceuticals such as strontium-89 or samarium-153 can be used to help relieve bone pain in patients who no longer respond to hormonal therapy or standard chemotherapy. However, because of cumulative myelotoxicity, radiopharmaceutical agents are generally reserved for palliation in patients for whom additional systemic therapy is contraindicated.

Prostate Cancer Recurrence after Definitive Therapy

Up to 50% of prostate cancer recurrences occur within the first 2 years after completion of definitive therapy, 75% develop within 5 years, and 95% develop within 9 years. Digital rectal examination is recommended yearly for all patients after completing definitive therapy. A serum PSA level should also be obtained every 6 to 12 months for the first 5 years after treatment. A rising PSA level indicates biochemical recurrence, and estimates of survival can be made from the time of completion of treatment to the rise in the PSA, the rate of that rise, and the initial Gleason score. Although recurrent disease after definitive therapy of early-stage prostate cancer is incurable, significant palliation can be achieved with hormone deprivation therapy and chemotherapy.

KEY POINTS

- Both radical prostatectomy, with or without pelvic lymph node dissection, and radiation therapy are equally effective treatment options for patients with early-stage prostate cancer.

- Expectant observation may be warranted for some patients with prostate cancer and an anticipated overall survival of less than 10 years based on age and comorbid disorders.

- Chemical castration is as effective as surgical castration in reducing testosterone levels in patients with prostate cancer.

- Docetaxel-based therapy improves median overall survival in patients with hormone-refractory metastatic prostate cancer.

Testicular Cancer

Testicular cancer is generally considered a highly curable malignancy. About 7920 new cases of testicular cancer were diagnosed in the United States in 2007, with only 380 deaths. Ninety-five percent of malignancies arising in the testes are germ cell tumors. The overall incidence of germ cell tumors is increasing in the United States, and germ cell malignancies are the most common solid tumors in male patients between 15 and 34 years of age. These tumors may also occur in extragonadal primary sites, such as the retroperitoneum and mediastinum, but are still treated as testicular germ cell tumors.

The primary risk factors for development of testicular cancer are the presence of Klinefelter syndrome and a family history of testicular neoplasms. Patients with cryptorchidism also have an increased risk of developing germ cell neoplasms. This risk is reduced, but not eliminated, following surgical correction of cryptorchidism. Approximately 25% of germ cell tumors in patients with cryptorchidism occur in the normal descended testis. A premalignant lesion, intratubular germ cell neoplasia, is often found adjacent to germ cell cancers and has been noted in about 1% of men undergoing testicular biopsy for the evaluation of infertility as well as in patients with cryptorchidism or Klinefelter syndrome.

Germ cell tumors are classified as seminomas or non-seminomatous testicular germ cell tumors (nonseminomas). Nonseminomas include several different histologic types, such as embryonal cell tumors, choriocarcinomas, yolk sac tumors, and teratomas. Patients with pure seminomas have a better prognosis than those with nonseminomas. Several serum tumor markers, including α-fetoprotein (AFP), lactate dehydrogenase (LDH), and human chorionic gonadotropin (hCG), are useful for determining the prognosis and following the patient's clinical course. An elevated serum AFP level always indicates that the tumor has a nonseminomatous component, as this marker is produced by embryonal or yolk sac tumor cells, whereas hCG may be present in seminomatous or nonseminomatous tumors. Any testicular cancer that has a nonseminomatous component based on histologic examination or the presence of an elevated serum AFP level is considered a nonseminoma and is treated as such.

Diagnosis and Staging

Patients typically present with a painless solid testicular mass or a testicular mass associated with mild discomfort or swelling. Approximately 10% of patients have acute testicular pain, and another 10% may have cough, dyspnea, bone pain, or other symptoms due to metastatic disease. All patients with a palpable mass require testicular ultrasonography. Staging studies include a CT scan of the abdomen and pelvis, chest radiograph, and measurement of serum AFP, LDH, and hCG levels.

Testicular cancer is staged according to the American Joint Committee on Cancer TNM staging system. The extent of the primary tumor is determined by pathologic study of surgical samples obtained during radical orchiectomy (which is the first-line treatment for all testicular tumors). T1 tumors

are limited to the testes and epididymides, T2 tumors have vascular or lymphatic invasion or extend into the tunica vaginalis, T3 tumors invade the spermatic cord, and T4 tumors invade the scrotum. Lymph node metastases are classified as N1 to N3, based on the size of the involved regional lymph nodes. For example, metastases in a regional lymph node measuring 2 cm or less with no other regional lymph nodes measuring more than 2 cm are classified as N1 tumors. The M stage is determined by the spread of metastases to nonregional lymph nodes or to the lung or other distant sites.

The presence of serum tumor markers is also used to classify testicular tumors. The designation "S" is a special classification used only for testicular cancers. Lesions associated with normal serum tumor markers are classified as S0, whereas tumors associated with increasingly abnormal levels of serum LDH, hCG, and AFP are classified as S1 to S3.

Testicular cancers are further staged into groups based on the TNM classification plus the degree of serum tumor marker elevation. These groups range from stage I (early-stage) to stage III (late-stage) disease. There is no stage IV classification for testicular cancer. Patients are also classified according to risk. The risk classification for patients with seminomas and nonseminomas is shown in **Table 38**.

Treatment

Seminomatous Tumors

After initial surgical resection (radical orchiectomy), patients with low-risk, early-stage seminomas (stage I disease) are usually treated with radiation therapy to include the paraaortic lymph nodes and often the ipsilateral ilioinguinal lymph nodes. Patients in whom postoperative irradiation is contraindicated can generally be followed with close observation because, even without adjuvant radiation therapy, only 15% to 20% relapse, and most relapses occur within the first year. However, radiation therapy is recommended for patients with intermediate disease (stage IIA or IIB). Alternatively, four cycles of etoposide and cisplatin can be administered. For patients with more advanced disease (stage IIC or III), standard chemotherapy with four cycles of etoposide and cisplatin is recommended. This regimen is as effective as three cycles of bleomycin, etoposide, and cisplatin and avoids the acute and chronic pulmonary toxicity associated with administration of bleomycin. However, four cycles of bleomycin, etoposide, and cisplatin are still advised for intermediate-risk patients with nonpulmonary visceral metastases. Non-bleomycin–containing chemotherapeutic regimens are currently being evaluated for most patients who require chemotherapy.

Aggressive surveillance is required after treatment for seminoma. Follow-up care should include a history and physical examination, chest radiograph, and tumor marker assays every 2 months for the first year, as early detection of recurrent disease and prompt treatment are thought to enhance the likelihood of cure. Thereafter, follow-up history and physical

TABLE 38 Risk Status for Patients with Nonseminomas and Seminomas

Risk Status	Nonseminoma	Seminoma

Good	Testicular or retroperitoneal primary tumor *and*
	No nonpulmonary visceral metastases *and*
	Good tumor markers – all of the following:
	  AFP <1000 ng/mL (1000 µg/L)
	  hCG <5000 U/L
	  LDH <1.5 × upper limit of normal
		Any primary site *and*
		No nonpulmonary visceral metastases *and*
		Tumor markers:
		  Normal AFP
		  Any hCG value
		  Any LDH value

Intermediate	Testicular or retroperitoneal primary tumor *and*
	No nonpulmonary visceral metastases *and*
	Intermediate tumor markers – any of the following:
	  AFP 1000–10,000 ng/mL (1000-10,000 µg/L)
	  hCG 5000–50,000 U/L
	  LDH <1.5–10 × upper limit of normal
		Any primary site *and*
		No nonpulmonary visceral metastases *and*
		Tumor markers:
		  Normal AFP
		  Any hCG value
		  Any LDH value

Poor	Mediastinal primary tumor *or*
	Nonpulmonary visceral metastases *or*
	Poor tumor markers – any of the following:
	  AFP >10,000 ng/mL
	  hCG >50,000 U/L
	  LDH 10 × upper limit of normal
		No patients classified as having a poor prognosis

AFP = α-fetoprotein, hCG = human chorionic gonadotropin, LDH = lactate dehydrogenase.

Reprinted with permission from the International Germ Cell Cancer Collaborative Group International Germ Cell Consensus Classification: A Prognostic Factor-based Staging System for Metastatic Germ Cell Cancers. J Clin Oncol. 1997;15(2):594-603. Copyright 2008, The American Society of Clinical Oncology.

examination, chest radiograph, and tumor marker assays are recommended every 3 months for the second year, every 4 months for the third year, every 6 months for the fourth year, and then annually. A CT scan of the abdomen and pelvis should be scheduled annually for the first 3 years.

Nonseminomatous Tumors

Patients with nonseminomas have a poorer prognosis than those with seminomas and therefore require more aggressive treatment. As with seminomas, initial treatment of nonseminoma is radical orchiectomy. This is followed by surveillance alone or by retroperitoneal lymph node dissection to determine the presence of residual disease. Postoperative surveillance alone is an option for highly compliant patients with early-stage disease. About 20% to 30% of patients who decide on surveillance will relapse, and all patients therefore need to be followed closely. More often, a nerve-sparing retroperitoneal lymph node dissection is performed by an experienced surgeon. The cure rate with either approach is 95%. If metastases are found during retroperitoneal lymph node dissection, chemotherapy is usually recommended with etoposide and cisplatin or etoposide, cisplatin, and bleomycin. Patients with elevated serum tumor marker levels postoperatively but without radiographic evidence of disease should also receive chemotherapy.

Patients with more advanced disease and those with extragonadal primary tumors, such as retroperitoneal or mediastinal lesions, are treated primarily with chemotherapy. Cure rates in good-risk patients approach 90%. However, 20% to 30% of intermediate-risk and poor-risk patients are not cured with conventional cisplatin-based therapy. Nonpulmonary visceral metastases, high serum tumor marker levels, and mediastinal primary tumor sites are considered poor prognostic features, and only about 50% of patients with these findings are cured despite aggressive chemotherapy.

If radiographic evidence of residual disease is found after completing chemotherapy and serum tumor marker levels have normalized, aggressive surgery to remove these lesions is warranted. Although the lesions may only be necrotic debris, they may also be mature teratomas, which do not respond to chemotherapy. If viable tumor is found at resection, two additional cycles of chemotherapy are administered. Salvage therapy is indicated for patients who have an incomplete response to first-line therapy or who develop disease recurrence. In addition to etoposide, cisplatin, and bleomycin, agents used for salvage therapy include ifosfamide (together with cisplatin), vinblastine, and paclitaxel. Autologous stem cell transplantation may also be indicated, and durable complete responses have been reported in 15% to 20% of patients following this procedure.

As in patients with seminomas, patients with nonseminomas should adhere to strict follow-up guidelines. Frequent chest radiographs, serum tumor marker assays, and CT scans of the abdomen and pelvis are recommended because of the potential for cure even in patients with recurrent disease.

KEY POINTS

- Testicular germ cell malignancies (seminomas and nonseminomas) are the most common solid tumors in male patients 15 to 34 years of age.
- Seminomas and nonseminomas are highly curable and are often associated with a good prognosis even when disseminated.
- Radical orchiectomy is the initial treatment for both seminomas and nonseminomas.

Bladder Cancer

Approximately 67,200 new cases of bladder cancer are diagnosed in the United States each year, and about 13,750 deaths due to this disease occur annually. About 80% of all bladder cancers are diagnosed in patients over 60 years of age. Men are affected four times more often than women. Bladder cancer is considered a smoking-related malignancy with a two- to threefold increased risk in smokers compared with nonsmokers. Other environmental exposures, such as chemicals used in textile industries, may account for up to 20% of all bladder cancers. In other parts of the world, schistosomiasis is also associated with the development of this neoplasm.

Diagnosis and Staging

Because patients typically present with symptoms suggestive of urinary tract infection, interstitial cystitis, or prostatitis, the diagnosis of bladder cancer is often delayed. The most common presenting symptom is hematuria, which is frequently macroscopic and painless. Tumors that are locally advanced or metastatic may cause suprapubic, perineal, or flank pain due to obstruction. Bladder cancer commonly metastasizes to bone, and bone pain can be a presenting sign of advanced disease. In addition to pain and irritation, patients may have difficulty voiding that may be accompanied by systemic symptoms such as fatigue, weight loss, and poor appetite.

Bladder cancer is usually diagnosed by cystoscopy and biopsy. Transurethral resection of a bladder tumor will help determine the histologic subtype and depth of invasion. Most urothelial cancers are transitional cell carcinomas. Less common histologic subtypes include adenocarcinomas, squamous cell tumors, and small cell tumors. Once the diagnosis is established, additional staging studies may include intravenous pyelography to evaluate the upper urinary tract, CT scan of the abdomen and pelvis, and, possibly, a bone scan if the patient has an elevated serum alkaline phosphatase level or bone pain.

Bladder cancer is staged using the TNM staging system. Ta tumors are noninvasive papillary carcinomas. T1 tumors invade the subepithelial connective tissue, T2 tumors invade muscle, T3 tumors invade perivesical tissue, and T4 tumors invade adjacent organs such as the prostate, uterus, vagina, pelvic wall, or abdominal wall. Lymph node involvement is classified as N1 to N3, based on the number and size of involved nodes. Distant metastases are classified as either absent (M0) or present (M1).

Treatment

Therapy for superficial bladder cancer is primarily managed by urologic oncologists. After transurethral resection of the bladder tumor, patients may receive intravesical therapy with bacillus Calmette-Guérin or other agents such as mitomycin C. Because of the high likelihood of recurrence of bladder cancer, patients are followed with repeat cystoscopy and urine cytologic studies every 3 months.

Advanced or Recurrent Bladder Cancer

Cystectomy is recommended for treating patients with bladder carcinoma in situ or T1 disease that recurs following therapy with bacillus Calmette-Guérin or other intravesical agents. Radical cystectomy is recommended for patients who have a tumor that invades muscle. Ongoing studies are evaluating the role of preoperative chemotherapy and radiation therapy so that patients may undergo bladder-preserving surgical techniques with reasonable outcomes.

Patients with locally advanced disease (stage T3b or T4) or with regional lymph node metastases have 5-year survival rates that are generally less than 20% and should receive postoperative radiation therapy or adjuvant chemotherapy. The effectiveness of cisplatin-based adjuvant chemotherapy has been studied in several controlled clinical trials. Results varied, as some studies found a survival benefit, whereas others showed no overall benefit. The studies that did not report a benefit may have enrolled insufficient numbers of patients or used suboptimal chemotherapy regimens. Nonetheless, compared with observation alone, adjuvant chemotherapy appears to delay tumor progression at the very least. However, there is no widely accepted standard of care for patients with advanced bladder cancer, and the same treatment regimens used to treat advanced bladder cancer are also used in the adjuvant setting.

Metastatic Disease

A regimen that includes methotrexate, vinblastine, doxorubicin, and cisplatin (MVAC) was previously considered the standard of care for treatment of metastatic bladder cancer. However, this regimen is quite toxic. A recent randomized phase III trial compared the effectiveness of MVAC therapy with that of gemcitabine plus cisplatin. The gemcitabine-cisplatin regimen was better tolerated and had a similar response rate (49% versus 46%) and similar time-to-treatment failure (5.8 months versus 4.6 months). Median overall survival for both arms of the study was comparable (13.8 months versus 14.8 months). Carboplatin is a slightly better tolerated agent that can be substituted for the more emetogenic and ototoxic cisplatin. Other active agents for treatment of metastatic bladder cancer include paclitaxel and docetaxel. Newer agents such as cetuximab, a monoclonal antibody targeting the epidermal growth factor receptor, are currently being evaluated in clinical trials.

KEY POINTS

- Bladder cancer is a smoking-related malignancy.
- The diagnosis of bladder cancer is often delayed because symptoms may be similar to those of urinary tract infection, cystitis, or prostatitis.
- Treatment of superficial bladder cancer involves transurethral resection of the bladder tumor followed by intravesical administration of bacillus Calmette-Guérin or other agents.
- Treatment of advanced or recurrent bladder cancer involves cystectomy and adjuvant chemotherapy.

Renal Cancer

Although cancer of the kidneys and pelvis accounts for only 3% of all adult malignancies in the United States, the incidence has been increasing over the past several years. Approximately 51,200 new cases of kidney and renal pelvis cancer are diagnosed in this country each year, and about 12,900 cancer-related deaths occur annually. The typical age of onset is 50 to 70 years, and men are affected more often than women. Tobacco and hereditary factors contribute to the risk for developing renal cancer. Most renal cancers are of the clear cell type associated with the von Hippel–Lindau (VHL) gene mutation. About 15% are of the papillary cell type. Because any of the histologic subtypes may have sarcomatoid features, renal cancer is a fairly aggressive malignancy.

Patients with von Hippel–Lindau disease (an inherited disorder characterized by various benign and malignant tumors) are prone to cancers of the kidney, brain, spinal cord, adrenal glands, pancreas, and epididymis. About 40% of these patients develop multiple bilateral tumors or cysts in the kidneys.

Diagnosis and Staging

Hematuria is the most common symptom in patients with renal cancer. Flank pain may also occur but usually develops only in those with more advanced disease. Many patients are asymptomatic, and the cancer is found incidentally during imaging studies for other disorders. The diagnosis is generally established by a CT scan of the abdomen and pelvis. Additional imaging studies may also be indicated to detect the presence of possible metastases.

Renal cancer is staged using the TNM staging system. The TNM findings are then grouped to determine the stage of disease (stage I to stage IV). Stage I tumors are small lesions that are limited to the kidney without lymph node involvement or metastatic spread. Stage IV tumors are characterized by involvement of two or more regional lymph nodes, tumor that extends beyond Gerota's fascia, or the presence of distant metastatic lesions.

Five-year overall survival rates are 95% for patients with stage I renal cancer, 88% for stage II disease, 60% for stage III disease, and 20% for stage IV disease. Risk factors associated with a poorer prognosis include the presence of disease-related symptoms, time from diagnosis to development of metastatic disease of less than 1 year, a hemoglobin level of 13.0 g/dL (130 g/L) or less in men and 11.5 g/dL (115 g/L) or less in women, a corrected serum calcium level greater than 10 mg/dL (2.5 mmol/L), and an elevated serum lactate dehydrogenase level. Patients with metastatic disease (Stage IV disease) with no risk factors have a median survival of 29 months, patients with one or two risk factors have a median survival of 14 months, and those with three or more risk factors have a median survival of 4 months.

Treatment

Early-stage localized renal cancer is managed surgically by either partial or radical nephrectomy. Treatment of advanced or metastatic disease is evolving. Immunotherapeutic agents such as interleukin-2 and interferon alfa provide a very modest survival benefit for patients with late-stage disease but are associated with considerable toxicity. Immunotherapy has now generally been supplanted by targeted therapy, which has resulted in a radical change in the treatment of renal cancer. Several targets that play an important role in renal cancer development and progression include vascular endothelial growth factor (VEGF), vascular endothelial growth factor receptor (VEGFR), and the mammalian target of rapamycin (mTOR). Recent developments in understanding the tumor biology that influences the growth of renal cell cancers have resulted in the development of targeted agents that have proved to be effective in large randomized clinical trials. Three agents (sunitinib, sorafenib, and temsirolimus) were recently approved for treatment of metastatic renal cell carcinoma and at least 15 new agents are currently being studied.

Sunitinib is a small-molecule-receptor tyrosine kinase inhibitor that inhibits VEGFR, platelet-derived growth factor receptor (PDGFR), c-*kit*, and fluorothymidine-3 (FLT-3). A large phase III study randomized 690 patients to receive either interferon alfa or sunitinib as first-line therapy for metastatic disease. The sunitinib arm of the study was associated with a significantly increased response rate (31% versus 5%) and a 6-month increase in progression-free survival. Sorafenib is the second small-molecule-receptor tyrosine kinase inhibitor that was recently approved for use in patients with advanced disease. This oral agent inhibits VEGFR-2, VEGFR-3, FLT-3, PDGFR, c-*kit*, and Raf kinase. In a phase III study, the median progression-free survival for patients enrolled in the sorafenib arm was 24 weeks compared with 6 weeks for the placebo. Temsirolimus is the third recently approved targeted agent. This agent inhibits mTOR, which is an intermediate in the phosphoinositide-3 kinase/Akt pathway. Poor-risk patients with advanced metastatic renal cell carcinoma were randomized to receive interferon alfa alone, temsirolimus alone, or interferon alfa plus temsirolimus. Both overall and progression-free survival improved in patients receiving temsirolimus alone.

The agents discussed above and other new targeted therapies are now being evaluated in the postoperative setting in hopes of decreasing the risk of relapse and ultimately improving the chance for cure in patients with advanced renal cancer.

KEY POINTS

- Most renal cancers are of the clear cell type associated with the von Hippel–Lindau (VHL) mutation.
- Early-stage renal cancer is treated surgically.
- Three new targeted agents (sunitinib, sorafenib, and temsirolimus) have recently been approved that prolong the time to disease progression in patients with renal cancer.

Bibliography

D'Amico AV, Whittington R, Malkowicz SB, et al. Predicting prostate specific antigen outcome preoperatively in the prostate specific antigen era. J Urol. 2001;166(6): 2185-2188. [PMID: 11696732]

Freedland SJ, Humphreys EB, Mangold LA, et al. Risk of prostate cancer-specific mortality following biochemical recurrence after radical prostatectomy. JAMA. 2005;294(4):433-439. [PMID: 16046649]

Hudes G, Carducci M, Tomczak P, et al; Global ARCC Trial. Temsirolimus, interferon alfa, or both for advanced renal-cell carcinoma. N Engl J Med. 2007;356(22):2271-2281. [PMID: 17538086]

International Germ Cell Consensus Classification: a prognostic factor-based staging system for metastatic germ cell cancers. International Germ Cell Cancer Collaborative Group. J Clin Oncol. 1997;15(2): 594-603. [PMID: 9053482]

Motzer RJ, Bacik J, Murphy BA, Russo P, Mazumdar M. Interferon-alfa as a comparative treatment for clinical trials of new therapies against advanced renal cell carcinoma. J Clin Oncol. 2002;20(1):289-296. [PMID: 11773181]

Motzer RJ, Bosl GJ. High-dose chemotherapy for resistant germ cell tumors: recent advances and future directions. J Natl Cancer Inst. 1992;84(22):1703-1709. [PMID: 1331482]

Petrylak DP, Tangen CM, Hussain MH, et al. Docetaxel and estramustine compared with mitoxantrone and prednisone for advanced refractory prostate cancer. N Engl J Med. 2004;351(15):1513-1520. [PMID: 15470214]

Ratain MJ, Eisen T, Stadler WM, et al. Phase II placebo-controlled randomized discontinuation trial of sorafenib in patients with metastatic renal cell carcinoma. J Clin Oncol. 2006;24(16):2505-2512. [PMID: 16636341]

Tannock IF, de Wit R, Berry WR, et al; TAX 327 Investigators. Docetaxel plus prednisone or mitoxantrone plus prednisone for advanced prostate cancer. N Engl J Med. 2004;351(15):1502-1512. [PMID: 15470213]

Trainer TD. Mortality following prostate cancer recurrence after radical prostectomy. JAMA. 2005;294(23):2969. [PMID: 16414939]

Lymphadenopathy and Lymphoid Malignancies

Lymphadenopathy

Although most lymphadenopathy is self-limited, caused by upper respiratory tract illness, or not determined, there is a broad differential diagnosis in patients with this finding. Malignancy is the underlying cause of lymphadenopathy in less than 1% of patients in a primary care setting, although the risk increases with advancing age and chronicity of the findings.

Key initial components of the workup are a detailed medical history, physical examination, selected laboratory and radiographic studies, and, occasionally, a lymph node biopsy. The history should guide the investigation of a patient's symptoms, especially those suggesting associated infection or systemic illness; occupation and travel history; sexual behavior; and medication use. The examination should provide clues to the underlying cause of the lymphadenopathy, such as the size, number, tenderness, consistency, and location of enlarged lymph nodes; signs of associated infection; evidence of masses in other sites; or the presence of splenomegaly or

skin lesions. A complete blood count with review of the peripheral blood smear, evaluation of antibody titers against viral and other infectious agents, evaluation for connective tissue disease markers, and microbial cultures are also appropriate as clinically warranted. A chest radiograph is used to identify hilar lymph nodes, and a chest CT is used to evaluate mediastinal lymphadenopathy and pulmonary disease. More sophisticated imaging studies are appropriate as clinically indicated. Usually, a workup should be initiated in patients with progressively enlarging lymph nodes or persistently enlarged nodes for greater than 2 weeks.

KEY POINTS

- Malignancy is the underlying cause of lymphadenopathy in less than 1% of patients in primary care, although the risk increases with advancing age and the chronicity of the findings.
- The physical examination in patients with lymphadenopathy should focus on the size, number, consistency, and location of enlarged lymph nodes; signs of associated infection; evidence of masses in other sites; and the presence of splenomegaly or skin lesions.
- Laboratory tests in the setting of lymphadenopathy might include a complete blood count with review of the peripheral smear, evaluation of antibody titers against viral and other infectious agents, evaluation for connective tissue disease markers, and microbial cultures as indicated.

Malignant Lymphoma

Epidemiology

Approximately 56,000 new cases of non-Hodgkin lymphoma (NHL) are diagnosed in the United States annually, with approximately 24,000 people dying from this disease each year. The incidence of NHL increases exponentially with age and is greater in men than women and in whites than blacks.

Hodgkin lymphoma is a relatively rare cancer, with approximately 7400 cases diagnosed and 1300 deaths from this disease in the United States annually. Most cases occur among patients 15 to 40 years of age. This disease has an unusual bimodal peak of incidence, with an initial peak among patients 15 to 34 years and a second peak among patients 55 to 70 years. Incidence is highest among white men.

Risk Factors

Autoimmune disease and immunodeficiency states have a known association with NHL. NHL may also be caused by viruses (see Cancer Risk section). Several chemicals, such as organochlorine agents (for example, DDT), have been weakly associated with an increased risk for NHL. Farming is one of the few occupations that consistently shows an association with an increased risk for NHL, which is often thought to be related to the use of pesticides. Three large population-based studies have now failed to link the use of hair dye to risk for lymphoma.

There is a suggested link between Hodgkin lymphoma and delayed exposure to common childhood infections because patients with this disease tend to have grown up in smaller families with a higher socioeconomic status. The second peak of incidence in Hodgkin lymphoma may be a consequence of latent virus reactivation with age-related decline in immunity, or it may represent a truly distinct disease entity. Epstein-Barr virus has long been suspected as being a leading contributing cause to Hodgkin lymphoma (see Cancer Risk section).

There is an increased risk for Hodgkin lymphoma among first-degree relatives, especially siblings of the same sex. Monozygotic twins have a significantly higher risk of developing Hodgkin lymphoma compared with dizygotic twins. Although familial clustering of NHL has been reported, familial aggregation studies do not provide evidence of a strong genetic basis for NHL independent of environmental factors, and no specific genetic marker for NHL has been identified.

KEY POINT

- Chemicals used in farming, such as organochlorine agents, have been associated with an increased risk for non-Hodgkin lymphoma, but the use of hair dye has not.

Classification, Staging, and Prognostic Factors

The current system for classification of NHL is that derived by the World Health Organization, which currently incorporates immunophenotyping and genetic information into the classification scheme (**Figure 33**). Lymphoid tumors are classified into three groupings: B-cell neoplasms, T- and NK-cell neoplasms, and Hodgkin lymphoma. Approximately 80% to 85% of non-Hodgkin lymphoid neoplasms in adults are of B-cell origin; most of the remainder are derived from T cells. Lymphomas are grouped into categories of indolent, aggressive, or highly aggressive based on their biology and natural history (**Table 39**). Indolent NHLs are considered incurable (except for the few patients with stage I disease [disease confined to one lymph node group] that can be eradicated by radiotherapy). The median survival of patients with indolent NHL (most of whom present with advanced disease) is 7 to 10 years. Patients with aggressive or highly aggressive NHL potentially are curable with combination chemotherapy. Immunophenotyping of these malignant cells is routinely performed in the diagnosis of NHL. All B-cell–derived NHLs are CD19+ and CD20+. Characteristic cytogenetic markers may be found in patients with some forms of NHL, and the differential diagnosis of NHL can be narrowed by using a panel of monoclonal antibodies and genetic markers (**Table 40**).

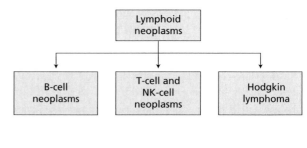

Classification criteria

- Morphology

- Clinical features

- Genetic features

- Immunophenotype

FIGURE 33.
World Health Organization classification of lymphoid malignancies.

TABLE 39 B-cell Lymphomas

Indolent	Aggressive	Highly Aggressive
Small lymphocytic	Diffuse large cell	Burkett
Follicular	Mantle cell	Lymphoblastic
Marginal zone		AIDS-related
MALT		
Splenic		
Nodal		

MALT = mucosa-associated lymphoid tissue.

In general, disease in indolent NHL is characterized by extensive lymph node involvement at presentation; more aggressive NHL is more likely to involve extranodal organs. The National Cancer Center Network recommends obtaining a biopsy to establish the initial diagnosis of NHL rather than relying solely on fine-needle aspiration. Once the diagnosis of lymphoma is confirmed by microscopy and flow cytometry and fluorescent in-situ hybridization or cytogenetics, the staging workup can proceed. Laboratory studies in the staging of NHL include complete blood count; measurement of serum lactate dehydrogenase, uric acid, and β2 microglobulin; comprehensive metabolic panel; and a hepatitis panel and HIV testing. Imaging studies include CT of the neck, chest, abdomen, and pelvis; an echocardiogram or multigated nuclear medicine study to assess cardiac function if an anthracycline-based regimen is being considered; and, often, positron emission tomography. Patients also should undergo a bone marrow biopsy. In certain circumstances (for example, in patients with sinus, bone marrow, testicular, ocular,

TABLE 40 Immunophenotype and Genetic Markers for Low-Grade Non-Hodgkin Lymphoma Translocation

	CD5	CD10	CD20	CD23	Chromosomal Marker	Oncogene
Follicular	-	+	+	-	t(14:18)	bcl-2
SLL/CLL	+	-	Dim	+	trisomy 12	-
Mantle Cell	+	-	+	-	t(11:14)	bcl-1 (cyclin D$_1$)
MZL/MALT	-	-	+	-	t(1:18) t(1:14)	API-2; MALTI bcl-10

SLL/CLL = small lymphocytic lymphoma/chronic lymphocytic leukemia; MZL/MALT = marginal-zone lymphoma/mucosa-associated lymphoid tissue lymphoma.

paravertebral, or parameningeal involvement), a lumbar puncture is indicated to exclude central nervous system involvement requiring additional forms of therapy, because there is a higher incidence of central nervous system involvement when large-cell lymphoma is found in any of these sites.

Patients with NHL who have the same stage of disease per the Ann Arbor staging system may have very different clinical outcomes (**Figure 34**). The International Prognostic Index (IPI) was developed as a predictive model of outcome for patients with diffuse large cell lymphoma. The index is based on five pretreatment characteristics found to be independent predictors of death (**Table 41**). The age-adjusted IPI was derived for patients younger than 60 years. For these patients, the age-adjusted factors are performance status, serum lactate dehydrogenase concentration, and stage.

Risk categories and corresponding survival rates are provided in Table 41 and **Figure 35**. The IPI was modified to be applied to follicular lymphoma and is referred to as the Follicular Lymphoma IPI (FLIPI). This index also includes five independent factors consisting of number of extranodal

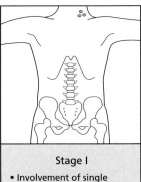

Stage I

- Involvement of single lymph node region; or
- Involvement of single extralymphatic site (stage IE)

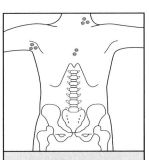

Stage II

- Involvement of ≥2 lymph node regions on same side of diaphragm
- May include localized extralymphatic involvement on same side of diaphragm (stage IIE)

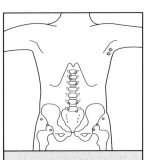

Stage III

- Involvement of lymph node regions on both sides of diaphragm
- May include involvement of spleen (stage IIIS) or localized extranodal disease (stage IIIE) or both (IIIE+S)

For Hodgkin lymphoma:

III1

- Disease limited to upper abdomen — spleen, splenic hilar, celiac, or portahepatic nodes

III2

- Disease limited to lower abdomen — periaortic, pelvic or inguinal nodes

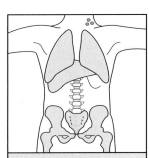

Stage IV

- Disseminated (multifocal) extralymphatic disease involving one or more organs (e.g., liver, bone, marrow, lung, skin), +/- associated lymph node involvement; or
- Isolated extralymphatic disease with distant (nonregional) lymph node involvement

FIGURE 34.
Ann Harbor Staging System for Hodgkin and non-Hodgkin lymphoma.

TABLE 41 Prognostic Indices for non-Hodgkin Lymphoma			
FLIPI		**IPI (for Large Cell Lymphoma)**	
Age >60 yr		Age >60 yr	
Ann Arbor stage (III or IV)		Stage I or II	
Hemoglobin level <12 g/dL (120 g/L)		Performance status 0 or 1	
Number of nodal[a] areas >4		Extranodal involvement >1 site	
Serum LDH level above normal		Serum LDH level >1X normal	
Risk Categories (Factors)	**5-/10-yr Overall Survival (%)**	**Risk Categories (Factors)**	**5-yr Overall Survival (%)**
Low (0-1)	90/70	Low (0-1)	73
Intermediate (2)	77/50	Low Intermediate (2)	51
High (>3)	52/35	High Intermediate (3)	43
—	—	High (4-5)	26

FLIPI = Follicular Lymphoma International Prognostic Index; IPI = International Prognostic Index; LDH = lactate dehydrogenase.

[a]The nodal categories are cervical, mediastinal, axillary, mesenteric, para-aortic, inguinal, epitrochlear, and popliteal.

Part of this research was based on and originally published in Blood. Solal-Céligny P, Roy P, Colombat P, et al. Follicular Lymphoma International Prognostic Index. Blood. 2004;104(5):1258-1265. [PMID: 15126323] Copyright 2004, American Society of Hematology; and A predictive model for aggressive non-Hodgkin's lymphoma. The International Non-Hodgkin's Lymphoma Prognostic Factors Project. N Engl J Med. 1993;329(14):987-994. [PMID: 8141877]

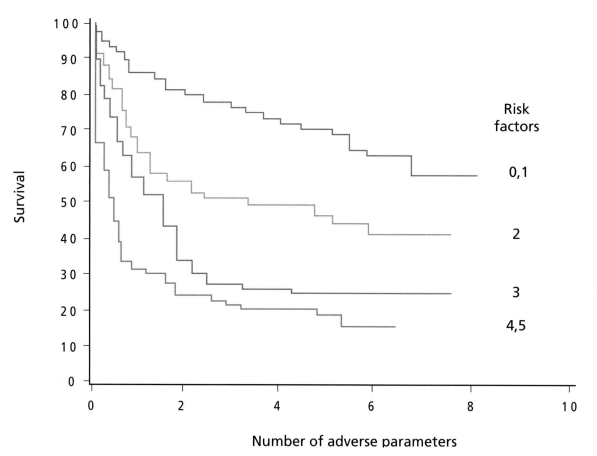

FIGURE 35.

Survival according to the International Prognostic Index for aggressive large B-cell non-Hodgkin lymphoma.

Data used with permission from Solal-Céligny P, Roy P, Colombat P, et al. Follicular lymphoma International Prognostic Index. Blood. 2004;104(5):1258-1265. [PMID: 15126323] Copyright 2004, American Society of Hematology.

sites, serum lactate dehydrogenase concentration, age, stage, and hemoglobin concentration, which replaces performance status in this scheme.

Patients with high-risk IPI scores are destined to have a poor prognosis. Whether more aggressive treatment such as high-dose chemotherapy with hematopoietic cell support as part of front-line therapy will improve the outcome of such patients is unknown. The National Cancer Center Network guidelines recommend that these patients be considered for clinical trials (preferred) evaluating new approaches or standard cyclophosphamide, doxorubicin, vincristine, prednisone, and rituximab (R-CHOP). Similarly, patients with follicular lymphoma with a high-risk FLIPI score are candidates for clinical trials or treatment with standard regimens such as R-CVP (cyclophosphamide, vincristine, prednisone, rituximab) or R-CHOP. There are no data from randomized, prospective trials using these prognostic indices to guide therapeutic decisions. In the future, prognostication will be further refined with the use of DNA micro-array technology, which shows which genes are over- or underexpressed in a given tumor.

KEY POINT

- Diagnosis of non-Hodgkin lymphoma should be established by biopsy, not fine-needle aspiration, and confirmed by microscopy and flow cytometry and fluorescent in-situ hybridization or cytogenetics.

Overview and Treatment of Indolent Lymphoma

Follicular Lymphoma

Follicular lymphoma, the most common indolent lymphoma, constitutes approximately 40% of cases of NHL in the United States and occurs equally among men and women (median age, 60 years). Disease in NHL is assigned one of three grades, with grade 3 being the most aggressive. The immunophenotypes of follicular lymphomas are CD20+ and CD10+ (see Table 40). Most patients are asymptomatic at diagnosis despite having disseminated disease, often with bone marrow involvement. This type of lymphoma is characterized by a relatively long survival (median survival, 8 to 12 years) but, overall, is considered incurable except for those patients whose disease is localized at presentation and can be irradiated.

Standard treatment is controversial and ranges from a watch-and-wait approach, to treatment with a monoclonal antibody (alone or tagged with a radionuclide), to combination chemotherapy. Rituximab is a chimeric (approximately two thirds human/one third murine) monoclonal antibody raised against the CD20 protein on the surface of most cells of the B-lymphocyte lineage. It has a single-agent response rate of approximately 50% in patients with recurrent follicular NHL. Overall response rate, complete response rate, and

time to progression were improved when rituximab was administered in combination with cyclophosphamide, vincristine, and prednisone (CVP) compared with CVP alone. The response rate of patients receiving anti-CD20 monoclonal antibody therapy was improved to approximately 80% as a single agent when labeled with a radionuclide of either iodine-131 (tositumomab I-131) or yttrium-90 (ibritumomab tiuxetan Y-90). An even more aggressive approach would be to add an anthracycline (doxorubicin) to CVP, forming the CHOP regimen, or purine analog–based treatment with fludarabine or cladribine in combination with rituximab.

The decision to initiate treatment is based on the presence of symptoms, threat to vital organ function, issues over appearance because of enlarged lymph nodes, and patient preference. Those for whom a watch-and-wait approach is chosen require close follow-up soon after their initial diagnosis to assess the pace of their illness as well as counseling about symptoms and signs warranting medical attention.

Patients with early-stage disease (stages IA and IIA) often are treated with radiation therapy if the disease is readily encompassed within a reasonably sized irradiation field. At least 50% of these patients will be disease-free at 10 years. Most patients whose disease recurs will have a recurrence outside the radiation field, suggesting that current staging studies are suboptimal. Patients with disseminated disease need systemic treatment once the decision is made to abandon watchful waiting. Emerging data suggest that rituximab, as a maintenance treatment, prolongs progression-free and overall survival. An ongoing large randomized trial is evaluating whether continuing rituximab as a maintenance treatment after induction is superior to no maintenance treatment and restarting rituximab at the time of recurrence.

MALT Lymphoma

Mucosa-associated lymphoid tissue (MALT) lymphomas are classified in the World Health Organization system as marginal-zone lymphomas (see Table 40). Indolent forms are often localized in extranodal sites, such as the stomach, lung, thyroid or salivary glands, breast, or eye. Gastric MALT lymphoma often is associated with *Helicobacter pylori* infection. A combination of antibiotics, including metronidazole, amoxicillin, or clarithromycin, with proton pump inhibitor therapy, is used to eradicate the *H. pylori* infection that provides the antigenic drive for lymphocyte proliferation. This treatment often induces complete responses in 70% to 80% of patients with localized gastric MALT lymphoma. However, this approach is less well-established outside the stomach because the association with a specific causative agent often is unknown. There are conflicting data concerning the role of chlamydial infection in orbital MALT lymphoma. Radiation is often used to treat MALT lymphoma when an antibiotic approach is not successful or for sites other than the stomach.

For more extensive disease, the treatment choices are similar to those used in follicular lymphoma. Marginal-zone lymphomas can also present as a more aggressive lymphoma, with large cells having a higher mitotic rate than the more common indolent marginal-zone NHL, and are treated similarly to diffuse large cell lymphomas.

KEY POINTS

- Fifty percent of patients with early-stage follicular lymphoma who are able to receive radiation therapy are disease free after 10 years.

- A combination of antibiotics, including metronidazole, amoxicillin, or clarithromycin, with proton pump inhibitor therapy, is used to eradicate the *Helicobacter pylori* infection in patients with gastric mucosa-associated lymphoid tissue lymphoma.

- Radiation is often used to treat mucosa-associated lymphoid tissue lymphoma when an antibiotic approach is not successful or for sites other than the stomach.

Overview and Treatment of Aggressive Lymphomas

Diffuse Large Cell Lymphoma

Diffuse large cell lymphoma is the most common of the aggressive lymphomas, and the primary therapy for this malignancy is CHOP with rituximab for six cycles. A shorter course of chemotherapy may be used for localized (early-stage) disease when combined with involved-field radiation depending on the disease location. Patients with advanced disease and a high-risk IPI score may be candidates for additional therapy such as high-dose chemotherapy with autologous stem cell rescue. The risk for developing late toxicities from high-dose chemotherapy with stem cell rescue, including acute myeloid leukemia and myelodysplastic syndrome, needs to be balanced against any potential benefits of treatment and often is reserved for patients with chemotherapy-sensitive, relapsed, aggressive lymphoma. Patients who have a relapse may still be cured by stem cell transplantation consolidation after they respond to re-induction therapy with an aggressive combination-chemotherapy regimen.

High-grade lymphomas, namely lymphoblastic lymphoma and Burkitt lymphoma, are treated with highly complex regimens. Patients with lymphoblastic lymphoma receive the same regimens as those administered to patients with acute lymphocytic leukemia, which includes 2 to 3 years of maintenance therapy and intrathecally administered chemotherapy because of the high risk for central nervous system involvement in this disease. Patients who receive this approach may achieve complete response rates of approximately 80%, with long-term survival rates of approximately 45%. Patients with Burkitt lymphoma receive a brief, high-intensity regimen, also with central nervous system treatment, with high cure rates for affected adults in the United States.

Mantle Cell Lymphoma

Mantle cell lymphoma is characterized by the worst features of indolent and aggressive lymphomas. This disease is considered incurable (as are disseminated indolent lymphomas) but has a shorter median survival than disseminated indolent lymphomas of approximately 3 years. Patients with mantle cell lymphoma often present with disseminated disease, including gastrointestinal involvement. In these patients, cell-cycle protein cyclin D_1 is expressed as a result of an 11;14 chromosomal translocation activating the *bcl-1* gene (see Table 40). These patients often respond to chemotherapy, but duration of responses is short with regimens such as R-CHOP. More intensive regimens, such as with cyclophosphamide, vincristine, doxorubicin, dexamethasone, cytarabine, and methotrexate (hyper C-VAD-AM) combined with rituximab, have improved both response rate and duration of response but still do not cure patients. Stem cell transplantation during first remission has yielded encouraging results.

Hodgkin Lymphoma

Hodgkin lymphoma is regarded as a highly curable cancer. The emphasis of current research is on developing less-toxic therapies without compromising efficacy. The most concerning of these toxicities is the development of secondary malignancies.

All forms of classical Hodgkin lymphoma are treated similarly. Prior to the early 1990s, patients with clinically apparent early-stage Hodgkin lymphoma who were being considered for treatment with radiation therapy alone underwent a staging laparotomy with the attendant risk of postsplenectomy sepsis. The need for performing a staging laparotomy has disappeared with the advent of combined-modality treatment consisting of chemotherapy and smaller (involved) fields of radiotherapy. Patients with early-stage disease (IA and IIA) should be treated with a short course of chemotherapy, such as doxorubicin, bleomycin, vinblastine, and dacarbazine (ABVD), and irradiation to involved lymph node sites. Patients with bulky stage I or II disease or B symptoms should receive a full course of chemotherapy (ABVD) followed by radiation therapy to initially bulky areas. Patients with higher-stage disease often are treated with chemotherapy (ABVD) or the Stanford V regimen. For patients with high-risk disease as defined by the International Prognostic Factor Project (**Table 42**), a more intensive regimen consisting of bleomycin, etoposide, doxorubicin, cyclophosphamide, vincristine, procarbazine, and prednisone (BEACOPP) may be considered. Patients who relapse after initial therapy are treated with radiation, chemotherapy, or high-dose chemotherapy with hematopoietic stem cell rescue depending on the clinical situation.

Patients with the lymphocyte-predominant variant of Hodgkin lymphoma are treated differently than are patients with other subtypes of this disease. Those with early-stage disease are preferentially treated with involved-field or regional radiation. A watch-and-wait approach is appropriate for patients who cannot tolerate radiation. The treatment of

TABLE 42 Hodgkin Lymphoma International Prognostic Factor Project[a]		
Number of Factors	Freedom from Progression (%)	5-Year Overall Survival (%)
0	84	89
1	77	90
2	67	81
3	60	78
4	51	61
5	42	56

[a]Prognostic factors: Age ≥45 years; stage IV; male sex; leukocyte count ≥15,000 μL (15 × 10^9/L); lymphocyte count <600 cells/μL or <8%; albumin <4 g/dL (40 g/L); hemoglobin <10.5 g/dL (105 g/L).

choice for patients with B symptoms or more disseminated disease is the same as that used in treating those with classical Hodgkin lymphoma. Observation or rituximab may be used in selected patients who are not candidates for chemotherapy because this type of lymphoma expresses CD20⁺, differentiating it from the other forms of Hodgkin lymphoma, (that is, it is more akin to a low-grade NHL).

Hairy Cell Leukemia

Hairy cell leukemia derives its name from its morphologic appearance, which consists of atypical lymphocytes with thread-like cytoplasmic projections from the cell surface (**Figure 36**). It occurs most commonly in older adults and is more common in men than women (approximately 5:1). This disease is characterized by significant bone marrow involvement, pancytopenia, and splenomegaly, but not lymphadenopathy. The tumor in hairy cell leukemia has B-cell immunophenotypic features (SIg⁺, CD20⁺) and expresses CD11⁺ and CD103⁺ on flow cytometry.

The mainstay of treatment currently is cladribine. One course of a 7-day continuous infusion of this agent induces durable complete remissions in 82% of patients. Interferon, fludarabine, and rituximab also have been shown to be active in affected patients.

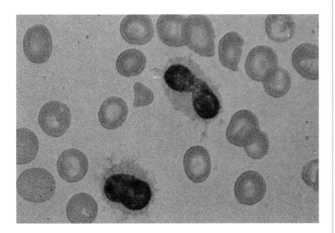

FIGURE 36.
Hairy cell leukemia depicted by atypical lymphocytes with thread-like cytoplasmic projections from the cell surface.

Mycosis Fungoides

CD4⁺ T-cell leukemia that is characterized by major skin involvement is known as mycosis fungoides. When the leukemic phase is also prominent, it is referred to as Sézary syndrome. The cells in mycosis fungoides have a folded or cerebriform nucleus morphology. The only definitive test for determining clonality is to evaluate for T-cell receptor gene rearrangements, because there are no immunologic markers for T-cell clonality.

Skin involvement in patients with mycosis fungoides ranges from patchy areas to diffuse erythroderma, and early skin manifestations may be difficult to distinguish clinically from benign skin disease. Infection of skin lesions is common, and infection leading to sepsis is the leading cause of death in these patients. Treatment of early-stage disease is directed at the skin. Topical agents, such as corticosteroids, mechlorethamine, and carmustine; and retinoids, such as bexarotene gel, have been used. More extensive skin involvement responds well to electron-beam radiation. Phototherapy with ultraviolet light and oral psoralen also is effective in patients with mycosis fungoides. Combination chemotherapy or immunotherapy with purine nucleoside-based or CHOP-like regimens; monoclonal antibody–based treatment (denileukin diftitox, an anti-interleukin-2 receptor monoclonal antibody linked to diphtheria toxin); interferon-alfa; or alemtuzumab (an anti-CD52 monoclonal antibody) are useful in treating mycosis fungoides in the setting of disseminated disease. Vorinostat or suberoylanilide hydroxamic acid recently has been approved by the U.S. Food and Drug Administration for the treatment of cutaneous T-cell lymphoma. Its mechanism of action is that of a histone deacetylase inhibitor that affects epigenetic regulation of DNA activity.

Chronic Lymphocytic Leukemia

Chronic lymphocytic leukemia (CLL) is the most common form of leukemia in adults in the Western world. The median age of onset of CLL is 70 years, with more than 80% of patients older than 60 years of age at diagnosis. Exposure to ionizing radiation, toxic chemicals, or viruses has not been associated with the development of CLL. A familial basis may account for 5% to 10% of cases of CLL, although no specific gene has been implicated in this disease.

Approximately 50% of patients with CLL are asymptomatic at diagnosis. The most common physical findings are lymphadenopathy and splenomegaly, with fewer patients presenting with hepatomegaly.

The diagnosis of CLL is often established from analysis of peripheral blood by flow cytometry with cells expressing the appropriate B-cell CLL immunophenotype (see Table 40). The natural history of CLL is highly variable. Patients are stratified into risk groups based on presenting features. This risk stratification constitutes the staging criteria, which includes the presence of lymphadenopathy, hepatosplenomegaly, anemia, or thrombocytopenia (excluding idiopathic thrombocytopenic purpura). Risk may be further assessed by the presence of a short doubling time of the lymphocyte count (<12 months), cytologic atypia, increased β_2 microglobulin concentration, and increased expression of soluble CD23.

Genetic risk factors for CLL include the *p53* mutation, 17p deletion, and 11q deletion, which are associated with shortened survival. Patients with trisomy 12q, a normal karyotype, and 13q deletions have relatively longer survival rates. The presence of unmutated *IgVH* genes is also a poor prognostic sign in patients with CLL and is associated with zap-70 expression, an intracellular protein tyrosine kinase important in T-cell signaling (**Figure 37**).

Criteria for initiating treatment in patients with CLL include B symptoms (fever, weight loss, and night sweats);

symptoms due to lymph node enlargement; hepatosplenomegaly; or worsening cytopenia. No treatment short of allogeneic stem cell transplantation has curative potential in affected patients. This form of treatment is applicable only to a few patients because the median age of patients with CLL is 70 years. The risk of graft-versus-host disease and other toxicities increases with age and often precludes its use.

Several randomized trials have shown the superiority of purine-based regimens over alkylating agent–based chemotherapy in patients with CLL. The highest response rates have been achieved with a regimen consisting of fludarabine, cyclophosphamide, and rituximab. Therapy may be complicated by a high infection rate, including opportunistic infections requiring prophylaxis against *Pneumocystis* species and herpesvirus infections. Patients with *p53* mutations have a short duration of response to chemotherapy and seem to respond better to induction therapy with alemtuzumab, an anti-CD52 monoclonal antibody. Patients who achieve a complete response are more likely to have prolonged progression-free and overall survival.

Clinically detectable hemolytic anemia occurs in 3% to 37% of patients with CLL, usually in those with advanced-stage disease. This form of anemia does not confer a negative impact on overall survival. Most cases of hemolytic anemia in this setting involve a warm IgG antibody against Rh antigens, although anemia with cold IgM autoantibodies that fix complement also can occur. This complication is treated independently of the underlying CLL with high-dose

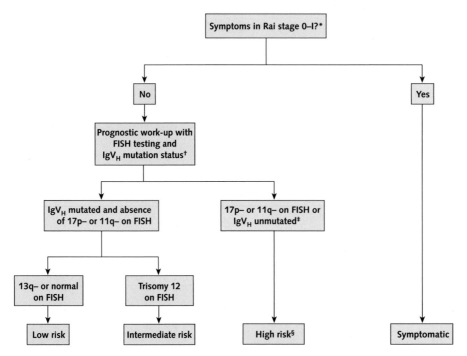

FIGURE 37.
Narrative Review: Initial Management of Newly Diagnosed, Early-Stage Chronic Lymphocytic Leukemia.

FISH = flourescent in situ hybridization; IgVH = immunoglobulin variable region heavy chain gene. *Fever, weight loss, night sweats, and fatigue not due to another cause. †If available at center. ‡Less than or equal to 2% mutated compared with germline sequence. §Although high Z-chain–associated protein kinase-70 expression may be used to characterize patients with early-stage disease as high risk in the future, this assay cannot be recommended for routine clinical use until it can be standardized and shown to have reliable intralaboratory reproducibility.

Reprinted with permission from Shanafelt TD, Byrd JC, Call TG, Zent CS, Kay NE. Ann Intern Med. 2006;145(6):435-447. [PMID: 16983131] Copyright 2006, American College of Physicians.

corticosteroids, and in refractory patients, intravenous gamma globulin, splenectomy, or treatment of the CLL may be necessary. Patients with CLL also may develop immune thrombocytopenia that needs to be distinguished from thrombocytopenia secondary to malignant infiltration of the bone marrow or from that induced by treatment toxicity. Treatment of these patients may include corticosteroids, intravenous immune globulin, or more aggressive chemotherapy directed at the underlying lymphoproliferative disease.

It is estimated that up to 70% of patients with CLL will develop infection, of which up to 55% of patients will die. Immunosuppression is caused by CLL therapy as well as the underlying disease. Patients are often hypogammaglobulinemic and may require intravenous immune globulin infusions when threatened by repetitive pulmonary infections.

Second malignancies occur more frequently in patients with CLL compared with the general population and most commonly include Kaposi sarcoma; melanoma; and cancer of the head and neck, bladder, stomach, lung, or brain. Given the long survival of patients with CLL, they should be carefully monitored and urged to avoid exposure to carcinogens, such as tobacco and excessive sunlight. Development of acute myeloid leukemia/myelodysplastic syndromes is rare.

Disease in a few patients with CLL transforms into a more aggressive form of cancer, either prolymphocytic leukemia or Richter syndrome (large cell lymphoma). Treatment for these diseases usually consists of R-CHOP, the therapy most often used in NHL, and frequently is followed by some form of hematopoietic stem cell transplantation.

KEY POINTS

- The primary treatment for diffuse large cell lymphoma is cyclophosphamide, doxorubicin, vincristine, and prednisone (CHOP) with rituximab.

- Patients with early-stage Hodgkin lymphoma should be treated with a short course of chemotherapy and irradiation to any involved areas.

- The mainstay of treatment for patients with hairy cell leukemia is cladribine.

- Treatment for early-stage mycosis fungoides is directed at the skin and includes topical corticosteroids, mechlorethamine, carmustine, and retinoids.

- Criteria for initiating treatment in patients with chronic lymphocytic leukemia include fever, weight loss, and night sweats; symptoms due to lymph node enlargement; hepatosplenomegaly; or worsening cytopenia.

- No treatment short of allogeneic stem cell transplantation has curative potential in patients with chronic lymphocytic leukemia.

- Fludarabine, cyclophosphamide, and rituximab therapy has yielded the highest response rates in patients with chronic lymphocytic leukemia.

Bibliography

Ansell SM, Armitage J. Non-Hodgkin Lymphoma: Diagnosis and Treatment. Mayo Clin Proc. 2005;80(8):1087-1097. [PMID: 16092591]

Ansell SM, Armitage JO. Hodgkin Lymphoma: Diagnosis and Treatment. Mayo Clin Proc. 2006;81(3):419-426. [PMID: 16529147]

Archuleta TD, Armitage JO. Advances in follicular lymphoma. Semin Oncol. 2004;31(2 Suppl 4):66-71. [PMID: 15124137]

Coiffier B, Lepage E, Briere J, et al. CHOP chemotherapy plus rituximab compared with CHOP alone in elderly patients with diffuse large-B-cell lymphoma. N Engl J Med 2002;346(4):235-242. [PMID: 11807147]

Else M, Ruchlemer R, Osuji N, et al. Long remissions in hairy cell leukemia with purine analogs: A report of 219 patients with a median follow-up of 12.5 years. Cancer. 2005;104(11):2442-2448. [PMID: 16245328]

Hasenclever D, Diehl V. A prognostic score for advanced Hodgkin's disease. International Prognostic Factors Project on Advanced Hodgkin's Disease. N Engl J Med. 1998;339(21):1506-1514. [PMID: 9819449]

Hoppe RT, Advani RH, Bierman PJ, et al; National Comprehensive Cancer Network. J Natl Compr Canc Netw. 2006;4(3):210-230. [PMID: 16507269]

Miller TP, Dahlberg S, Cassady JR, et al. Chemotherapy alone compared with chemotherapy plus radiotherapy for localized intermediate- and high-grade non-Hodgkin's lymphoma. N Engl M Med. 1998;339(1):21-26. [PMID: 9647875]

Rosenwald A, Wright G. Chan WC, et al; Lymphoma/Leukemia Molecular Profiling Project. The use of molecular profiling to predict survival after chemotherapy for diffuse large-B-cell lymphoma. N Engl J Med. 2002;346(25):1937-1947. [PMID: 12075054]

Solal-Céligny P, Roy P, Colombat P, et al. Follicular lymphoma international prognostic index. Blood. 2004;104:1258-1265. [PMID: 15126323]

The International NHL Prognostic Factors Project. A predictive model for aggressive non-Hodgkin's lymphoma. N Engl J Med. 1993;329(14);987-994. [PMID: 8141877]

Yee KWL, O'Brien SM. Chronic Lymphocytic Leukemia: Diagnosis and Treatment. Mayo Clin Proc. 2006;81(8):1105-1129. [PMID: 16901035]

Zelenetz AD, Advani RH, Buadi F, et al; National Comprehensive Cancer Network. Non-Hodgkin's lymphoma. Clinical Practice guidelines in oncology. J Natl Compr Canc Netw. 2006;4(3):258-310. [PMID: 16507273]

Cancer of Unknown Primary Site

Overview

Cancer of unknown primary site (CUP) accounts for 3% of all cancer diagnoses, accounting for more than 45,000 cancer-related deaths in the United States in 2007. Patients with CUP remain a heterogeneous group, having a variety of clinical presentations and pathologic findings. Unfortunately, the diagnosis of CUP usually represents a far-advanced malignancy that is rarely curable and is usually refractory to even palliative chemotherapy. Tumors that are potentially responsive to chemotherapy are found in only about 20% of all patients with CUP. Better radiographic imaging and improved pathologic techniques have led to a decrease in the incidence of cancer of truly "unknown" primary site.

Diagnostic and Prognostic Considerations

A patient is considered to have CUP when a tumor is detected at one or more metastatic sites, and routine evaluation fails to define a primary site. The initial workup of patients presenting with presumed CUP should not be exhaustive but should focus on evaluation of likely primary sites. This initial evaluation should include, at a minimum, a thorough history and physical examination (including a pelvic examination in women and a prostate examination in men), complete blood count, urinalysis, chemistries, a chest radiograph or CT scan of the chest, and CT of the abdomen and pelvis. Mammography should be considered in women with a clinical presentation compatible with metastatic breast cancer.

Pathologic confirmation of malignancy should be performed early in the diagnostic evaluation. Optimal pathologic evaluation, including special stains that might reveal tissue of origin, help to distinguish carcinoma from other cancer types, determine histologic type, and identify specific treatment target characteristics. Measurement of common tumor markers (carcinoembryonic antigen, CA 19-9, CA 15-3, and CA-125) should not be used as diagnostic or prognostic tests; however, some of these concentrations are frequently elevated in the serum of patients with adenocarcinoma of unknown primary site, and serial measurement may be useful in monitoring the response to therapy.

Radiologic evaluation may include CT scans and positron emission tomography (PET). The prognosis of patients with CUP is unaffected by whether the primary lesion is ever found. Unfavorable prognostic features include involvement of multiple metastatic sites, well-differentiated or moderately differentiated adenocarcinoma histology, older age, and lower performance status. All efforts to manage patients with CUP should aim to differentiate the few patients who have treatment-responsive disease and to not inflict unnecessary, invasive, and costly studies on the majority of patients who have disease that is refractory to most therapy.

KEY POINTS

- Patients with cancer of unknown primary site should receive a thorough history and physical examination focusing on the head and neck, rectum, pelvis, and breasts.
- In patients with suspected metastatic cancer and no obvious primary site, biopsy of the most accessible site should be performed before specialized laboratory studies are done.

- Although not useful as a diagnostic or prognostic test in patients with cancer of unknown primary site, measurement of common tumor markers such as CA-125 may be useful in monitoring the response to therapy.
- Unfavorable prognostic features in patients with cancer of unknown primary site include involvement of multiple metastatic sites, well-differentiated or moderately differentiated adenocarcinoma histology, older age, and lower performance status.

Subsets of Treatable CUP

Axillary Lymphadenopathy in Women

Women who present with axillary lymphadenopathy without other findings should be treated for stage II breast cancer. An occult primary tumor is identified on mastectomy in 50% to 60% of these patients, even when the physical examination and mammogram are normal. MRI of the breast can often identify a primary site even if mammography is normal and can often lead to breast conservation. Patients who have CUP with axillary lymphadenopathy only and who are found to have breast cancer have the same survival rate as patients with stage II disease.

Inguinal Lymphadenopathy

Identification of a primary site in the perineal area is important in patients with inguinal lymphadenopathy, because curative therapy is available for some patients, even in those with metastases to inguinal lymph nodes. Primary sites characterized by unilateral lymphadenopathy of the groin are the skin, anus, rectum, pelvis, and lower urinary tract. If no primary site is found on examination, a superficial groin lymph node dissection is appropriate. Half of patients treated with excisional biopsy or superficial groin dissection alone appear to live for more than 2 years. A significant proportion of these patients have unclassifiable carcinomas that are likely amelanotic melanomas.

Cervical Lymphadenopathy

Patients with cervical lymphadenopathy that reveals squamous cell carcinoma and no clinically apparent primary tumor should be treated as if they had a primary tumor site in the head or neck. Upper-airway panendoscopy, which consists of laryngoscopy, bronchoscopy, and esophagoscopy, and dedicated CT of the head and neck, must be performed as part of the diagnostic evaluation. Concurrent treatment with chemotherapy and radiation can lead to long-term survival rates as high as 60% to 70%, with the extent of cervical lymphadenopathy as the most important prognostic factor in these patients. Patients with lower cervical or supraclavicular lymphadenopathy are more likely to have tumors of adenocarcinoma histology and tend to have a much poorer prognosis than those with upper cervical lymphadenopathy and tumors with squamous cell histology.

Peritoneal Carcinomatosis in Women

In women presenting with a combination of peritoneal carcinomatosis and malignant ascites, ovarian cancer should be strongly considered. If no extraovarian site is determined, these patients should be treated as though they had stage III ovarian cancer, with initial cytoreductive surgery followed by chemotherapy. In these patients, measurement of serum CA-125 can be useful in monitoring the response to therapy. Approximately 15% to 20% of these patients survive 5 years.

Poorly Differentiated Carcinoma

This heterogeneous group of patients includes a few with highly responsive neoplasms and therefore requires special attention in the initial clinical and pathologic evaluation. Young men with a predominant tumor location in the mediastinum and retroperitoneum may have the extragonadal germ-cell cancer syndrome. Serum levels of human chorionic gonadotropin and α-fetoprotein should be measured, and these patients should be treated as though they had poor-prognosis testicular cancer, with chemotherapy administration and surgical resection of residual radiographic abnormalities. Some of these patients have poorly differentiated neuroendocrine tumors of unknown primary site. These tumors, which are almost always characterized by liver metastases, are distinct from well-differentiated neuroendocrine tumors in their biology and treatment. Up to 15% of these patients will experience durable complete remissions with chemotherapy.

Systemic therapy for patients not included in any specific treatable subgroup of patients with CUP, which includes most patients with CUP, is difficult. Current empiric chemotherapy regimens have improved the treatment results for this group of patients, with a median survival of 10 to 12 months.

KEY POINTS

- Women who present with metastatic axillary lymphadenopathy without other findings should be treated for stage II breast cancer.
- Patients with cervical lymphadenopathy that reveals squamous cell carcinoma and no clinically apparent primary tumor should be treated as if they had a primary tumor site in the head or neck.
- Women with a combination of peritoneal carcinomatosis and malignant ascites without other findings should be treated as though they had stage III ovarian cancer.
- Young men with a predominant tumor location in the mediastinum and retroperitoneum and elevated serum levels of human chorionic gonadotropin and α-fetoprotein should be treated as though they had poor-prognosis testicular cancer.

Bibliography

Bugat R, Bataillard A, Lesimple T, et al; FNCLCC. Summary of the Standards, Options, and Recommendations for the management of patients with carcinoma of unknown primary site (2002). Br J Cancer. 2003;89(Suppl 1):S59-66. [PMID: 12915904]

Hainsworth JD, Erland JB, Kalman LA, Schreeder MT, Greco FA. Carcinoma of unknown primary site: treatment with 1-hour paclitaxel, carboplatin, and extended-schedule etoposide. J Clin Oncol. 1997;15(6):2385-2393. [PMID: 9196154]

Hainsworth JD, Greco FA. Treatment of patients with cancer of an unknown primary site. N Engl J Med. 1993;329(4):257-263. [PMID: 8316270]

Lenzi R, Hess KR, Abbruzzese MC, Raber MN, Ordoñez NG, Abbruzzese JL. Poorly differentiated carcinoma and poorly differentiated adenocarcinoma of unknown origin: Favorable subsets of patients with unknown primary carcinoma. J Clin Oncol. 1997;15(5):2056-2066. [PMID: 9164218]

Orel SG, Weinstein SP, Schnall MD, et al. Breast MR imaging in patients with axillary node metastases and unknown primary malignancy. Radiology. 1999;212(2):543-9. [PMID: 10429716]

Pavlidis N, Briasoulis E, Hainsworth J, Greco FA. Diagnostic and therapeutic management of cancer of an unknown primary. Eur J Cancer. 2003;39(14):1990-2005. [PMID: 12957453]

Oncologic Urgencies and Emergencies

Structural Urgencies and Emergencies

Superior Vena Cava Syndrome

Superior vena cava (SVC) syndrome, an oncologic urgency, is an often missed and, consequently, delayed diagnosis. This syndrome is caused by obstruction of blood flow through the SVC, which is the major vessel through which blood drains from the head, neck, upper extremities, and upper thorax. The most common cause of SVC syndrome is lung cancer, accounting for approximately 70% of cases. Other malignant causes include lymphoma and tumors metastatic to the mediastinum.

SVC syndrome typically has an insidious onset, with dyspnea the most common presenting symptom. Other symptoms include cough, upper extremity swelling, chest pain, and dysphagia. It is sometimes difficult to determine whether symptoms result from the SVC obstruction or invasion or compression of other structures in that area by the tumor. Common physical examination findings in SVC syndrome include venous distention of the neck and chest wall, facial edema, plethora, and cyanosis. These signs and symptoms are often exacerbated by lying down, stooping, or bending forward. The most common radiographic abnormalities in SVC syndrome are superior mediastinal widening and pleural effusion. CT is useful in providing detailed information about the SVC and its tributaries as well as the bronchi and lungs. Radionuclide imaging or contrast venography may also be useful in determining the patency of the SVC.

The treatment goals in patients with SVC syndrome are palliation and, if possible, cure of the primary causative process; the primary disorder in SVC syndrome determines treatment. Radiation therapy is the mainstay of treatment, but chemotherapy may also be used for typically chemoresponsive tumors, such as small cell lung cancer, non-Hodgkin lymphoma, and germ cell neoplasms. The role of anticoagulation for patients with SVC obstruction and thrombosis is controversial but may be warranted, especially in patients with chemoresponsive tumors. Endovascular angioplasty and stenting, as well as thrombolysis, may be used to provide symptomatic relief before more specific therapy is administered.

KEY POINTS

- The most common cause of superior vena cava syndrome is lung cancer; other malignant causes are lymphoma and tumors metastatic to the mediastinum.
- Superior vena cava syndrome develops insidiously, with dyspnea the most common presenting symptom; other symptoms are cough, upper extremity swelling, chest pain, and dysphagia.
- Radiation therapy is the mainstay of treatment of superior vena cava syndrome.

Brain Metastases with Increased Intracranial Pressure

Primary and metastatic brain tumors may lead to increased intracranial pressure (ICP). Headache is the most common symptom of increased ICP and is often severe and persistent despite analgesia and of maximum intensity in the morning on awakening.

Although a severe morning headache may occur as a sign of increased ICP, nonspecific headaches, cognitive changes, focal neurologic findings, and seizures may all be manifestations. Funduscopic examination may reveal papilledema (**Figure 38**).

Imaging studies, such as CT and MRI, are useful in confirming the diagnosis of increased ICP and brain metastases. Lumbar puncture may precipitate brain herniation in patients with space-occupying lesions of the central nervous system and increased ICP and, in general, should not be performed. Increased ICP may initially be managed with corticosteroids administered at moderate (dexamethasone, 6 to 10 mg every 6 hours) to high (dexamethasone, up to 100 mg/d) doses, although an improved response has not been established for higher doses, and the risk for adverse events increases with higher doses. Corticosteroids should be avoided in patients in whom a primary central nervous system lymphoma is suspected until a diagnosis is established. Osmotic diuresis with hyperosmolar agents such as mannitol may also be helpful in the initial management of increased ICP. Symptomatic, obstructive hydrocephalus is a neurosurgical emergency requiring immediate drainage. Ultimately, however, the

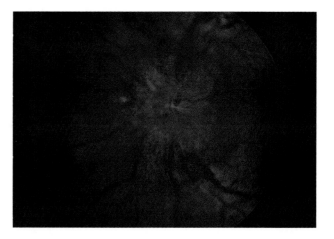

FIGURE 38.
Funduscopic examination results indicating papilledema in a patient with brain metastases characterized by increased intracranial pressure.

definitive treatment of increased ICP depends on the primary diagnosis and may include neurosurgical resection, chemotherapy, and radiation therapy. Surgical resection is the standard approach for patients with a resectable, single metastasis to the brain. A randomized trial showed a survival benefit for such patients treated with resection plus whole-brain radiation therapy compared with whole-brain radiation therapy alone.

KEY POINTS

- Headache is the most common symptom of increased intracranial pressure and is often severe and persistent despite analgesia and of maximum intensity in the morning on awakening.
- Lumbar puncture should be avoided in patients with space-occupying lesions of the central nervous system and increased intracranial pressure because it may precipitate brain herniation.
- Increased intracranial pressure may initially be managed with corticosteroids, except in those in whom a primary central nervous system lymphoma is suspected, until a diagnosis is established.

Spinal Cord Compression

The most common cause of spinal cord compression is tumor metastasis to a vertebral body, resulting in direct extension into the epidural space or a pathologic fracture. Pain is the most common initial presenting symptom in patients with spinal cord compression, with neurologic symptoms typically evolving later. It is important to establish the diagnosis before the patient develops motor weakness or other neurologic deficits, because a significant percentage of patients with spinal cord compression fail to recover neurologic function. MRI of the entire spine is the most commonly used diagnostic test for evaluating spinal cord compression because multiple levels of spinal involvement may be present in up to 30%

of patients. Corticosteroids should be administered immediately in patients with suspected spinal cord compression for improved pain management and prevention of further neurologic impairment, with dexamethasone the most commonly used therapeutic regimen. When feasible, decompressive surgery followed by radiation therapy is more effective than radiation alone in treating selected patients with spinal cord compression caused by metastatic cancer. In patients not amenable to surgery, radiation therapy is the standard treatment. Systemic chemotherapy is useful in patients with highly chemosensitive tumors such as lymphoma.

KEY POINTS

- Establishing a diagnosis of spinal cord compression before motor weakness or other neurologic deficits occur is important to avoid permanent loss of neurologic function.

- MRI of the entire spine is the most commonly used diagnostic test for evaluating spinal cord compression.

- Corticosteroids should be administered immediately in patients with suspected spinal cord compression for improved pain management and prevention of further neurologic impairment.

- Radiation therapy is the most commonly used definitive therapy for patients with spinal cord compression.

Metabolic Urgencies and Emergencies

Tumor Lysis Syndrome

Tumor lysis syndrome occurs when spontaneous or treatment-induced lysis of malignant cells results in the release of intracellular products, causing hyperkalemia, hyperuricemia, hyperphosphatemia, hypocalcemia, acute renal failure, and disseminated intravascular coagulation. Typically, tumor lysis syndrome occurs within 1 to 5 days of treatment and develops most commonly in patients with hematologic malignancies or other rapidly dividing tumors, such as acute leukemia and high-grade lymphoma; this syndrome occurs much less commonly in patients with solid tumors. Risk factors for tumor lysis syndrome include bulky disease, a high leukocyte count, high pretreatment levels of lactate dehydrogenase or uric acid, compromised renal function, and use of nephrotoxic agents.

Tumor lysis syndrome and its complications can be prevented and managed by aggressive hydration with diuresis and use of allopurinol and rasburicase. Although urine alkalinization is widely used, it remains somewhat controversial because it increases the precipitation of calcium phosphate complexes.

Hyperkalemia and other metabolic abnormalities of this condition should be aggressively treated. If acute renal failure develops, hemodialysis may be indicated.

KEY POINTS

- Tumor lysis syndrome can typically occur within 1 to 5 days of treatment in patients with hematologic malignancy or other rapidly dividing tumors.

- Risk factors for tumor lysis syndrome are bulky disease, a high leukocyte count, high pretreatment levels of lactate dehydrogenase or uric acid, compromised renal function, and use of nephrotoxic agents.

Hypercalcemia

Hypercalcemia occurs most commonly in patients with breast, kidney, lung, and head and neck cancer and in those with multiple myeloma. Its incidence and severity are decreasing because of the routine use of bisphosphonates in patients with solid tumors metastatic to bone and in those with multiple myeloma. Hypercalcemia may occur as a result of osteolytic activity in bone or more often as a paraneoplastic syndrome mediated by factors produced by malignant cells, such as parathyroid hormone–related protein. Symptoms of hypercalcemia include nausea, vomiting, constipation, polyuria, and mental status changes.

Intravenous hydration with isotonic saline, forced diuresis/calciuresis with furosemide (after rehydration), and administration of bisphosphonates are the mainstays of treatment of hypercalcemia of malignancy. The most commonly used bisphosphonates to treat this condition are pamidronate and zoledronate. Agents such as gallium nitrate, plicamycin, and calcitonin are used less frequently. Corticosteroids are also used to lower serum calcium levels in patients whose underlying tumor is corticosteroid responsive, such as those with lymphoma or myeloma.

KEY POINTS

- Hypercalcemia occurs most frequently in patients with breast, kidney, lung, and head and neck cancer and in those with multiple myeloma.

- Symptoms of hypercalcemia include nausea, vomiting, constipation, polyuria, and mental status changes.

- Intravenous hydration with isotonic saline, forced diuresis/calciuresis with furosemide (after rehydration), and administration of bisphosphonates are the mainstays of treatment of hypercalcemia of malignancy.

Chemotherapy-Related Toxicities

Chemotherapy and antitumor biologic agents can produce various organ toxicities (**Table 43**), and some of these may be true medical emergencies, such as cytotoxic chemotherapy-induced neutropenic fever. The prompt administration of empiric antibiotics has significantly lowered the mortality rate in affected patients. Diarrhea resulting from capecitabine, 5-fluorouracil, and irinotecan can lead to life-threatening volume

TABLE 43 Chemotherapy-induced Toxicities

Chemotherapy Toxicities	Representative Chemotherapeutic Agents
Myelosuppression	Most cytotoxic drugs
Emesis	Cisplatin, doxorubicin, cyclophosphamide
Diarrhea	5-FU, capecitabine, irinotecan
Alopecia	Doxorubicin, paclitaxel, cyclophosphamide
Stomatitis	Doxorubicin, methotrexate
Vesicant	Doxorubicin, mitomycin
Peripheral neuropathy	Paclitaxel, docetaxel, cisplatin, vincristine
Pulmonary toxicity	Bleomycin, mitomycin
Renal toxicity	Cisplatin, ifosfamide
Cardiac toxicity	Doxorubicin
Gonadal toxicity	Alkylating agents (e.g., cyclophosphamide)
Carcinogenicity	Alkylating agents, etoposide, and doxorubicin (AML), cyclophosphamide (bladder cancer), tamoxifen (endometrial cancer)
Biologicals and Targeted Therapy	**Representative Biologicals and Targeted Therapy Toxicities**
Infusion reactions	Rituximab, trastuzumab, bevacizumab
Rash	Cetuximab, erlotinib
Fatigue	Sorafenib, sunitinib
Thrombosis/bleeding	Bevacizumab
Reactivation of viral diseases	Rituximab (hepatitis B), alemtuzumab (cytomegalovirus)
Reversible posterior leukoencephalopathy	Rituximab

5-FU = 5-fluorouracil; AML = acute myeloid leukemia.

depletion, and even death, in some patients, particularly the elderly. Severe anaphylactic-type infusion reactions can occur with certain chemotherapeutic agents such as paclitaxel and carboplatin and may occur commonly with monoclonal antibodies such as rituximab. Chemotherapy infusion centers must be aware of and prepared to treat these potential reactions. Anthracycline, nitrogen mustard, and mitomycin are vesicants, and extravasation may lead to severe ulceration. Prompt diagnosis and treatment in affected patients, and early plastic surgery consultation are crucial to avoid extensive skin damage and injury to the deep structures of the arm or hand. Bleomycin, methotrexate, gemcitabine, and mitomycin may cause acute pulmonary pneumonitis with respiratory failure. The recognition and treatment of these pulmonary syndromes with corticosteroids may result in rapid improvement.

KEY POINTS

- Gastrointestinal side effects, mucositis, and hematologic side effects are common chemotherapy-induced toxicities.
- Prompt recognition and treatment of anthracycline- and vinca alkaloid agent–induced extravasation injury are necessary to avoid severe skin damage in patients receiving chemotherapy.

Bibliography

Altman A. Acute tumor lysis syndrome. Semin Oncol. 2001;28(2 suppl 5):3-8. [PMID: 11343271]

Baeksgaard L, Sorensen JB. Acute tumor lysis syndrome in solid tumors-a case report and review of the literature. Cancer Chemother Pharmacol. 2003;51(3):187-192. [PMID: 12655435]

Forsyth PA, Posner JB. Headaches in patients with brain tumors: a study of 111 patients. Neurology. 1993;43(9):1678-1683. [PMID: 8414011]

Levack P, Graham J, Collie D, et al; Scottish Cord Compression Study Group. Don't wait for a sensory level-listen to the symptoms: a prospective audit of the delays in diagnosis of malignant cord compression. Clin Oncol (R Coll Radiol). 2002;14(6):472-480. [PMID: 12512970]

Patchell RA, Tibbs PA, Regine WF, Payne R, Saris S, Kryscio RJ, Mohiuddin M, Young B. Direct decompressive surgical resection in the treatment of spinal cord compression caused by metastatic cancer: a randomised trial. Lancet. 2005;366(9486):643-648. [PMID: 16112300]

Rowell NP, Gleeson FV. Steroids, radiotherapy, chemotherapy and stents for superior vena caval obstruction in carcinoma of the bronchus: a systematic review. Clin Oncol (R Coll Radiol). 2002;14(5):338-351. [PMID: 12555872]

Schiff D, O'Neill BP, Wang CH, O'Fallon JR. Neuroimaging and treatment implications of patients with multiple epidural spinal metastases. Cancer. 1998;83(8):1593-1601. [PMID: 9781953]

Sørensen S, Helweg-Larsen S, Mouridsen H, Hansen HH. Effect of high-dose dexamethasone in carcinomatous metastatic spinal cord compression treated with radiotherapy: a randomized trial. Eur J Cancer. 1994;30A(1):22-7. [PMID: 8142159]

Effects of Cancer and Cancer Therapy

Cardiac Issues

Asymptomatic and symptomatic abnormalities in left ventricular function have been associated with all of the anthracycline agents, which are widely used in the treatment of childhood and adult malignancies. The risk for developing doxorubicin-induced cardiomyopathy is dose related. Trastuzumab can result in heart failure; however, unlike anthracycline-related heart failure, trastuzumab-induced heart failure may be at least partially reversible with or without medical treatment and does not appear to be dose related.

Radiation therapy to the mediastinum (as in the treatment of Hodgkin lymphoma) may result in progressive cardiac sequelae including inflammation and fibrosis of all structures in the heart, leading to abnormalities in left ventricular function and mass, valvular dysfunction, and premature coronary artery disease (see Cardiovascular Disease syllabus).

KEY POINTS

- Asymptomatic and symptomatic abnormalities in left ventricular function have been associated with all of the anthracycline agents.
- Patients with cancer who received trastuzumab may develop heart failure.
- Abnormalities in valvular function and left ventricular size and function may occur in long-term survivors of Hodgkin lymphoma who have undergone radiation therapy.

Pulmonary Issues

Bleomycin, commonly used to treat germ cell tumors and lymphoma (especially Hodgkin lymphoma), may result in pulmonary toxicity, most commonly bleomycin-induced pneumonitis (BIP). Risk factors that predispose patients to BIP include a cumulative dose of bleomycin, advanced age, tobacco use, renal dysfunction, mediastinal radiation therapy, and oxygen administration. There is a possibility of severe anesthesia risk after bleomycin if high concentrations of oxygen are given. Although BIP typically begins during therapy, it may develop after completion of therapy. BIP resolves in most patients after discontinuation of bleomycin and corticosteroids; however, pulmonary fibrosis develops in a small percentage of patients.

Radiation-induced pneumonitis has been described in patients treated with radiation therapy to the mediastinum and thorax. Factors increasing the risk for radiation pneumonitis include concomitant chemotherapy, prior radiation therapy, and recent withdrawal of corticosteroids.

KEY POINTS

- Risk factors for bleomycin-induced pneumonitis include a cumulative dose of bleomycin, advanced age, tobacco use, renal dysfunction, mediastinal radiation therapy, and oxygen administration.
- Bleomycin-induced pneumonitis resolves in most patients after discontinuation of bleomycin and corticosteroids.
- Factors increasing the risk for radiation pneumonitis include concomitant chemotherapy, prior radiation therapy, and recent withdrawal of corticosteroids.

Reproductive Issues

Infertility due to chemotherapy or radiation therapy is a common issue for cancer survivors. It may occur transiently, during treatment, or permanently. Fertility in women may be impaired despite regular menses. Infertility may present later as premature ovarian failure. The risk for infertility varies depending on the cancer treatment regimen. Fertility preservation options in men and women undergoing cancer treatment are an active area of research. The American Society of Clinical Oncology recommends that fertility preservation methods be considered as early as possible during cancer treatment planning. For men, freezing/storing sperm prior to chemotherapy is an option. For women with partners, storing of embryos is an option. In addition to infertility, both men and women may experience severe symptoms from hormone deprivation for the treatment of breast cancer and prostate cancer, resulting in major impairment of their quality of life. Impotence may also occur after surgery and/or radiation therapy for prostate cancer. The incidence of congenital anomalies or fetal wastage among cancer survivors who are able to conceive is no higher than that in the general population.

KEY POINTS

- Freezing or storing sperm prior to chemotherapy is an option for men in managing potential cancer therapy–related reproductive issues.
- For women with partners, storing of embryos is an option for managing potential cancer therapy–related reproductive issues.
- The incidence of congenital anomalies or fetal wastage among cancer survivors who are able to conceive is no higher than that in the general population.

Cognitive Issues

Some cancer survivors report cognitive impairment during and after chemotherapy. Women treated with endocrine therapy for breast cancer also report this issue. This is a relatively new area of research, and there are many difficulties in interpreting the published data because of a lack of pretreatment assessments and appropriate control groups, variation in measuring instruments, and use of inconsistent criteria for defining cognitive impairment. A further complicating factor is that cognitive dysfunction is often reported in cancer patients prior to therapy.

Other Issues

In general, patients who have received extensive corticosteroid exposure as part of their chemotherapy regimen are at risk for aseptic necrosis of the hips/ankles, cataracts, and osteoporosis.

Radiation to the cervical lymph nodes or neck significantly increases the risk for hypothyroidism. Patients who have received such therapy should be monitored for hypothyroidism.

KEY POINTS

- Some cancer survivors report cognitive impairment during and after chemotherapy.

- Patients who have received radiation therapy to the cervical lymph nodes or neck should be evaluated for hypothyroidism.

Secondary Malignancies

Secondary malignancies can result from cancer therapy. An increased risk for breast cancer has been identified in patients who have received mantle radiation therapy for Hodgkin lymphoma. Cancer survivors who were treated at age 25 years with chest radiation therapy have an estimated cumulative risk of breast cancer by ages 35, 45, and 55 years of 1.4%, 11.1%, and 29%, respectively. Although still very rare, the incidence of soft-tissue sarcoma is also increased following radiation therapy. Chemotherapy can also cause secondary malignancies (See Table 43 from Oncologic Urgencies and Emergencies section).

Information on supportive and palliative care for patients with cancer is available to physicians and patients at the National Cancer Institute Web site (www.cancer.gov/cancertopics/pdq/supportivecare).

KEY POINT

- Cancer survivors who were treated at age 25 years with chest radiation therapy have an estimated cumulative risk of breast cancer at ages 35, 45, and 55 years of 1.4%, 11.1%, and 29%, respectively.

Bibliography

Adams MJ, Lipsitz SR, Colan SD, et al. Cardiovascular status in long-term survivors of Hodgkin's disease treated with chest radiotherapy. J Clin Oncol. 2004;22(15):3139-3148. [PMID: 15284266]

Carver JR, Shapiro CL, Ng A, et al; ASCO Cancer Survivorship Expert Panel. American Society of Clinical Oncology clinical evidence review on the ongoing care of adult cancer survivors: cardiac and pulmonary late effects. J Clin Oncol. 2007;25(25): 3991-4008. [PMID: 17577017]

Ewer MS, Vooletich MT, Durand JB, et al. Reversibility of trastuzumab-related cardiotoxicity: new insights based on clinical course and response to medical treatment. J Clin Oncol. 2005;23(31):7820-7826. [PMID: 16258084]

Ganz PA. Monitoring the physical health of cancer survivors: a survivorship-focused medical history. J Clin Oncol. 2006;24(32):5105-5111. [PMID: 17093271]

Hermelink K, Untch M, Lux MP, et al. Cognitive function during neoadjuvant chemotherapy for breast cancer: results of a prospective, multicenter, longitudinal study. Cancer. 2007;109(9):1905-1913. [PMID: 17351951]

Hillner BE, Ingle JN, Chlebowski RT, et al; American Society of Clinical Oncology. American Society of Clinical Oncology 2003 update on the role of bisphosphonates and bone health issues in women with breast cancer. J Clin Oncol. 2003;21(21):4042-4057. [PMID: 12963702]

Lee, SL, Schover LR, Partridge AH, et al; American Society of Clinical Oncology. American Society of Clinical Oncology Recommendations on fertility preservation in cancer patients. J Clin Oncol. 2006;24(18):2917-31. [PMID: 16651642]

National Cancer Institute. Facing Forward: Life After Cancer Treatment. www.cancer.gov/cancertopics/life-after-treatment. Accessed July 21, 2008.

O'Sullivan JM, Huddart RA, Norman AR, Nicholls J, Dearnaley DP, Horwich A. Predicting the risk of bleomycin lung toxicity in patients with germ-cell tumors. Ann Oncol. 2003;14(1):91-96. [PMID: 12488299]

Sleijfer S. Bleomycin-induced pneumonitis. Chest. 2001;120(2):617-624. [PMID: 11502668]

Travis LB, Hill DA, Dores GM, et al. Cumulative absolute breast cancer risk for young women treated for Hodgkin lymphoma. J Natl Cancer Inst. 2005;97(19):1428-1437. [PMID: 16204692]

Vardy J, Rourke S, Tannock IF. Evaluation of cognitive function associated with chemotherapy: a review of published studies and recommendations for future research. J Clin Oncol. 2007;25(17):2455-2463. [PMID: 17485710]

Self-Assessment Test

This self-assessment test contains one-best-answer multiple-choice questions. Please read these directions carefully before answering the questions. Answers, critiques, and bibliographies immediately follow these multiple-choice questions. The American College of Physicians is accredited by the Accreditation Council for Continuing Medical Education (ACCME) to provide continuing medical education for physicians.

The American College of Physicians designates MKSAP 15 Hematology and Oncology for a maximum of 14 *AMA PRA Category 1 Credits*™. Physicians should only claim credit commensurate with the extent of their participation in the activity. Separate answer sheets are provided for each book of the MKSAP program. Please use one of these answer sheets to complete the Hematology and Oncology self-assessment test. Indicate in Section H on the answer sheet the actual number of credits you earned, up to the maximum of 14, in ¼-credit increments. (One credit equals one hour of time spent on this educational activity.)

Use the self-addressed envelope provided with your program to mail your completed answer sheet(s) to the MKSAP Processing Center for scoring. Remember to provide your MKSAP 15 order and ACP ID numbers in the appropriate spaces on the answer sheet. The order and ACP ID numbers are printed on your mailing label. If you have *not* received these numbers with your MKSAP 15 purchase, you will need to acquire them to earn CME credits. E-mail ACP's customer service center at custserv@acponline.org. In the subject line, write "MKSAP 15 order/ACP ID numbers." In the body of the e-mail, make sure you include your e-mail address as well as your full name, address, city, state, ZIP code, country, and telephone number. Also identify where you have made your MKSAP 15 purchase. You will receive your MKSAP 15 order and ACP ID numbers by e-mail within 72 business hours.

CME credit is available from the publication date of July 31, 2009, until July 31, 2012. You may submit your answer sheets at any time during this period.

Self-Scoring Instructions:

Hematology and Oncology

Compute your percent correct score as follows:

Step 1: Give yourself 1 point for each correct response to a question.

Step 2: Divide your total points by the total number of questions: 100.

The result, expressed as a percentage, is your percent correct score.

	Example	Your Calculations
Step 1	85	
Step 2	85 ÷ 100	÷ 100
% Correct	85%	%

Hematology Questions

Item 1

A 72-year-old man is hospitalized because of dyspnea, anginal chest pain, and new-onset anemia. Chronic lymphocytic leukemia was diagnosed 2 years ago. He has not received specific therapy and has never required a blood transfusion.

On physical examination, the patient appears pale. Blood pressure is 110/80 mm Hg, pulse rate is 112/min, and respiration rate is 24/min. Diffuse cervical, axillary, and inguinal lymphadenopathy is present. There is no jugular venous distention. The lungs are clear. Abdominal examination reveals splenomegaly. There is no peripheral edema.

Laboratory studies:

Hemoglobin	6.0 g/dL (60 g/L)
Leukocyte count	55,000/µL (55 × 10⁹/L) with 90% lymphocytes
Platelet count	115,000/µL (115 × 10⁹/L)
Reticulocyte count	12% of erythrocytes
Total bilirubin	2.8 mg/dL (47.9 µmol/L)
Direct bilirubin	0.6 mg/dL (10.26 µmol/L)
Direct antiglobulin (Coombs test)	Positive for IgG
ABO/Rh blood type	A positive

A peripheral blood smear shows microspherocytes.

Corticosteroid therapy is begun, and a cross-match for two units of packed erythrocytes is ordered. However, no compatible units are available in the blood bank.

Which of the following is the most appropriate management at this time?

(A) Begin erythropoietin
(B) Schedule splenectomy
(C) Transfuse one unit of A-positive packed erythrocytes
(D) Transfuse one unit of O-negative packed erythrocytes
(E) Withhold transfusion until a compatible unit of blood is available

Item 2

A 70-year-old man is evaluated for a 2-week history of a progressive burning sensation in his hands and feet and constant discomfort and dull pain in his legs. Medical history is significant for symptomatic multiple myeloma that developed 2 years ago and was treated with oral thalidomide and dexamethasone. He recently experienced a relapse of myeloma and has completed four cycles of therapy with bortezomib and dexamethasone. He also has type 2 diabetes mellitus that has been well controlled for 10 years with oral hypoglycemic agents.

On physical examination, he is afebrile; blood pressure is 138/80 mm Hg, pulse rate is 70/min, and respiration rate is 15/min. There is no evidence of retinopathy, organomegaly, lymphadenopathy, or skin changes. Neurologic examination discloses bilateral loss of ankle-stretch reflexes and hyperesthesia in a "stocking-glove" distribution to the ankles and wrists bilaterally. Vibratory and position sensation are intact, and muscle strength is normal. The remainder of the physical examination is normal.

Laboratory studies:

Hemoglobin	11.0 g/dL (110 g/L)
Calcium	9.2 mg/dL (2.3 mmol/L)
Creatinine	1.4 mg/dL (106.8 µmol/L)
Hemoglobin A₁c	6%
Albumin	3.8 g/dL (38 g/L)

Which of the following is the most likely cause of this patient's current symptoms?

(A) Bortezomib toxicity
(B) Diabetic neuropathy
(C) Multiple myeloma–induced neuropathy
(D) POEMS syndrome

Item 3

A 27-year-old black man is admitted to the hospital following his first episode of diabetic ketoacidosis. The patient has also had bacterial sinusitis for which he has been taking trimethoprim-sulfamethoxazole for the past 4 days. He has also noticed that his urine is dark. Additional medications are lispro and glargine insulins.

On physical examination, the patient appears to be uncomfortable. He has scleral icterus. Temperature is 37.8 °C (100.2 °F), blood pressure is 127/66 mm Hg, pulse rate is 112/min, and respiration rate is 25/min. Tachycardia is heard on cardiac auscultation, but cardiac examination is otherwise unremarkable. Abdominal examination discloses diffuse abdominal tenderness but no hepatosplenomegaly.

Laboratory studies:

Hemoglobin	10.2 g/dL (102 g/L)
Reticulocyte count	11% of erythrocytes
Lactate dehydrogenase	1145 U/L
Total bilirubin	5.1 mg/dL (87.2 µmol/L)
Indirect bilirubin	4.6 mg/dL (78.7 µmol/L)
Urinalysis	3+ ketones, 3+ bilirubin

A peripheral blood smear is shown.

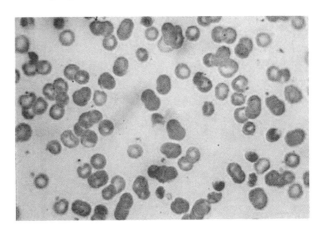

Which of the following is the most likely diagnosis?

(A) Glucose 6-phosphate dehydrogenase (G6PD) deficiency
(B) Hereditary spherocytosis
(C) Microangiopathic hemolytic anemia
(D) Warm antibody–mediated hemolytic anemia

Item 4

A 67-year-old man comes for a routine physical examination. The patient has hypertension treated with hydrochlorothiazide.

On physical examination, temperature is normal, blood pressure is 140/85 mm Hg, pulse rate is 88/min, and respiration rate is 16/min. The patient has a ruddy complexion. There is no jugular venous distention. Cardiopulmonary examination is normal. The spleen tip is palpable just below the left costal margin.

Laboratory studies:

Hematocrit	61%
Leukocyte count	11,200/µL (11.2 × 10^9/L)
Platelet count	405,000/µL (405 × 10^9/L)
Erythropoietin	10 mU/mL (10 U/L)
Arterial oxygen saturation	96% (on ambient air)

Cytogenetic studies show a *JAK2* mutation.

Which of the following is the most appropriate treatment?

(A) Therapeutic phlebotomy
(B) Therapeutic phlebotomy plus anagrelide
(C) Therapeutic phlebotomy plus aspirin
(D) Therapeutic phlebotomy plus hydroxyurea

Item 5

An 18-year old man is evaluated 5 hours after a routine tooth extraction in which he experienced excessive bleeding that the dentist was able to control. The patient is healthy and takes no medications, including aspirin or NSAIDs. Medical history includes easy bruisability and occasional nose bleeds that are easily controllable. The patient was circumcised at birth and recalls his mother saying that he had more bleeding than expected from the circumcision site. His father also has easy bruisability.

Physical examination is unremarkable, with no evidence of petechiae, ecchymoses, or abnormal vasculature.

Laboratory studies:

Hemoglobin	14.2 g/dL (142 g/L)
Platelet count	195,000/µL (195 × 10^9/L)
INR	1.1
Activated partial thromboplastin time (aPTT)	41 s
aPTT mixing study	Corrects to normal
Thrombin time	16 s (control, 15 s)
Fibrinogen	266 mg/dL (2.66 g/L)
D-dimer assay	Negative
Bleeding time	10 min
Factor VIII activity	60% (normal, 65%-120%)

Which of the following is the most likely diagnosis?

(A) Factor XI deficiency
(B) Hemophilia A (factor VIII deficiency)
(C) Presence of a lupus inhibitor
(D) Vitamin K deficiency
(E) von Willebrand disease

Item 6

A 63-year-old man is evaluated during a follow-up visit after a recent diagnosis of immune thrombocytopenic purpura. His initial platelet count at diagnosis was 10,000/µL for which he was given corticosteroid therapy and experienced an initial increase to 15,000/µL (15 × 10^9/L) followed by an increase to 60,000/µL (60 × 10^9/L) over 1 week before the platelet count returned to 10,000/µL (10 × 10^9/L) 3 months after the corticosteroids were tapered and withdrawn. The corticosteroid treatment was then repeated, but the platelet count once again decreased to the 10,000/µL (10 × 10^9/L) range 3 months after an initial response.

The patient's other medical problems include obesity and a 10-year history of type 2 diabetes mellitus, hypertension, and heart failure. Each time the patient receives corticosteroids, his blood glucose becomes more difficult to control, resulting in symptomatic hyperglycemia requiring the use of basal and short-acting insulin. His current medications include aspirin, glipizide, metformin, metoprolol, lisinopril, and hydrochlorothiazide.

On physical examination, vital signs are normal. BMI is 31. The patient has petechiae on the lower extremities, and there is evidence of gingival bleeding and recent epistaxis. Cardiopulmonary examination reveals an S$_3$ and clear lungs. There is trace pedal edema. The remainder of the physical examination is noncontributory.

The patient's blood type is A negative.

After discussing the risks and benefits of various treatment options, the patient declines splenectomy and additional courses of corticosteroids.

Which of the following is the most appropriate next step in treatment to achieve a prompt increase of his platelet count?

(A) Azathioprine
(B) Cyclophosphamide
(C) Danazol
(D) Intravenous immune globulin
(E) Platelet transfusion

Item 7

A 42-year-old man is hospitalized because of hematuria. The patient has a mechanical mitral valve and has been taking warfarin, 5 mg/d.

On physical examination, he is alert and appears pale. Blood pressure is 105/65 mm Hg, pulse rate is 96/min, and respiration rate is 16/min. The lungs are clear.

Laboratory studies:

Hemoglobin	8.0 g/dL (80 g/L)
Platelet count	200,000/µL (200 × 10^9/L)

INR	7.0
Activated partial thromboplastin time	28 s
Urinalysis	Gross blood

Three units of fresh frozen plasma are transfused over the next 4 hours. Halfway through the third unit, the patient develops severe dyspnea without chest pain or cough. Temperature is normal, blood pressure is 115/70 mm Hg, pulse rate is 104/min, and respiration rate is 28 min. Arterial oxygen saturation on ambient air is 86%. Bibasilar crackles are auscultated. There is no S_3 on cardiac examination, jugular venous distention, or peripheral edema.

A chest radiograph shows bilateral pulmonary infiltrates. Serum B-type-natriuretic peptide level is normal.

Which of the following is the most likely diagnosis?

(A) Anaphylaxis
(B) Aspiration pneumonia
(C) Pulmonary embolism
(D) Heart failure
(E) Transfusion-related acute lung injury

Item 8

A 58-year-old man is evaluated for increasing fatigue of 2 months' duration. The patient has hypertension and hyperlipidemia treated with lisinopril and atorvastatin. A sister has hypothyroidism.

On physical examination, temperature is normal, blood pressure is 135/80 mm Hg, pulse rate is 72/min, and respiration rate is 18/min. There is no lymphadenopathy or peripheral edema. The spleen is palpable 4 cm below the left costal margin.

Laboratory studies:

Hemoglobin	12.1 g/dL (121 g/L)
Leukocyte count	55,200/μL (55.2 × 10⁹/L)
Platelet count	105,000/μL (105 × 10⁹/L)

A peripheral blood smear shows an increased number of granulocytic cells in all phases of development but no Auer rods in the blasts. Bone marrow examination shows hypercellular marrow (80% cellularity) with marked granulocytic hyperplasia, a left shift in the granulocytes, and 3% myeloblasts. Cytogenetic testing reveals a *BCR/ABL* translocation.

Which of the following is the most appropriate next step in managing this patient?

(A) Administration of imatinib
(B) HLA typing of the patient and his sister
(C) Leukapheresis
(D) Observation with monthly follow-up office visits

Item 9

A 19-year-old female college student is treated for a deep venous thrombosis, which occurred after she took a long flight on her return from school. Her only medication is an oral contraceptive she began taking 6 months prior to the diagnosis.

The patient is instructed to stop taking oral contraceptives and is given therapy with low-molecular-weight heparin followed by warfarin to achieve a target INR of 2.5.

Which of the following is the best duration of anticoagulation for this patient?

(A) Lifelong anticoagulation
(B) 12 months
(C) 3 to 6 months
(D) 4 to 6 weeks

Item 10

A 64-year-old man is evaluated during a routine examination. Medical history is significant for osteoarthritis, for which he takes aspirin and acetaminophen.

On physical examination, pallor is absent. Blood pressure is 116/72 mm Hg, with no orthostatic changes, and pulse rate is 68/min. The remainder of the examination is normal.

Laboratory studies:

Hemoglobin	9.7 g/dL (97 g/L)
Leukocyte count	5800/μL (5.8 × 10⁹/L)
Platelet count	265,000/μL (265 × 10⁹/L)
Mean corpuscular volume	72 fL
Reticulocyte count	0.5% of erythrocytes
Lactate dehydrogenase	80 U/L
Iron	40 μg/dL (7.2 μmol/L)
Total iron-binding capacity	200 μg/dL (35.8 μmol/L)
Ferritin	210 ng/mL (210 mg/L)

Results of the peripheral blood smear are normal.

Which of the following is the most likely diagnosis?

(A) Inflammatory anemia
(B) Hemoglobin C disease
(C) Iron deficiency
(D) Thalassemia

Item 11

A 66-year-old woman is evaluated for a 1-month history of gradually increasing headache, blurred vision, and episodes of confusion. Medical and family histories are unremarkable. She takes no medications.

On physical examination, she is afebrile; blood pressure is 150/80 mm Hg, and pulse rate is 90/min. Ophthalmoscopic examination reveals dilated, segmented, and tortuous retinal veins. On cardiopulmonary auscultation, an S_3 is heard, and the lungs are clear. Abdominal examination discloses hepatosplenomegaly.

Laboratory studies:

Hemoglobin	8.5 g/dL (85 g/L)
Leukocyte count	14,000/μL (14 × 10⁹/L), with 80% lymphocytes
IgM	4800 mg/dL (48 g/L)
Lactate dehydrogenase	80 U/L

A chest radiograph shows cardiac enlargement. A CT scan of the abdomen and pelvis shows an enlarged liver and spleen and many enlarged retroperitoneal lymph nodes. Bone marrow aspirate and biopsy reveals 70% replacement with lymphoplasmacytic cells.

Which of the following is the most appropriate next therapeutic option?

(A) Blood transfusion

(B) Furosemide

(C) Plasma exchange

(D) Intravenous immune globulin

Item 12

A 26-year-old woman is admitted to the hospital for treatment of deep venous thrombosis of the right lower extremity confirmed by duplex Doppler ultrasonography. Medical history is noncontributory, and her only medication is an oral contraceptive.

On physical examination, there is mild scleral icterus. Temperature is 37.2° C (99.9 °F), blood pressure is 110/67 mm Hg, pulse rate is 100/min, and respiration rate is 16/min. Abdominal examination discloses mild splenomegaly.

Laboratory studies:

Hemoglobin	10.0 g/dL (100 g/L)
Leukocyte count	2700/μL (2.7 × 10⁹/L)
Platelet count	42,000/μL (42 × 10⁹/L)
Reticulocyte count	8% of erythrocytes
Mean corpuscular volume	70 fL
Total bilirubin	5.0 mg/dL (85.5 μmol/L)
Direct bilirubin	0.8 mg/dL (13.7 μmol/L)
Lactate dehydrogenase	1126 U/L

Alanine aminotransferase, aspartate aminotransferase, and alkaline phosphatase levels are normal. A bone marrow biopsy reveals hypocellular bone marrow, absent iron stores, and signs of early myelodysplasia. The results of a direct and indirect antiglobulin (Coombs) test are negative.

Which of the following is the most appropriate diagnostic test to determine the cause of this patient's hematologic abnormalities?

(A) Flow cytometry

(B) Hemoglobin electrophoresis

(C) Osmotic fragility study

(D) Parvovirus B19 serology

Item 13

A 29-year-old woman is evaluated for a petechial rash of the lower extremities of 3 weeks' duration. The patient reports no bleeding problems except for recent, occasional bleeding from her gums after brushing her teeth. Medical history is otherwise unremarkable, and she takes no medications.

Physical examination reveals petechiae limited mainly to both lower extremities, with a few similar spots noted on her forearms and abdomen. The remainder of the examination is normal.

Laboratory studies:

Hemoglobin	12.5 g/dL (125 g/L)
Leukocyte count	8500/μL (8.5 × 10⁹/L)
Platelet count	14,000/μL (14 × 10⁹/L)
Reticulocyte count	2.0% of erythrocytes
INR	1.0
Activated partial thromboplastin time	26 s
Liver chemistry studies	Normal
Creatinine	0.8 mg/dL (61.0 μmol/L)
Antinuclear antibody assay	Negative
HIV antibody	Negative

A peripheral blood smear is shown.

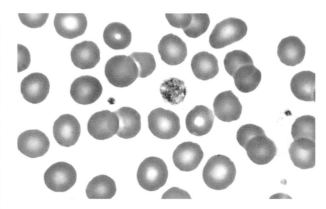

Which of the following is the most appropriate next step in management?

(A) Admit for urgent splenectomy

(B) Initiate corticosteroids

(C) Initiate platelet transfusion

(D) Observation alone

(E) Perform a bone marrow biopsy

Item 14

A 42-year-old woman is evaluated for swelling and discomfort of the right leg without an obvious precipitating event. She has no other medical problems.

On physical examination, vital signs are normal. Examination of the right lower extremity shows mild erythema, swelling, warmth, and tenderness to deep palpation of the calf. Cardiopulmonary and abdominal examinations are normal.

An ultrasound shows a right proximal, lower extremity, deep venous thrombosis.

Laboratory studies indicate a moderately elevated IgG anticardiolipin antibody level and the presence of a lupus inhibitor on coagulation testing.

The patient is treated with anticoagulation therapy. Repeat anticardiolipin antibody testing 12 weeks later confirms the previous results.

Which of the following is the most appropriate anticoagulation management for this patient?

(A) Anticoagulation therapy for a total of 12 months

(B) Anticoagulation therapy for a total of 6 months

(C) Cessation of anticoagulation therapy at 3 months

(D) Anticoagulation therapy indefinitely

Item 15

A 78-year-old woman has a 3-month history of increasing fatigue. She has no other medical problems and does not take any medications.

On physical examination, temperature is normal, blood pressure is 130/80 mm Hg, pulse rate is 72/min, and respiration rate is 16/min. The patient appears pale. Examination is unremarkable.

Laboratory studies:

Hemoglobin	7.8 g/dL (78 g/L)
Leukocyte count	2800/µL (2.8 × 10⁹/L)
Absolute neutrophil count	1200/µL (1.2 × 10⁹/L) (normal >1500/µL [1.5 × 10⁹/L])
Platelet count	560,000/µL (560 × 10⁹/L)
Erythropoietin	600 mU/mL (600 U/L)

Bone marrow examination shows hypercellular marrow with erythroid hyperplasia and dysplasia of the erythroid and granulocyte series. Megakaryocytes are increased with many hypolobulated cells. Iron stores are normal. Cytogenetic studies show deletion of the long arm of chromosome 5 [del(5q-)].

Which of the following is the most appropriate treatment?

(A) Azacitidine

(B) Danazol

(C) Lenalidomide

(D) Granulocyte colony-stimulating factor and recombinant erythropoietin

Item 16

A 58-year-old man is evaluated for preoperative clearance prior to elective hernia surgery after a prolonged activated partial thromboplastin time (aPTT) is found on laboratory studies. Personal and family history of abnormal bleeding is negative. Medical history is otherwise noncontributory, and the patient takes no medications.

The vital signs and general screening examination are normal.

The inhibitor mixing study corrects the prolonged aPTT, and factor assays indicate an isolated factor XI deficiency with a value of 47% of normal (normal, 70% to 120%).

Which of the following is the most appropriate management?

(A) Cancel surgery

(B) Proceed to surgery with no preoperative treatment

(C) Treat with factor VIII concentrate preoperatively

(D) Treat with cryoprecipitate preoperatively

(E) Treat with fresh frozen plasma therapy preoperatively

Item 17

A 62-year-old man undergoes a routine examination. The patient has a severe iron deficiency of many years' duration as well as hypertension. He also underwent a proximal small bowel resection 7 years ago necessitated by a gun shot injury. Current medications are ferrous sulfate, 325 mg/d, and atenolol, 50 mg/d.

On physical examination, he has pale conjunctivae. Temperature is 36.7 °C (98.0 °F), blood pressure is 136/75 mm Hg, pulse rate is 62/min, and respiration rate is 14/min.

Laboratory studies:

Hemoglobin	7.3 g/dL (73 g/L)
Mean corpuscular volume	58 fL
Reticulocyte count	0.2% of erythrocytes
Iron	13 µg/dL (2.3 µmol/L)
Total iron-binding capacity	427 µg/dL (76.4 µmol/L)
Ferritin	1 ng/mL (1 mg/L)

Which of the following is the most appropriate management?

(A) Add ascorbic acid to ferrous sulfate therapy

(B) Increase oral ferrous sulfate dosage to 650 mg/d

(C) Switch to deferoxamine

(D) Switch to intravenous iron

Item 18

A 54-year-old man is evaluated for increased lethargy and vague abdominal symptoms of 2 weeks' duration. His medical and family histories are noncontributory. He does not smoke cigarettes and takes no medications.

On physical examination, blood pressure is 136/82 mm Hg, pulse rate is 90/min, respiration rate is 18/min, and arterial oxygen saturation is 99% on ambient air. There is no clubbing or evidence of cyanosis. Cardiopulmonary examination is normal. The abdomen is soft, and there is no hepatosplenomegaly.

Laboratory studies:

Hemoglobin	20.2 g/dL (202 g/L)
Platelet count	312,000/µL (312 × 10⁹/L)
Leukocyte count	8200/µL (8.2 × 10⁹/L)
Erythropoietin	35 mU/mL (35 U/L)

Which of the following is the most appropriate next diagnostic test?

(A) Ultrasound of the abdomen

(B) Echocardiogram

(C) *JAK2* mutation analysis

(D) Erythrocyte mass study

Item 19

A 20-year-old black woman is evaluated in the hospital after admission 5 days ago with acute right hemispheric stroke. Medical history is significant for sickle cell disease complicated by multiple episodes of acute chest syndrome. Current medications are hydroxyurea and folic acid.

On physical examination, temperature is 37.5 °C (99.5 °F), blood pressure is 166/92 mm Hg, pulse rate is 112/min and regular, and respiration rate is 18/min. The cardiopulmonary examination is unremarkable. There are no carotid bruits. Right upper and lower extremity weakness and aphasia are noted on neurologic examination.

Laboratory studies indicate a hemoglobin level of 10.1 g/dL (101 g/L). An MRI shows an acute infarction in the territory of the right middle cerebral artery.

In addition to aspirin, which of the following is the most appropriate secondary prevention of stroke in this patient?

(A) Clopidogrel
(B) Dipyridamole
(C) Angiotensin-converting enzyme inhibitor
(D) Monthly erythrocyte transfusions

Item 20

A 72-year-old man undergoes preoperative evaluation 2 weeks prior to colonoscopy and polypectomy for a growth detected during an earlier procedure. Medical history is significant for a mechanical mitral valve. Medications include warfarin, metoprolol, and lisinopril.

Physical examination, including vital signs, is normal.

Which of the following is the most appropriate management of this patient?

(A) Continue with procedure without stopping warfarin
(B) Stop warfarin and begin low-molecular-weight-heparin preoperatively and resume both agents postoperatively
(C) Stop warfarin preoperatively and resume postoperatively
(D) Stop warfarin preoperatively, use fresh frozen plasma intraoperatively, and resume warfarin postoperatively
(E) Stop warfarin preoperatively, use vitamin K intraoperatively, and resume warfarin postoperatively

Item 21

A 42-year-old woman who is scheduled to undergo a hysterectomy for endometrial carcinoma comes for a preoperative evaluation. At the time of her initial evaluation, she was also discovered to have thrombocytosis. In addition to menorrhagia, the patient recently developed epistaxis and easy bruising. Her only medications are an oral contraceptive agent and an iron supplement.

On physical examination, temperature is normal, blood pressure is 110/70 mm Hg, pulse rate is 68/min, and respiration rate is 16/min. Examination is normal. No petechiae, ecchymoses, or splenomegaly is noted.

Repeat laboratory studies:

Hemoglobin	11.3 g/dL (113 g/L)
Leukocyte count	4600/µL (4.6 × 10⁹/L)
Platelet count	1,500,000/µL (1500 × 10⁹/L)

Platelet function studies show abnormal platelet aggregation with a decreased response to adenosine diphosphate and collagen. Cytogenetic studies reveal a *JAK2* mutation. Bone marrow examination shows hypercellular marrow with increased megakaryocytes in clusters.

Which of the following is the most appropriate treatment?

(A) Anagrelide beginning 2 days preoperatively
(B) Hydroxyurea beginning the night after surgery
(C) Low-dose aspirin postoperatively
(D) Platelet apheresis preoperatively and hydroxyurea postoperatively

Item 22

A 27-year-old woman undergoes follow-up evaluation 5 months after diagnosis of an idiopathic pulmonary embolism for which she was prescribed a 6-month course of anticoagulant therapy. Family history includes a maternal grandmother who took warfarin for many years for an unknown reason and an older brother with a history of deep venous thrombosis diagnosed at age 32 years. The patient takes no oral contraceptives or other medications and is otherwise healthy. The complete blood count is normal and the INR is 3.0.

Which of the following is the most appropriate next step in the evaluation of this patient?

(A) Immediate thrombophilic screening
(B) *JAK2* mutation analysis
(C) No further evaluation needed
(D) Thrombophilic screening at least 2 weeks after therapy cessation

Item 23

A 27-year-old woman is evaluated in the emergency department for a 2-day history of diffuse headache, fatigue, and gingival bleeding on brushing her teeth. She is otherwise healthy. Her only medication is an oral contraceptive, and medical and family histories are unremarkable.

On physical examination, she is alert and oriented but reports having a headache. Funduscopic examination is normal. There are a few scleral hemorrhages, and mild icterus is noted. Petechiae that had gone unnoticed by the patient are visible on the lower extremities. Cardiopulmonary and abdominal examinations are normal.

Laboratory studies:

Hemoglobin	8 g/dL (80 g/L)
Platelet count	34,000/µL (34 × 10⁹/L)
Reticulocyte count	12% of erythrocytes
INR	1.1
Activated partial thromboplastin time (aPTT)	32 s
Thrombin time	16 s (control, 15 s)
Lactate dehydrogenase	2000 U/L
Serum creatinine	0.8 mg/dL (61 µmol/L)
D-dimer assay	Negative

A peripheral blood smear is shown on the next page.

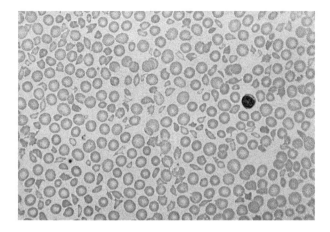

Which of the following is the most appropriate next step in management?

(A) aPTT mixing study
(B) Direct antiglobulin (Coombs) test
(C) Intravenous immune globulin
(D) Plasma exchange
(E) Platelet antibody test

Item 24

A 19-year-old black man is evaluated in the emergency department for a 2-day history of pain in the upper and lower extremities and back. His medical history includes episodes of achy pain in his extremities and back, but this is the first time his pain was severe enough to seek medical attention. Medical history is also remarkable for anemia of unknown cause. Family history is positive for anemia. Other than poor exercise tolerance, the patient has no other medical problems, no allergies, and takes no medications.

On physical examination, there are mildly icteric sclerae. Temperature is 37.2 °C (99.0 °F), blood pressure is 126/62 mm Hg, pulse rate is 112/min, and respiration rate is 18/min; BMI is 22. There is no splenomegaly or hepatomegaly on abdominal examination.

Laboratory studies:

Hemoglobin	10.2 g/dL (102 g/L)
Leukocyte count	8600/µL (8.6 × 10⁹/L)
Mean corpuscular volume	70 fL
Total bilirubin	5.7 mg/dL (97.5 µmol/L)
Direct bilirubin	0.3 mg/dL (5.1 µmol/L)

The peripheral blood smear shows rare sickled erythrocytes and target cells.

Hemoglobin electrophoresis:

Hemoglobin S	67% (0%)
Hemoglobin F	3% (0-2%)
Hemoglobin A	25% (94.8%-97.8%)
Hemoglobin A₂	5% (2.2 %-3.2%)

Which of the following is the most likely diagnosis?

(A) Sickle cell trait (AS)
(B) Sβ+ thalassemia

(C) Hemoglobin SC disease
(D) Hemoglobin S with hereditary persistence of fetal hemoglobin

Item 25

A 37-year-old man with HIV infection has a 1-week history of increasing fatigue and dyspnea on exertion. He is receiving highly active antiretroviral therapy and trimethoprim-sulfamethoxazole.

On physical examination, temperature is normal, blood pressure is 120/70 mm Hg, pulse rate is 72/min, and respiration rate is 24/min. The patient appears pale but does not have jaundice or a rash. Examination is unremarkable. There is no lymphadenopathy, organomegaly, or edema. A stool sample is negative for occult blood.

Laboratory studies:

Hemoglobin	7.2 g/dL (72 g/L)
Leukocyte count	4600/µL (4.6 × 10⁹/L)
Platelet count	346,000/µL (346 × 10⁹/L)
Reticulocyte count	0.3% of erythrocytes
Erythropoietin	500 mU/mL (500 U/L)
Haptoglobin	72 mg/dL (720 mg/L)
Ferritin	55 ng/mL (55 mg/L)
Iron	135 µg/dL (24.2 µmol/L)
Transferrin saturation	65%
Lactate dehydrogenase	124 U/L
Direct antiglobulin (Coombs) test	Negative

A peripheral blood smear shows normocytic, normoblastic erythrocytes without inclusion bodies. Bone marrow examination reveals a mildly hypocellular marrow with giant pronormoblasts. Parvovirus B19 DNA is present in the serum and bone marrow. There are no IgG antibodies to parvovirus.

Which of the following is the most appropriate treatment?

(A) Erythrocyte transfusion, antithymocyte globulin, and cyclosporine
(B) Erythrocyte transfusion, cytarabine, and an anthracycline
(C) Erythrocyte transfusion and intravenous immune globulin
(D) Recombinant erythropoietin

Item 26

A 37-year-old man undergoes follow-up evaluation after a recent diagnosis of an idiopathic deep venous thrombosis (DVT) for which he has been receiving oral anticoagulant therapy consisting of warfarin for the past 6 months. This was his first episode, and he has had no postthrombotic symptoms and is doing well. He wishes to avoid ongoing anticoagulation if his risk of a recurrent venous thrombosis is acceptably low.

Physical examination is normal.

The patient stops taking warfarin at the end of his 6-month treatment regimen.

Which of the following is most helpful in identifying this patient's risk for recurrent DVT?

(A) C-reactive protein measurement

(B) D-dimer measurement

(C) Homocysteine measurement

(D) Methylenetetrahydrofolate reductase genotype analysis

Item 27

A 77-year-old man has a 1-year history of increasing fatigue. He has not seen a physician for at least 3 years. Medical and family histories are unremarkable, and he takes no medications.

On physical examination, the patient appears pale. Temperature is normal, blood pressure is 140/85 mm Hg, pulse rate is 72/min, and respiration rate is 16/min. There is no scleral icterus or jugular venous distention. Cardiopulmonary examination is normal. The spleen is palpable 6 cm below the left costal margin.

Laboratory studies:

Hemoglobin	7.6 g/dL (76 g/L)
Leukocyte count	11,200/μL (11.2 × 10⁹/L)
Platelet count	104,000/μL (104 × 10⁹/L)
Haptoglobin	Elevated
Direct antiglobulin (Coombs) test	Negative

A bone marrow aspiration reveals a "dry tap." A peripheral blood smear and bone marrow biopsy are shown.

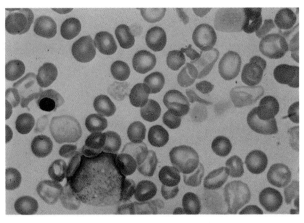

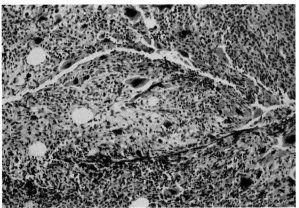

Cytogenetic studies are negative for the Philadelphia chromosome.

Which of the following is the most likely diagnosis?

(A) Aplastic anemia

(B) Chronic myeloid anemia

(C) Myelofibrosis

(D) Pure red cell aplasia

Item 28

A 25-year-old man is evaluated for the recent onset of fever, fatigue, dyspnea, easy bruising, and bleeding gums. Medical and family histories are unremarkable, and he takes no medications.

On physical examination, temperature is 38.8 °C (101.8 °F), blood pressure is 105/60 mm Hg, pulse rate is 120/min, and respiration rate is 24/min. Petechiae are present on the buccal mucosa and extremities. Cervical and axillary lymphadenopathy is noted. Cardiopulmonary examination is normal. The liver edge and spleen tip are palpable. There is bilateral peripheral edema.

Laboratory studies:

Hemoglobin	8.5 g/dL (85 g/L)
Leukocyte count	104,000/μL (104 × 10⁹/L)
Absolute neutrophil count	600/μL (0.6 × 10⁹/L) (normal >1500/μL [1.5 × 10⁹/L])
Platelet count	17,000/μL (17 × 10⁹/L)
Reticulocyte count	0.3% of erythrocytes
Lactate dehydrogenase	2200 U/L
Uric acid	11.5 mg/dL (0.68 mmol/L)

A chest radiograph shows a mediastinal mass. Bone marrow examination reveals hypercellular marrow that is virtually replaced with large blasts containing prominent nucleoli and abundant basophilic cytoplasm. The blasts do not contain Auer rods. Sudan black and myeloperoxidase stains are negative; periodic acid-Schiff stain is positive. Blasts are also positive for terminal deoxynucleotidyl transferase (TdT). Immunophenotyping shows CD2, CD3, CD7, and CD38. No *BCR/ABL* translocation is present.

Which of the following is the most likely diagnosis?

(A) Acute lymphoblastic leukemia

(B) Acute myeloid leukemia

(C) Chronic lymphocytic leukemia

(D) Hodgkin lymphoma

Item 29

A 59-year-old man is evaluated for a 4-day history of progressive worsening of fatigue, forgetfulness, constipation, excessive thirst, and increased urination. He has no pain. The patient has hypertension, treated with hydrochlorothiazide, and type 2 diabetes mellitus, controlled by diet. He developed right lower lobe streptococcal pneumonia 3 months ago.

On physical examination, he appears somnolent but is easily arousable. Temperature is 37.1 °C (98.8 °F), blood pressure is 110/70 mm Hg, pulse rate is 120/min, and respiration rate is 17/min. The oral mucosa is dry, and the conjunctivae are pale. The lungs are clear.

Laboratory studies:

Hemoglobin	8.9 g/dL (89 g/L)
Platelet count	150,000/µL (150 × 10⁹/L)
Leukocyte count	2500/µL (2.5 × 10⁹/L)
Calcium	13.6 mg/dL (3.4 mmol/L)
Creatinine	2.9 mg/dL (221.3 µmol/L)
Total protein	7.6 g/dL (76 g/L)
Albumin	3.3 g/dL (33 g/L)
Urinalysis	Negative for protein

A peripheral blood smear shows normochromic, normocytic erythrocytes with rouleaux formation, and no evidence of tear drop erythrocytes or immature myeloid and erythroid cells.

A chest radiograph shows osteopenia of all ribs. No pulmonary parenchymal infiltrates are seen.

The patient is hospitalized and responds to intravenous hydration with normal saline. He undergoes bone marrow aspiration while results of other laboratory tests are pending. Results are shown.

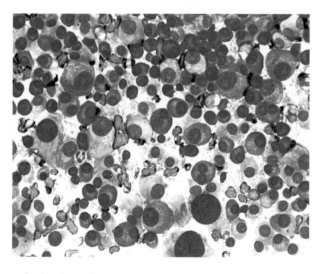

Which of the following is the most likely diagnosis?

(A) Acute myeloid leukemia
(B) Chronic lymphocytic leukemia
(C) Metastatic small cell lung cancer
(D) Multiple myeloma

Item 30

A 46-year-old black man is evaluated in the emergency department with swelling of the feet and ankles and a 2-month history of worsening dyspnea. The patient has homozygous sickle cell disease and a history of lower extremity ulcers and episodes of acute chest syndrome. Current medications are hydroxyurea and folic acid. There are no known drug or other allergies.

On physical examination, temperature is normal, blood pressure is 145/85 mm Hg, pulse rate is 98/min, and respiration rate is 28/min; BMI is 22. Jugular venous pressure is elevated and is associated with large *a* and *v* waves. On cardiac examination, there is a heave, fixed splitting of S₂ with a palpable P₂, and a systolic murmur at the lower left sternal border that increases with respiration. The lungs are clear. Examination of the lower extremities shows 2+ edema bilaterally.

The chest radiograph reveals enlargement of the central pulmonary arteries with clear lung fields. Echocardiography discloses a normal left ventricular ejection fraction, right ventricular enlargement and hypertrophy, right atrial enlargement, tricuspid regurgitation, and paradoxical bulging of the septum into the left ventricle during systole.

Which of the following is the most likely cause of this patient's findings?

(A) Constrictive pericarditis
(B) Giant cell myocarditis
(C) Pulmonary hypertension
(D) Hypertrophic cardiomyopathy

Item 31

A 33-year-old woman who recently completed chemotherapy for Hodgkin lymphoma requires an urgent tooth extraction. She does not have bruising or bleeding.

Physical examination is unremarkable; no petechiae or purpura is present. The platelet count is 25,000/µL (25 × 10⁹/L).

Transfusion with which of the following is most appropriate before the dental procedure?

(A) One bag of apheresis platelets
(B) Two bags of apheresis platelets
(C) One unit of fresh frozen plasma
(D) One unit of platelet concentrate

Item 32

A 55-year-old man has a 1-year history of fatigue, daytime hypersomnolence, and frequent nighttime awakenings. The patient has hypertension and a 48-pack-year smoking history. His only medication is lisinopril. His family history is noncontributory.

On physical examination, temperature is normal, blood pressure is 135/85 mm Hg, pulse rate is 88/min, and respiration rate is 28/min. BMI is 35. Examination is otherwise unremarkable.

Laboratory studies:

Hematocrit	59%
Leukocyte count	5700/µL (5.7 × 10⁹/L)
Platelet count	345,000/µL (345 × 10⁹/L)
Erythropoietin	30 mU/mL (30 U/L)
Arterial oxygen saturation (on ambient air)	95%

Hematocrit measurements prior to 5 years ago were all normal.

Cytogenetic studies are negative for the *JAK2* gene mutation.

Which of the following is the most likely cause of the patient's elevated hematocrit?

(A) Relative polycythemia
(B) High-oxygen–affinity hemoglobin
(C) Polycythemia vera
(D) Secondary polycythemia

Item 33

A 37-year-old woman undergoes preoperative evaluation prior to a hysterectomy for worsening menstrual bleeding of several years' duration caused by uterine fibroids. She has a recent history of recurrent epistaxis and bleeding after recent dental work but denies thromboembolism and a family history of unusual bleeding. The patient is otherwise healthy. Her only medication is an occasional aspirin.

The pelvic examination reveals a slightly enlarged, irregular uterus. The remainder of the physical examination is normal.

Laboratory studies:

Hemoglobin	11 g/dL (110 g/L)
Platelet count	182,000/µL (182 × 10⁹/L)
INR	1.1
Activated partial thromboplastin time (aPTT)	52 s

Which of the following is the most appropriate next diagnostic test?

(A) Anticardiolipin antibody assay
(B) aPTT mixing study
(C) Factor VIII assay
(D) von Willebrand factor assay

Item 34

An asymptomatic 35-year-old man comes for a routine annual examination. Medical and family histories are unremarkable, and his only medication is a daily multivitamin.

On physical examination, temperature is normal, blood pressure is 120/70 mm Hg, pulse rate is 64/min, and respiration rate is 14/min. There are no abnormal findings.

Laboratory studies:

Hemoglobin	9.1 g/dL (91 g/L)
Leukocyte count	2100/µL (2.1 × 10⁹/L)
Platelet count	135,000/µL (135 × 10⁹/L)
Lactate dehydrogenase	890 U/L
Uric acid	11.6 mg/dL (0.68 mmol/L)

A peripheral blood smear shows circulating blasts and promyelocytes. Bone marrow examination shows hypercellular marrow with 80% myeloblasts and promyelocytes. Cytogenetic studies reveal translocation of chromosomes 15 and 17 [t(15;17)].

In addition to hydration and allopurinol, which of the following is the most appropriate management at this time?

(A) Broad-spectrum antibiotics
(B) Chemotherapy
(C) Chemotherapy plus all-*trans*-retinoic acid
(D) HLA typing

Item 35

A 33-year-old woman who has been trying to become pregnant for 8 years is evaluated after receiving positive pregnancy test results. Medical history is significant for three miscarriages 6 years ago, 3 years ago, and 1 year ago, each of which occurred early in her pregnancies. Following her last miscarriage, laboratory studies indicated the presence of a lupus inhibitor and antiphospholipid antibodies. She has no history of venous thromboembolism. Her last menstrual period was approximately 5 weeks ago.

Physical examination, including vital signs and abdominal examination, is normal.

Which of the following is the most appropriate anticoagulation regimen for the duration of this patient's pregnancy?

(A) Full-dose unfractionated heparin
(B) Low-dose aspirin
(C) Prophylactic-dose low-molecular-weight heparin (LMWH) plus low-dose aspirin
(D) Prophylactic-dose LMWH
(E) Warfarin

Item 36

A 27-year-old man is evaluated for new-onset anemia that was found during a routine complete blood count this morning. The patient has hereditary nephritis (Alport syndrome) and received a kidney transplant 2 months ago. Medications are cyclosporine, mycophenolate, prednisone, and trimethoprim-sulfamethoxazole. He has no other medical problems.

On physical examination, conjunctivae are pale. Temperature is 37.5 °C (99.5 °F), blood pressure is 136/82 mm Hg, pulse rate is 112/min, and respiration rate is 18/min. Petechiae are noted on the lower extremities. A nontender right pelvic kidney, with a well-healed surgical scar, is also noted.

Laboratory studies:

Hemoglobin	8.1 g/dL (81 g/L)
Platelet count	12,000/µL (12 × 10⁹/L)
Leukocyte count	8200/µL (8.2 × 10⁹/L)
Lactate dehydrogenase	1430 U/L
Creatinine	3.2 mg/dL (244.2 µmol/L)
Direct and indirect antiglobulin (Coombs) tests	Negative

A peripheral blood smear is shown on the next page.

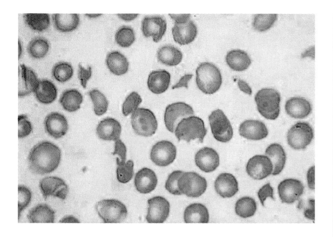

Which of the following medications is most likely responsible for this patient's findings?

(A) Cyclosporine
(B) Mycophenolate
(C) Prednisone
(D) Trimethoprim-sulfamethoxazole

Item 37

A 70-year-old malnourished man with a 4-year history of Alzheimer dementia is admitted to the intensive care unit from the emergency department for treatment of community-acquired pneumonia and impending respiratory failure. He is inattentive and confused and has a weak productive cough. His only medications are donepezil and memantine.

Temperature was 38.3 °C (101.0 °F), blood pressure 100/62 mm Hg, pulse rate 110/min, and respiration rate 26/min; BMI was 18. Arterial oxygen saturation on ambient air was 92%. Pulmonary examination revealed crackles in the right lower lobe. A chest radiograph confirmed an extensive right lower lobe pneumonia.

The patient was treated with ceftriaxone and azithromycin, oxygen, and low-dose unfractionated heparin, 5000 U, three times daily. During the subsequent 48 hours he had several episodes of hypotension and oxygen desaturation that responded to intubation, mechanical ventilation, and intravenous fluids. By day 4, his serum creatinine level increased to 4.0 mg/dL (305.2 μmol/L) before returning to his hospital-admission value of 1.2 mg/dL (91.6 μmol/L) by day 7. On day 8 he was successfully extubated and transferred to the medicine ward. His wife agreed to his transfer to a nursing home.

At day 10 of hospitalization he is ready for transfer, but he is eating little and develops new bruising on his extremities and gross hematuria.

Day 10 laboratory studies:

Platelet count	152,000/μL (152 × 10⁹/L)
INR	7.7
Activated partial thromboplastin time	46 s
Thrombin time	16 s (control, 15 s)
Fibrinogen	450 mg/dL (4.5 g/L)
D-dimer assay	Mildly elevated
Mixing study	Corrects to near normal

Which of the following is the most likely diagnosis?

(A) Disseminated intravascular coagulation
(B) Heparin toxicity
(C) Presence of a lupus inhibitor
(D) Vitamin K deficiency

Item 38

An 86-year-old woman is evaluated for a 6-month history of increasing fatigue and paresthesias of her toes. Medical history is significant for type 2 diabetes mellitus and hypertension. Current medications are metformin, lisinopril, and aspirin.

On physical examination, temperature is 36.6 °C (98.0 °F), blood pressure is 127/74 mm Hg, pulse rate is 97/min, and respiration rate is 12/min. Neurologic examination discloses normal vibratory sense and proprioception in the toes and fingers. Monofilament testing for foot sensation is intact. The remainder of the neurologic and general physical examination is normal.

Laboratory studies:

Hemoglobin	11.8 g/dL (118 g/L)
Platelet count	102,000/μL (102 × 10⁹/L)
Reticulocyte count	0.8% of erythrocytes
Mean corpuscular volume	106 fL
Vitamin B₁₂	220 pg/mL (162.4 pmol/L)
Folate (serum)	22 ng/mL (49.8 nmol/L)
Lactate dehydrogenase	470 U/L

A peripheral blood smear shows macro-ovalocytes but no other abnormality.

Which of the following is the most appropriate next diagnostic test?

(A) Bone marrow biopsy
(B) Erythrocyte folate measurement
(C) Methylmalonic acid and homocysteine measurement
(D) Parietal cell antibody assay

Item 39

A 23-year-old black man with sickle cell disease is hospitalized because of fever, bone pain, and increasing jaundice. His most recent blood transfusion was 2 weeks ago, when he underwent hip replacement surgery for avascular necrosis.

On physical examination, the patient appears uncomfortable and has scleral icterus. Temperature is 38.4 °C (100.1 °F); other vital signs are normal. The remainder of the examination is unremarkable. There is no evidence of bleeding.

Hemoglobin concentration is 7.0 g/dL (70 g/L) compared with a measurement of 1 week ago of 9.0 g/dL (90 g/L). Platelet and leukocyte counts are normal. Results of the direct and indirect antiglobulin (Coombs) tests are positive, and a new erythrocyte alloantibody is identified by the blood bank.

Which of the following is the most likely diagnosis?

(A) Autoimmune hemolytic anemia
(B) Aplastic crisis
(C) Delayed hemolytic transfusion reaction
(D) Vaso-occlusive crisis

Item 40

A 57-year-old woman is brought to the emergency department because of fever and shaking chills of 8 hours' duration. The patient has a 1-year history of myelodysplastic syndrome treated with azacitidine.

On physical examination, temperature is 39.2 °C (102.6 °F), blood pressure is 100/70 mm Hg, pulse rate is 110/min, and respiration rate is 20/min. Examination is unremarkable. There is no rash, lymphadenopathy, costovertebral angle tenderness, abdominal tenderness, or splenomegaly.

Laboratory studies:
Hemoglobin	10.6 g/dL (106 g/L)
Leukocyte count	33,600/µL (33.6 × 10⁹/L)
Platelet count	88,000/µL (88 × 10⁹/L)
Urinalysis	Normal

Chest radiograph is normal.
A peripheral blood smear is shown.

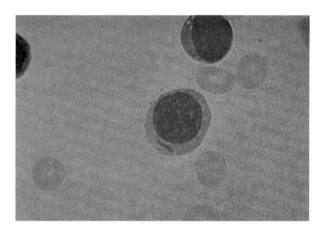

Which of the following is the most likely diagnosis?

(A) Acute lymphoblastic leukemia
(B) Acute myeloid leukemia
(C) Acute promyelocytic leukemia
(D) Chronic myeloid leukemia

Item 41

A 24-year-old black woman with sickle cell disease is admitted to the hospital with a typical painful crisis involving pain in the back and legs. The patient is 12 weeks' pregnant with her first child. She also has dysuria and urinary frequency and urgency. Her only medication is folic acid.

On physical examination, the patient is in obvious discomfort. Temperature is 38.7 °C (101.8 °F), blood pressure is 130/64 mm Hg, pulse rate is 112/min, and respiration rate is 22/min. Arterial oxygen saturation on ambient air is 95%. The patient has a gravid uterus appropriate for gestation. Her lungs are clear, and there is no costovertebral-angle tenderness.

Laboratory studies:
Hemoglobin	7.2 g/dL (72 g/L)
Leukocyte count	13,200/µL (13.2 × 10⁹/L)
Urinalysis	Positive for leukocyte esterase

A chest radiograph is normal.
She is treated with intravenous hydration, amoxicillin, and analgesics and does well and is now ready for discharge.

Which of the following medications is contraindicated in this patient?

(A) Oxycodone
(B) Acetaminophen
(C) Inactivated influenza vaccine
(D) Folic acid
(E) Hydroxyurea

Item 42

A 67-year-old woman is admitted to the hospital from the emergency department for a new diagnosis of left lower extremity, deep venous thrombosis confirmed by positive results on duplex ultrasonography. Medical history is significant for a 2-day hospitalization 4 weeks ago for a non-ST elevation myocardial infarction for which she underwent cardiac catheterization and was given low-molecular-weight heparin. Her current medications include aspirin, clopidogrel, pravastatin, and lisinopril.

On physical examination, the left thigh is swollen and tender. Complete blood count, electrolytes, and liver chemistry tests are unremarkable except for a platelet count of 102,000/µL (102 × 10⁹/L).

Unfractionated heparin is administered. Twelve hours later, the patient's platelet count is 27,000/µL (27 × 10⁹/L).

Which of the following is the most appropriate next step in treatment?

(A) Continue heparin and administer a platelet transfusion
(B) Continue heparin and initiate high-dose corticosteroid therapy
(C) Stop heparin and initiate argatroban
(D) Stop heparin and initiate warfarin

Item 43

A 27-year-old woman (gravida 1, para 0) at 12 weeks' gestation is evaluated for a platelet count of 72,000/µL (72 × 10⁹/L); her complete blood count, including differential and peripheral blood smear, is otherwise normal. Her platelet count at the beginning of gestation was 102,000/µL (102 × 10⁹/L). There is no known history of thrombocytopenia, petechiae, bleeding, or induced or spontaneous abortions. Current medications include a prenatal vitamin only.

Physical examination, including vital signs and abdominal examination, is normal.

Which of the following is the most appropriate management?

(A) Corticosteroids
(B) Observation
(C) Plasma exchange
(D) Platelet transfusion
(E) Intravenous immune globulin

Item 44

A 57-year-old woman with chronic lymphocytic leukemia (CLL) is evaluated in the emergency department because of a 2-week history of increasing malaise, decreased exercise tolerance, and darkened urine. Her CLL was last treated 2 months ago with fludarabine, cyclophosphamide, and rituximab.

On physical examination, the patient has scleral icterus. Temperature is 37.3 °C (99.2 °F), blood pressure is 142/82 mm Hg, pulse rate is 117/min, and respiration rate is 18/min. Shotty lymphadenopathy is palpated in the cervical area. Cardiopulmonary examination discloses a regular tachycardia and crackles at the bases of both lungs. Splenomegaly is found on abdominal examination.

Laboratory studies:

Hemoglobin	6.9 g/dL (69 g/L)
Platelet count	250,000/µL (250 × 10⁹/L)
Leukocyte count	6500/µL (6.5 × 10⁹/L)
Reticulocyte count	10% of erythrocytes
Total bilirubin	6.3 mg/dL (107.7 µmol/L)
Direct bilirubin	0.5 mg/dL (8.6 µmol/L)
Lactate dehydrogenase	357 U/L
Direct antiglobulin (Coombs) test	Positive for IgG

A peripheral blood smear is shown.

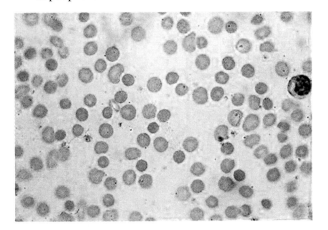

Which of the following is the most likely diagnosis?

(A) α-Thalassemia
(B) Autoimmune hemolytic anemia
(C) Hemoglobin C disease
(D) Microangiopathic hemolytic anemia

Item 45

A 50-year-old woman is evaluated in the emergency department for a 4-day history of pain, swelling, and erythema of the left leg. There is no history of recent immobilization, cancer, surgery, or deep venous thrombosis.

On physical examination, temperature is 37.7 °C (100.0 °F), blood pressure is 132/82 mm Hg, pulse rate is 65/min, and respiration rate is 16/min. Examination of the left leg discloses warmth and circumscribed erythema and tenderness limited to the posterior tibial portion of the leg. The circumference of the left leg is 1 cm greater than the right when measured 10 cm below the tibial tuberosity. Localized tenderness along the distribution of the deep venous system and pitting edema are absent as are venous varicosities.

Which of the following is the most appropriate next step in diagnosis?

(A) CT of the leg
(B) D-dimer assay
(C) Duplex ultrasonography
(D) MRI of the leg
(E) Venography

Item 46

A 28-year-old woman has a 3-month history of easy bruising and bleeding gums. She feels otherwise well. Medical and family histories are unremarkable, and she takes no medications.

On physical examination, temperature is normal, blood pressure is 110/70 mm Hg, pulse rate is 64/min, and respiration rate is 14/min. Petechiae are present on the buccal mucosa and pretibial areas, and ecchymoses are noted on the upper thighs. There is no lymphadenopathy or splenomegaly.

Laboratory studies:

Hemoglobin	10.4 g/dL (104 g/L)
Leukocyte count	5200/µL (5.2 × 10⁹/L)
Absolute neutrophil count	1200/µL (1.2 × 10⁹/L) (normal >1500/µL [1.5 × 10⁹/L])
Platelet count	18,000/µL (18 × 10⁹/L)
Reticulocyte count	0.9% of erythrocytes
Direct antiglobulin (Coombs) test	Negative

A peripheral blood smear shows no circulating blasts. The platelets are decreased and are not clumped, enlarged, or bizarre in appearance. Bone marrow examination shows hypoplastic marrow (<20% cellularity) with trilineage normoblastic maturation and normal iron stores. There are no findings suggesting an infiltrative disease and no increases in CD34 blasts or reticulin fibrosis.

Which of the following is the most likely diagnosis?

(A) Acute myeloid leukemia
(B) Aplastic anemia
(C) Immune thrombocytopenic purpura
(D) Myelodysplastic syndrome

Item 47

A 57-year-old woman is evaluated in the emergency department for a 1-week history of swelling and pain in the left lower extremity. She has had two normal pregnancies and no miscarriages. There is no family or personal history of thromboembolic disease. The patient is otherwise healthy.

A proximal deep venous thrombosis is confirmed on ultrasound. Unfractionated heparin is given as an initial bolus followed by a continuous infusion at a dose to prolong the activated partial thromboplastin time to two times the control value. Warfarin, 5 mg daily, is also initiated.

Which of the following is the most appropriate heparin therapy for this patient?

(A) Minimum of 5 days, with 2 INR measurements of ≥2, 24 h apart

(B) Minimum of 2 weeks, with 4 INR measurements of ≥2, 24 h apart

(C) Minimum of 3 days, with 1 INR measurement of ≥2

(D) Minimum of 24 hours, with 1 INR measurement of ≥2

Item 48

A 74-year-old woman is evaluated after a high serum total protein level was found during routine laboratory testing. Medical history is noncontributory except for hypertension treated with ramipril.

On physical examination, temperature is 37.0 °C (98.6 °F), blood pressure is 120/80 mm Hg, and pulse rate is 80/min. Examination is unremarkable; there is no organomegaly or lymphadenopathy.

Laboratory studies:

Hemoglobin	13.5 g/dL (135 g/L)
Leukocyte count	5500/µL (5.5 × 10⁹/L)
Platelet count	230,000/µL (230 × 10⁹/L)
Calcium	9.0 mg/dL (2.3 mmol/L)
Total protein	10.1 g/dL (101 g/L)
Albumin	4.0 g/dL (40 g/L)
Creatinine	1.0 mg/dL (76.3 µmol/L)

Serum protein electrophoresis shows a monoclonal spike of 1.8 g/dL, further identified as IgG-κ by serum immunofixation. Bone marrow aspirate reveals 6% plasma cells. Skeletal survey does not show any lytic lesions.

Which of the following is the most appropriate next step in this patient's management?

(A) Administration of bisphosphonates

(B) Administration of thalidomide and dexamethasone

(C) Positron emission tomography

(D) Repeat laboratory studies in 3 to 6 months

Item 49

A 22-year-old black man is evaluated for worsening of chronic anemia. His medical history is significant for sickle cell anemia complicated by frequent painful crises, cholecystitis, and one episode of acute chest syndrome that occurred 2 years ago with an accompanying stroke. To prevent stroke recurrence, he initially underwent monthly exchange transfusions, which were subsequently stopped owing to nonadherence. His current medications include hydroxyurea, folate, and oxycodone as needed for pain. The patient admits to difficulty remembering to take his medications, particularly since his stroke.

On physical examination, the patient has pale conjunctivae. Temperature is 36.6 °C (97.9 °F), blood pressure is 116/82 mm Hg, pulse rate is 112/min, and respiration rate is 18/min. Cardiopulmonary examination discloses tachycardia and an S₄; the lungs are clear. Examination of the abdomen shows a healed cholecystectomy scar. Neurologic examination reveals right-sided weakness with dysarthria. Vibratory sensation and position sense are intact.

Laboratory studies:

Hemoglobin	4.1 g/dL (41 g/L)
Leukocyte count	8200/µL (8.2 × 10⁹/L)
Platelet count	197,000/µL (197 × 10⁹/L)
Corrected reticulocyte count	0.7% of erythrocytes
Mean corpuscular volume	107 fL

Which of the following is the most likely diagnosis?

(A) Anemia of chronic disease

(B) Cobalamin deficiency

(C) Folate deficiency

(D) Hyperhemolysis

Item 50

A 50-year-old woman with advanced multiple myeloma diagnosed 6 months ago undergoes a follow-up visit. Treatment includes daily oral thalidomide and pulse dexamethasone. The patient now feels well.

Laboratory studies indicate a serum monoclonal protein concentration of 3.0 g/dL (30 g/L). Hemoglobin concentration, serum calcium level, and renal function studies are normal. A bone marrow aspirate shows reduction in plasma cells from 50% to 10%.

Which of the following is the most appropriate treatment to optimize this patient's disease-free and overall survival?

(A) Autologous stem cell transplantation

(B) Continuation of oral thalidomide

(C) Initiation of parenteral bisphosphonates

(D) Initiation of oral melphalan

Item 51

A 53-year-old woman presents for follow-up evaluation 2 years after undergoing matched-related–donor allogeneic stem cell transplantation for acute leukemia. The patient is scheduled to undergo right knee arthroplasty for osteoarthritis, and her orthopedic surgeon requests advice about use of perioperative blood transfusions. The patient feels well except for fatigue and right knee pain, and her leukemia is in complete remission. There is no record of any transfusion reactions during the stem cell transplantation 2 years ago. She has no other medical problems.

Physical examination is unremarkable except for hypertrophic changes of the right knee associated with a small effusion. The hemoglobin concentration is 10.0 g/dL (100 g/L).

Which of the following types of blood transfusion should be recommended intraoperatively and postoperatively, if needed?

(A) Autologous blood donation
(B) Leukoreduced irradiated blood
(C) Leukoreduced nonirradiated blood
(D) Washed blood

Item 52

A 28-year-old woman has an 8-month history of refractory immune (idiopathic) thrombocytopenia with resulting intermittent bleeding. Treatment with prednisone, intravenous immune globulin, and rituximab has been ineffective.

On physical examination, temperature is normal, blood pressure is 105/70 mm Hg, pulse rate is 72/min, and respiration rate is 16/min. Petechiae are present on the buccal mucosa and extremities. There is no splenomegaly.

Laboratory studies:

Hemoglobin	12.5 g/dL (125 g/L)
Leukocyte count	5800/µL (5.8 × 10⁹/L)
Platelet count	12,000/µL (12 × 10⁹/L)
Antinuclear antibody	Negative

A peripheral blood smear shows giant platelets. No platelet clumps or schistocytes are seen.

Which of the following is the most appropriate treatment?

(A) Dexamethasone by pulse administration
(B) Plasmapheresis
(C) Recombinant thrombopoietin
(D) Thrombopoietin receptor agonists (romiplostim or eltrombopag)

Item 53

A 54-year-old woman is evaluated because of gradually increasing swelling of both legs. She also has fatigue, dyspnea on exertion, easy bruising, and postural dizziness.

On physical examination, temperature is 36.9 °C (98.4 °F), blood pressure is 110/70 mm Hg reclining and 80/60 mm Hg standing, and pulse rate is 90/min. Examination findings of her tongue are shown.

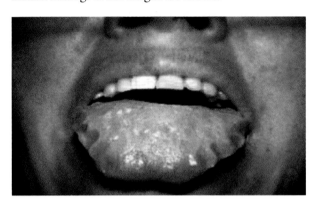

The submandibular glands are enlarged. No organomegaly is present. There is +3 bilateral pitting edema of both lower extremities.

Laboratory studies:

Hemoglobin	12.8 g/dL (128 g/L)
Leukocyte count	8000/µL (8 × 10⁹/L)
Platelet count	230,000/µL (230 × 10⁹/L)
INR	1.9
Activated partial thromboplastin time	28 s
Urinalysis	4+ protein; no erythrocytes or erythrocyte casts

Serum protein electrophoresis shows a 0.6-g/dL monoclonal protein spike, further identified as IgG-λ by serum immunofixation.

Which of the following is the most likely diagnosis?

(A) AL amyloidosis
(B) POEMS syndrome
(C) Multiple myeloma
(D) Monoclonal gammopathy of undetermined significance

Oncology Questions

Item 54

A 52-year-old woman undergoes evaluation for a recent abnormality of the right breast discovered on routine mammography. Her aunt died of breast cancer at age 85 years, but there is no other family history of breast or ovarian cancer. The patient is otherwise healthy.

Physical examination, including examination of the breasts and axillary lymph nodes, is normal. The complete blood count, metabolic profile, liver chemistry tests, urinalysis, and chest radiograph are normal.

A radiographic-guided needle biopsy reveals invasive ductal adenocarcinoma. The patient undergoes resection of the tumor and a sentinel lymph node biopsy of the right axilla. On pathologic examination, a 1.2-cm invasive ductal adenocarcinoma with free margins is confirmed, and the lymph node reveals no metastases.

Which of the following will be most helpful in directing the approach to management of this patient?

(A) Full right axillary lymph node dissection
(B) Genetic testing for the *BRCA1/2* mutation
(C) Tumor estrogen and progesterone receptor assay
(D) Whole-body positron-emission tomography

Item 55

Seven years ago, a 45-year-old man was diagnosed with a biopsy-proven mediastinal germ cell tumor. The patient was treated with combination chemotherapy (bleomycin, etoposide, and cisplatin) and had a complete radiographic response. He has been disease-free since completing therapy, and follow-up serum tumor marker measurements, chest radiographs, and CT scans of the abdomen and pelvis have been normal.

Which of the following is the most appropriate management at this time?

(A) Age- and sex-appropriate screening
(B) Audiometry
(C) Exercise stress test
(D) Pulmonary function tests
(E) Renal ultrasonography

Item 56

A 54-year-old man from Jamaica is evaluated because of a 2-month history of fatigue, indigestion, abdominal bloating, and early satiety. Over-the-counter antacids provide only minimal relief.

Physical examination reveals a thin, tired-appearing man who seems older than his stated age. Vital signs are normal. There is no supraclavicular lymphadenopathy. Abdominal examination discloses normal bowel sounds and no evidence of an abdominal mass, tenderness to palpation, or hepatomegaly.

A stool specimen obtained on rectal examination is positive for occult blood. The hemoglobin concentration is 9.8 g/dL (98 g/L).

Upper endoscopy shows gastric ulceration, and biopsy specimens document *Helicobacter pylori* organisms and moderately differentiated invasive adenocarcinoma. A CT scan of the abdomen and pelvis shows no evidence of distant disease. However, lymph nodes measuring up to 2.1 cm are seen in the retrocrural area. The liver appears normal.

Which of the following is the most appropriate treatment at this time?

(A) Chemotherapy
(B) Chemotherapy, radiation therapy, and surgical resection
(C) Omeprazole, amoxicillin, clarithromycin, and metronidazole
(D) Radiation therapy
(E) Surgical resection

Item 57

A 56-year-old man with a 9-year history of compensated cirrhosis secondary to alcoholism is evaluated because of new-onset, right upper-quadrant abdominal pain and an unexplained 2.2-kg (5-lb) weight loss. He has also recently developed a cough. He has no other medical problems and has abstained from drinking alcohol since his diagnosis of cirrhosis. Because his cirrhosis has been stable for many years, the patient elected to forgo routine follow-up and has not seen a physician for 3 years.

On physical examination, vital signs are normal. BMI is 24. There are numerous spider angiomas on the face, chest, and arms. Cardiopulmonary examination results are normal. The abdomen is slightly protuberant, and a nodular liver edge is easily palpable 4 cm below the right costal margin.

Laboratory studies:

Total bilirubin	1.7 mg/dL (29.1 µmol/L)
Alanine aminotransferase	80 U/L
Aspartate aminotransferase	125 U/L
α-Fetoprotein	550 ng/mL (550 µg/L)

A chest radiograph shows multiple pulmonary nodules. A CT scan of the chest and abdomen reveals a cirrhotic liver with diffuse nodules and periportal lymphadenopathy.

Which of the following is the most appropriate treatment at this time?

(A) Chemoembolization
(B) Doxorubicin
(C) Liver transplantation
(D) Sorafenib
(E) Surgical resection

Item 58

A 67-year-old postmenopausal woman has a 3-month history of vague abdominal discomfort and bloating and a

4.5-kg (10.0-lb) weight gain with increased abdominal girth. There is no change in appetite or bowel habits and no vaginal bleeding or discharge. The patient has a 20-pack-year smoking history but quit smoking 10 years ago. Results of a screening colonoscopy performed 7 years ago were normal. Her mother was diagnosed with breast cancer at age 72 years, and her father developed cardiovascular disease at age 76 years.

On physical examination, temperature is 37.2 °C (98.9 °F), blood pressure is 118/64 mm Hg, pulse rate is 64/min, and respiration rate is 16/min; BMI is 28. There is no palpable lymphadenopathy. The abdomen is soft and nontender with normal bowel sounds, mild distention, a fluid wave, and no organomegaly. Pelvic examination shows left adnexal fullness.

The hemoglobin level is 11.0 g/dL (110 g/L). Results of a complete metabolic panel are normal. Transvaginal ultrasonography shows a 10- × 11-cm left adnexal mass suspicious for ovarian cancer. Serum CA-125 level is 1786 U/mL (1786 kU/L) (normal range, 1.9-16.3 U/mL [1.9-16.3 kU/L]).

Which of the following is the most appropriate next step in management?

(A) Laparotomy with surgical cytoreduction and staging
(B) Left oophorectomy
(C) Initiation of carboplatin and paclitaxel
(D) Radiation therapy to the pelvis

Item 59

A 63-year-old woman is evaluated in the emergency department after the abrupt onset of left upper-extremity weakness. The patient denies any weight loss, headache, nausea, or vomiting. Until today, she has been active and able to completely care for herself. Medical history is significant for stage IIB non–small cell lung cancer (characterized by involvement of three of six peribronchial lymph nodes) diagnosed 1 year ago, for which she underwent right upper lobectomy followed by adjuvant cisplatin and vinorelbine chemotherapy. Mediastinoscopy results at the time were negative, and positron emission tomography showed no metastatic disease.

On physical examination, temperature is normal, blood pressure is 158/98 mm Hg, pulse rate is 96/min, and respiration rate is 22/min; BMI is 19. Cardiopulmonary examination is unremarkable. The patient is right-handed. Neurologic examination shows weakness of the left arm with hyperreflexia of the brachioradialis stretch reflex. Mental status, speech, visual fields, and gait are normal.

Results of complete blood count are normal. An MRI of the brain demonstrates a right parietal lesion measuring 1.5 cm, with evidence of significant edema. Further evaluation reveals no other evidence of extracranial disease. Dexamethasone is initiated.

Which of the following is the most appropriate next step in management?

(A) Best supportive care
(B) Initiation of erlotinib

(C) Initiation of temozolomide followed by radiation therapy
(D) Surgical resection of metastasis

Item 60

A 64-year-old man with a 3-year history of stage II, grade 1 follicular lymphoma is evaluated because of cervical and axillary lymph nodes that have been gradually enlarging since diagnosis. He is unable to wear a tie, cannot fasten the top button of his shirt, has trouble shaving, and is concerned about the appearance of the cervical lymph nodes. The enlarged axillary lymph nodes are also uncomfortable. The patient feels otherwise well and has not had night sweats, weight loss, or fevers.

On physical examination, temperature is 37.1 °C (98.8 °F), blood pressure is 124/68 mm Hg, pulse rate is 64/min, and respiration rate is 12/min; BMI is 24. Bilateral cervical lymphadenopathy (largest aggregate lymph node measuring 6 cm) and bilateral axillary lymphadenopathy (largest aggregate lymph node measuring 5 to 6 cm) are present. There is no palpable inguinal lymphadenopathy or organomegaly.

Laboratory studies:
Hemoglobin 12.0 g/dL (120 g/L)
Leukocyte count 9000/µL (9×10^9/L)
Platelet count 165,000/µL (165×10^9/L)

Contrast-enhanced CT scans of the neck, chest, abdomen, and pelvis show progressive axillary, mediastinal, and cervical lymphadenopathy. There are no measurable lymph nodes below the diaphragm.

Which of the following is the most appropriate next step in managing this patient?

(A) Cyclophosphamide, vincristine, and prednisone with rituximab
(B) High-dose chemotherapy followed by stem cell transplantation
(C) Fine-needle aspiration biopsy of a cervical lymph node
(D) Cyclophosphamide, vincristine, prednisone, and radiation therapy
(E) Observation with follow-up in 3 months

Item 61

A 20-year-old woman of Ashkenazi Jewish descent undergoes a routine annual examination. Family history includes her mother, who was diagnosed with breast cancer at age 45 years; her paternal grandmother, who was diagnosed with breast cancer at age 35 years and ovarian cancer at age 50 years; and her father, who was diagnosed with breast cancer at age 52 years.

Her physical examination is normal.

Which of the following is the most appropriate next step in management?

(A) Bilateral breast MRI
(B) Bilateral mastectomy and oophorectomy
(C) Genetic counseling and testing of the affected father
(D) Mammography

Item 62

A 29-year-old man has a 3-week history of a growing mass in the right supraclavicular region. He has not had fever, night sweats, or weight loss. The patient is otherwise healthy.

On physical examination, temperature is 37.1 °C (98.7 °F), blood pressure is 118/72 mm Hg, pulse rate is 84/min, and respiration rate is 16/min. A 4-cm mass is present in the right supraclavicular region. The remainder of the physical examination is normal.

The serum lactate dehydrogenase level is 695 U/L. Complete blood count, liver chemistry tests, and tests of renal function are normal. Integrated CT/positron emission tomography shows only the right supraclavicular mass. The results of a lymph node biopsy are consistent with large B-cell lymphoma. A bone marrow biopsy is negative.

Which of the following is the most appropriate treatment?

(A) Cyclophosphamide, doxorubicin, vincristine, and prednisone with rituximab for six cycles
(B) Cyclophosphamide, doxorubicin, vincristine, and prednisone with rituximab for three cycles followed by involved-field radiation therapy
(C) Involved-field radiation therapy
(D) Observation
(E) Rituximab

Item 63

A 24-year-old man is evaluated in the emergency department because of a 3-month history of a progressive nonproductive cough and increasing shortness of breath that did not improve after 14 days of antibiotics. The patient does not have fever, chills, or weight loss.

On physical examination, temperature is 37.1 °C (98.8 °F), blood pressure is 120/68 mm Hg, pulse rate is 72/min, and respiration rate is 18/min. The lungs are clear. The remainder of the physical examination is normal.

A chest radiograph shows multiple pulmonary nodules consistent with metastatic disease.

The patient is hospitalized. CT scan of the chest confirms metastatic lesions in the lungs and retroperitoneal lymphadenopathy. Testicular ultrasonography shows a slightly enlarged right testicle.

Laboratory studies:

Lactate dehydrogenase	310 U/L
α-Fetoprotein	1289 ng/mL (1289 µg/L)
β-Human chorionic gonadotropin	6247 mU/mL (normal <5 mU/mL)

Which of the following is the most appropriate treatment?

(A) Chemotherapy
(B) Radiation therapy
(C) Right radical orchiectomy followed by chemotherapy
(D) Right radical orchiectomy followed by retroperitoneal lymph node dissection

Item 64

A 64-year-old man is evaluated for a 3-month history of pain of increasing intensity in the left shoulder; the pain also radiates to the fourth and fifth digits and the medial aspect of the arm and forearm. Previous referral to a physical therapist for treatment of a suspected shoulder strain resulted in no improvement. The patient has a chronic cough with minimal sputum production and a 40-pack-year smoking history. The remainder of the medical history is noncontributory. He is currently taking ibuprofen for pain with minimal relief.

On physical examination, he is afebrile. Blood pressure is 140/80 mm Hg, pulse rate is 80/min, and respiration rate is 18/min. On examination of the shoulder, complete range of motion without exacerbation of the pain is noted. Neurologic examination reveals constriction of the right pupil and ptosis, in addition to weakness and atrophy of the intrinsic muscles of the hand.

Which of the following is the most appropriate next diagnostic test?

(A) CT of the chest
(B) Electromyography
(C) MRI of the brain
(D) MRI of the cervical spine
(E) MRI of the shoulder

Item 65

A 28-year-old woman has a 2-month history of vague discomfort in the left lower abdominal quadrant. Medical history is unremarkable, menses are normal, and she takes no medications.

On physical examination, temperature is 37.1 °C (98.7 °F), blood pressure is 110/72 mm Hg, pulse rate is 88/min, and respiration rate is 16/min; BMI is 22. Pelvic examination discloses fullness in the left adnexal region. A Pap smear is normal. Results of a complete blood count and comprehensive chemistry panel are normal. Serum CA-125 level is 70 U/mL (70 kU/L) (normal range, 1.9-16.3 U/mL [1.9-16.3 kU/L]). Ultrasonography of the abdomen and pelvis shows a solid left adnexal mass. A CT scan confirms the presence of an 8-cm adnexal lesion, as well as a 3-cm omental mass and a 2-cm mesenteric mass.

The patient undergoes exploratory laparotomy, during which the tumors are completely debulked. Histopathologic examination shows that all three lesions are serous tumors of low malignant potential with no invasive implants (stage IIIC).

Which of the following is the most appropriate management at this time?

(A) Genetic testing
(B) Intraperitoneal platinum-based chemotherapy
(C) Intravenous platinum-based chemotherapy
(D) Whole-abdomen radiation therapy
(E) Observation

Item 66

A 55-year-old man is evaluated in the emergency department because of midback pain that began 3 weeks ago and has been gradually increasing since then. Medical history is remarkable for metastatic prostate cancer diagnosed 18 months ago, which progressed on antiandrogen therapy and for which he is currently taking bicalutamide, zoledronic acid, docetaxel, and prednisone.

On physical examination, upper extremity strength is normal. The lower extremities are diffusely weak. Sensory examination shows diminished pinprick sensation from the nipples downward. Reflexes are 2+ in the biceps and triceps and 3+ in the knees and ankles. An extensor plantar response is present bilaterally. Anal sphincter tone is diminished.

Intravenous dexamethasone is administered.

Emergency MRI scan confirms epidural spinal cord compression at the level of the fourth thoracic vertebra.

Which of the following is the most appropriate next step in treatment?

(A) Addition of leuprolide
(B) Anterior surgical decompression
(C) Radiation therapy
(D) Substitution of paclitaxel for docetaxel

Item 67

Three years ago, a 67-year-old man underwent right hemicolectomy with adjuvant chemotherapy for stage III colon cancer. The patient has been followed with annual CT scans and measurement of serum carcinoembryonic antigen (CEA) levels. His most recent CEA level is 10.1 ng/mL (10.1 µg/L) (normal <2.0 ng/mL [2.0 µg/L]) compared with a value of 2.4 ng/mL (2.4 µg/L) 1 year ago. A restaging CT scan of the abdomen and pelvis shows a solitary lesion in the liver and is otherwise unremarkable.

Which of the following is the most appropriate initial treatment?

(A) Chemoembolization
(B) Chemotherapy
(C) Ethanol ablation
(D) Radiofrequency ablation
(E) Surgical resection

Item 68

A 72-year-old woman is evaluated for pain in her right upper extremity, right hip, and left lower extremity of 3 weeks' duration. She was diagnosed with stage I breast cancer 7 years ago for which she was treated with right lumpectomy, radiation therapy, and 5 years of tamoxifen therapy completed 1 year ago. She takes acetaminophen with codeine as needed for pain.

On physical examination, there is tenderness over the right humerus and left femur. Other than posttreatment effects, the breast examination and remainder of the physical examination are normal.

Results of a bone scan show increased uptake in multiple thoracic vertebrae, the right humerus, the left femur, and the right iliac bone. Plain radiographs of involved areas reveal lytic lesions in the right humerus, left femur, and multiple ribs but no impending fractures. Biopsy of a bone lesion reveals adenocarcinoma consistent with a primary breast tumor that is estrogen receptor–positive, progesterone receptor–negative, and *HER2*-negative.

Which of the following is the most appropriate next step in treatment?

(A) Anastrozole and alendronate
(B) Anastrozole and zoledronic acid
(C) Doxorubicin
(D) Tamoxifen and alendronate
(E) Tamoxifen and zoledronic acid

Item 69

A 60-year-old man is evaluated in the emergency department for weight loss, progressive cough, dyspnea, head fullness, and difficulty swallowing of 3 months' duration. Over the past 2 days he has also noted progressive facial swelling. He denies fever, chills, or sputum production. The patient has a 45-pack-year smoking history.

On physical examination, temperature is 37.1 °C (98.8 °F), blood pressure is 100/50 mm Hg, pulse rate is 120/min, and respiration rate is 20/min. The patient's face is edematous, and there is venous distention noted on the neck and chest wall. Cardiac examination reveals normal heart sounds without evidence of extra heart sounds, murmurs, or rubs. Faint expiratory wheezes but no crackles are heard on pulmonary auscultation. There is no hepatomegaly or peripheral edema.

A chest radiograph shows mediastinal widening and small, bilateral pleural effusions.

Which of the following is the most likely diagnosis?

(A) Heart failure
(B) Pneumonia
(C) Pulmonary embolism
(D) Superior vena cava syndrome

Item 70

A 20-year-old woman is evaluated for swelling of the neck and intermittent dysphagia that has progressively worsened over the past several months in addition to episodes of sweating and diarrhea. Her mother died suddenly at the age of 31 years of a hypertensive cerebral hemorrhage. The remainder of the family history is unremarkable.

On physical examination, temperature is normal, blood pressure is 180/96 mm Hg, and pulse rate is 110/min. A prominent nodular thyroid with a dominant 2-cm nodule on the right side is noted. Cardiopulmonary examination reveals a regular tachycardia with normal heart sounds and no extra sounds, murmurs, or rubs, as well as clear lungs. The abdominal examination is normal.

A fine-needle aspiration biopsy of the nodule reveals medullary thyroid carcinoma.

Which of the following is the most appropriate next step in management?

(A) Genetic screening for the *RET* mutation

(B) Levothyroxine therapy

(C) Mammography

(D) Radioactive iodine administration

Item 71

A 68-year-old woman is evaluated for a 4-month history of cough, dyspnea on exertion, and an 11.3-kg (25-lb) weight loss. She also has a long history of cigarette smoking.

On physical examination, vital signs are normal. Decreased breath sounds are heard throughout all lung fields on cardiopulmonary auscultation. Neurologic examination is normal. Abdominal examination discloses hepatomegaly 4 cm below the costal margin.

Laboratory studies indicate a normal complete blood count, a serum sodium level of 123 meq/L (123 mmol/L), and a serum albumin level of 3.2 g/dL (32 g/L).

A CT scan of the chest, abdomen, and pelvis shows a right hilar mass, a left adrenal mass, and multiple liver lesions. Small cell lung cancer is confirmed via bronchoscopic biopsy specimen.

An MRI of the brain reveals two small subcentimeter lesions that are suspicious for metastases.

Which of the following is the most appropriate next step in management?

(A) Best supportive care

(B) Bone marrow biopsy

(C) Cisplatin and etoposide

(D) Cisplatin and etoposide with chest radiation therapy

Item 72

A 36-year-old woman is evaluated 2 months after being diagnosed with breast cancer. Diagnostic mammogram and ultrasound confirmed the presence of a left breast mass, and a core biopsy revealed estrogen receptor–/progesterone receptor–negative invasive ductal carcinoma with *HER2* overexpression. A 3-cm tumor and six positive lymph nodes were found on lumpectomy and axillary lymph node dissection.

The patient is otherwise healthy and takes only acetaminophen as needed for postsurgical pain.

Physical examination is normal except for the healing lumpectomy site.

In addition to adjuvant therapy followed by radiation therapy, which of the following is the most appropriate treatment?

(A) Anastrozole

(B) Bevacizumab

(C) Tamoxifen

(D) Trastuzumab

Item 73

A 45-year-old man is brought from his job on a construction site to the emergency department because of acute-onset right-sided abdominal pain, nausea, and vomiting. A CT scan shows an inflamed area in the right lower abdominal quadrant, and the patient undergoes emergent appendectomy. Intraoperatively, he is found to have an obstructing lesion in the cecum. Frozen tissue section confirms the presence of high-grade adenocarcinoma, and right hemicolectomy and lymph node dissection are done. Biopsy specimens confirm stage III T3N2 colon cancer with 5 of 10 lymph nodes positive for metastatic disease. A postoperative CT scan of the abdomen and pelvis, chest radiograph, and complete colonoscopy show no synchronous lesions or distant metastases.

Which of the following is the most appropriate postoperative management?

(A) Chemotherapy

(B) Chemotherapy and radiation therapy

(C) Radiation therapy

(D) Observation

Item 74

A 38-year-old woman is evaluated for an asymptomatic thyroid nodule noticed by the patient's husband, a family physician. Medical history is otherwise noncontributory, and family history for malignancy and thyroid disease is negative.

On physical examination, temperature is normal, blood pressure is 116/68 mm Hg, pulse rate is 110/min, and respiration rate is 20/min. A palpable thyroid with a dominant, nontender 2-cm nodule is noted. There is no cervical lymphadenopathy. The lungs are clear. No masses or tenderness is noted on abdominal examination.

Results of a complete blood count and a comprehensive metabolic panel are normal. A serum thyroid-stimulating hormone level is normal. Fine-needle aspiration of the thyroid nodule reveals papillary carcinoma.

Which of the following is the most appropriate treatment?

(A) Administration of radioiodine-131

(B) External-beam radiation therapy

(C) Thyroidectomy alone

(D) Thyroidectomy and adjuvant chemotherapy

(E) Thyroidectomy followed by radioiodine-131

Item 75

An 80-year-old man is evaluated after a serum prostate-specific antigen (PSA) level of 5.7 ng/mL (5.7 µg/L) was noted during a community screening program. He has no symptoms related to the genitourinary system and denies bone pain, weight loss, or any change in his health status. The patient has hypertension and hypercholesterolemia and underwent four-vessel coronary artery bypass graft surgery

5 years ago. His current medications are hydrochlorothiazide, atenolol, lisinopril, pravastatin, and low-dose aspirin.

On physical examination, the patient is afebrile, blood pressure is 140/80 mm Hg, and the pulse rate is 72/min and regular. The lungs are clear, and the abdomen is soft and nontender. There is trace pedal edema in the lower extremities.

Which of the following is the most appropriate next step in management?

(A) Bone scan
(B) Repeat PSA
(C) Transrectal prostate biopsy
(D) Observation

Item 76

A 68-year-old woman is evaluated 3 weeks after pulmonary lobectomy for a lesion detected on chest radiography during hip arthroplasty preoperative evaluation. Staging chest CT showed a spiculated lesion in the right upper lobe, no mediastinal lymphadenopathy, and normal adrenal glands. Positron emission tomography showed uptake only in the primary lesion. The tumor was confirmed as a 2-cm moderately differentiated adenocarcinoma on pathologic examination. There was no pleural invasion, lymphovascular invasion, or necrosis. Eight lymph nodes were all found to be negative for tumor.

The patient experienced no complications following surgery and was free of pulmonary symptoms on initial detection of the lesion and remains asymptomatic now.

Which of the following is the most appropriate next step in management?

(A) Radiation therapy
(B) Cisplatin-based chemotherapy
(C) Erlotinib therapy
(D) Periodic physical examination and surveillance imaging

Item 77

A 56-year-old woman undergoes initial screening colonoscopy. An abnormality is found 10 cm from the anal verge. Biopsy specimens confirm the diagnosis of a moderately differentiated adenocarcinoma. Rectal ultrasonography shows that the tumor has extended into the perirectal fat, but no lymphadenopathy is noted. Chest radiograph and CT scan of the abdomen and pelvis show no metastatic disease.

Which of the following is the most appropriate treatment at this time?

(A) Surgical resection and adjuvant chemoradiation therapy
(B) Chemotherapy alone
(C) Radiation therapy alone
(D) Surgical resection alone
(E) Surgical resection and postoperative radiation therapy alone

Item 78

A 44-year-old Chinese woman is evaluated after presenting with an unremitting headache of 1 month's duration in addition to nasal congestion but no fever, rhinorrhea, or purulent discharge. Last week, the patient noticed an enlarged lymph node in her neck. The patient emigrated from China 30 years ago. She takes no medications and is otherwise healthy.

On physical examination, she is afebrile. Blood pressure is 120/70 mm Hg and pulse rate is 60/min. Right and left enlarged cervical lymph nodes are palpated. Both are mobile, nontender, and measure 2 cm in diameter. No other lymphadenopathy is noted, and no oropharyngeal or nasal lesions are found. No splenomegaly is noted on abdominal examination.

Laboratory studies, including complete blood count, serum lactate dehydrogenase level, metabolic profile, kidney function, and urinalysis, are normal.

Direct nasopharyngolaryngoscopy demonstrates a soft-tissue mass in the nasopharynx.

Which of the following is the most likely diagnosis?

(A) Burkitt lymphoma
(B) Hodgkin lymphoma
(C) Multiple myeloma
(D) Nasopharyngeal cancer

Item 79

A 58-year-old postmenopausal woman is evaluated after a recent diagnosis of ductal carcinoma in situ (DCIS) of the right breast. A 2-cm area of microcalcifications in the right breast was identified after a screening mammography. No palpable mass was noted. A stereotactic biopsy revealed high-grade, estrogen receptor–positive, progesterone receptor–positive DCIS with comedonecrosis. She was treated with wide-excision resection and 6 weeks of radiation therapy.

Physical examination discloses a well-healed right lumpectomy scar. No masses are palpated in either breast. There is no axillary or supraclavicular lymphadenopathy.

Which of the following is the most appropriate next step in treatment?

(A) Megestrol acetate
(B) Doxorubicin plus cyclophosphamide
(C) Raloxifene
(D) Tamoxifen

Item 80

A 19-year-old male college student has a 3-week history of a swollen left testicle. He plays rugby but has not had any recent injuries. He is sexually active with one female partner and usually uses condoms. Medical and family histories are noncontributory, and he takes no medications.

Physical examination is normal except for a minimally swollen and tender left testicle. The testes are both longitudinally oriented, and the affected testicle is not elevated. There is no penile discharge.

Laboratory studies:

Lactate dehydrogenase	80 U/L
α-Fetoprotein	62 ng/mL (62 µg/L)
β-Human chorionic gonadotropin	67 mU/mL (67 U/L) (normal <5 mU/mL [5 U/L])

Ultrasound shows a 5-cm mass in the left testicle.

Which of the following is the most likely diagnosis?

(A) *Neisseria gonorrhoeae* infection

(B) Nonseminoma

(C) Seminoma

(D) Testicular torsion

Item 81

A 62-year-old man is evaluated 4 months after diagnosis of limited-stage, small cell lung cancer. Treatment consisted of four cycles of chemotherapy and concurrent radiation, with significant tumor response confirmed by CT showing scarring only in the area of the primary tumor. The patient has excellent performance status and has stopped smoking cigarettes following his lung cancer diagnosis.

On physical examination, temperature is normal, blood pressure is 138/78 mm Hg, pulse rate is 80/min, and respiration rate is 22/min; BMI is 19. Pulmonary examination discloses decreased breath sounds throughout all lung fields and a few early crackles in the right upper chest. Neurologic examination results are normal.

A CT scan of the chest, abdomen, and pelvis reveals a right hilar scar and evidence of changes consistent with radiation pneumonitis in the right upper lobe.

Which of the following is the most appropriate next step in management?

(A) Maintenance topotecan

(B) Prophylactic cranial irradiation

(C) Right upper lobectomy and mediastinal lymph node dissection

(D) Expectant observation

(E) Small cell lung cancer vaccination

Item 82

A 72-year-old woman is evaluated in the emergency department for increasing dyspnea on exertion and bilateral lower extremity edema. She has a history of right-sided breast cancer, which was diagnosed 7 years ago and was treated with lumpectomy followed by local radiation therapy that did not include the internal mammary chain of lymph nodes. She received four cycles of doxorubicin and cyclophosphamide and 5 years of tamoxifen therapy, which was completed 2 years ago. She does not smoke and has no history of heart disease, diabetes mellitus, hypertension, or hyperlipidemia. Family history for heart disease is negative.

On physical examination, temperature is 36.7 °C (98.0 °F), blood pressure is 90/50 mm Hg, pulse rate is 120/min, and respiration rate is 28/min. A well-healed right lumpectomy scar is noted. No breast masses are palpated. There is no evidence of axillary or supraclavicular lymphadenopathy. There is jugular venous distention to the angle of the jaw with the patient sitting upright. Cardiac examination reveals a gallop rhythm and a systolic heart murmur best heard at the cardiac apex. The cardiac apex is displaced and diffuse. Heart rhythm is regular. The lungs reveal bibasilar crackles. Bilateral edema is noted.

An electrocardiogram shows a regular tachycardia with low voltage and no acute ST- or T-wave changes. A chest radiograph reveals vascular congestion and cardiomegaly.

An echocardiogram reveals a dilated left ventricle with global hypokinesis.

Which of the following is the most likely primary cause of this patient's findings?

(A) Cyclophosphamide

(B) Doxorubicin

(C) Radiation therapy

(D) Tamoxifen

Item 83

A 62-year-old man is evaluated for a 3-month history of hoarseness and odynophagia that has developed over the past 2 weeks. The patient has a 50-pack-year history of tobacco use.

On physical examination, vital signs, including temperature, are normal. There is no cervical or supraclavicular lymphadenopathy. The oral pharynx is normal to inspection and no masses are palpated. The cardiopulmonary examination is unremarkable.

Endoscopic examination reveals a 2-cm ulcerated lesion projecting from the right vocal cord. The lesion is friable, with some bleeding. The vocal cord is mobile.

Biopsy specimen of the vocal cord indicates squamous cell carcinoma. A CT scan of the neck and chest reveals no metastatic disease. A positron emission tomographic scan is also negative.

The patient would prefer not to lose his ability to speak and he is willing to stop smoking immediately.

Which of the following is the most appropriate next step in treatment?

(A) Cetuximab

(B) Chemotherapy

(C) External-beam radiation therapy

(D) Total laryngectomy

Item 84

A 42-year-old man is evaluated for a 3-week history of a nontender lump in his neck. Stage IIIA diffuse large B-cell non-Hodgkin lymphoma was diagnosed 2 years ago and treated with six cycles of cyclophosphamide, doxorubicin, vincristine, and prednisone with rituximab. He currently has no fevers, night sweats, weight loss, or fatigue.

On physical examination, temperature is 37.1 °C (98.8 °F), blood pressure is 128/70 mm Hg, pulse rate is

88/min, and respiration rate is 16/min; BMI is 25. The patient has a 5-cm mass in the right supraclavicular region plus a 4-cm mass in the left axilla and multiple 2-cm bilateral cervical lymph nodes. The lungs are clear, and cardiac examination is normal. On abdominal examination, the spleen is palpated 4 cm below the left costal margin. There is no hepatomegaly or peripheral edema.

Laboratory studies:
Hemoglobin   11.0 g/dL (110 g/L)
Leukocyte count   3200/µL (3.2 × 10⁹/L)
Platelet count   103,000/µL (103 × 10⁹/L)

Fine-needle aspiration biopsy of the cervical mass confirms the presence of monoclonal large B cells. Bone marrow biopsy shows non-Hodgkin lymphoma with diffuse large-cell histology involving 20% of the bone marrow. Contrast-enhanced CT scans of the chest and abdomen show multiple areas of lymphadenopathy and splenomegaly.

The patient is interested in pursuing curative therapy.

Which of the following is the most appropriate treatment at this time?

(A) Cyclophosphamide, doxorubicin, vincristine, and prednisone with rituximab
(B) Ifosfamide, carboplatin, and etoposide with rituximab followed by high-dose chemotherapy with autologous stem cell rescue
(C) Rituximab alone
(D) Whole-body radiation therapy with autologous stem cell rescue

Item 85

A 48-year-old postmenopausal woman is evaluated after a recent diagnosis of breast cancer. Her annual screening mammogram revealed dense breasts with a new 1.5-cm area of microcalcifications in the left breast without any associated mass. Stereotactic biopsy revealed grade 2, estrogen receptor–/progesterone receptor–negative and *HER2*-negative infiltrating ductal carcinoma. Her family history includes a maternal aunt with breast cancer diagnosed at age 50 years. She is otherwise healthy.

Her physical examination is normal except for ecchymosis at the biopsy site.

Which of the following is the most appropriate next step in management?

(A) Left lumpectomy with axillary lymph node dissection followed by breast irradiation
(B) Left lumpectomy with sentinel lymph node biopsy followed by breast irradiation
(C) Left lumpectomy with sentinel lymph node biopsy without breast irradiation
(D) Left modified radical mastectomy
(E) Left modified radical mastectomy and right simple mastectomy

Item 86

A 70-year-old man is evaluated because of increasing new-onset midback pain that is worse at night, interferes with his sleep, and does not improve with NSAIDs. The patient underwent radical prostatectomy for prostate cancer (Gleason score of 8) 2 years ago. He has had urinary incontinence since surgery, which has significantly increased over the past few weeks.

Physical examination findings include tenderness over the midthoracic vertebrae, mild flexor weakness, and hyperreflexia of the lower extremities.

Laboratory studies:
Hemoglobin   10.5 g/dL(105 g/L)
Alkaline phosphatase   1375 U/L
Other liver chemistry tests Normal

Which of the following diagnostic studies should be done next?

(A) Bone scan
(B) MRI of the brain
(C) MRI of the thoracolumbar spine
(D) Plain radiographs of the thoracic spine

Item 87

A 66-year-old man is evaluated because of an increasingly elevated serum prostate-specific antigen (PSA) level. He is currently asymptomatic. Prostate cancer was diagnosed 4 years ago (Gleason score of 8 and PSA level of 20 ng/mL [20 µg/L]). The patient underwent definitive radiation therapy, following which his PSA level became undetectable. A bone scan now shows multiple metastatic lesions.

Which of the following is the most appropriate management?

(A) Docetaxel plus prednisone
(B) Hospice care
(C) Leuprolide plus flutamide
(D) Samarium-153
(E) Observation

Item 88

A 43-year-old premenopausal woman is concerned about her risk for ovarian cancer after a friend was recently diagnosed with the disease. The patient is asymptomatic and has regular menses. Results of a pelvic examination and Pap smear 2 years ago were normal. She has hypertension that is treated with hydrochlorothiazide. There is no family history of ovarian, breast, uterine, or colon cancer.

Results of physical examination, including pelvic examination, are normal. Results of a complete blood count, cholesterol panel, complete metabolic panel, and Pap smear are normal.

Which of the following is the most appropriate screening recommendation for ovarian cancer in this patient?

(A) CT scan of the abdomen and pelvis

(B) Measurement of serum CA-125 level

(C) Transvaginal ultrasonography

(D) Transvaginal ultrasonography and measurement of serum CA-125 level

(E) No screening

Item 89

A 54-year-old man is evaluated because of right flank pain and abdominal fullness. He does not have fever, chills, or dysuria.

On physical examination, temperature is normal, blood pressure is 148/92 mm Hg, and pulse rate is 88/min. The cardiopulmonary examination is normal. The abdomen is not distended, and there are normal bowel sounds. There is a firm, right flank mass that moves with respiration. The remainder of the physical examination is normal.

Hematuria is present on urinalysis.

A CT scan of the abdomen and pelvis shows a 9.5-cm mass in the right kidney. A chest radiograph reveals multiple pulmonary nodules.

Right radical nephrectomy is done, and surgical biopsy specimens show clear cell renal carcinoma. The patient remains ambulatory, and his performance status is good.

Which of the following is the most appropriate treatment at this time?

(A) Hospice care

(B) Interferon alfa

(C) Sunitinib

(D) Trastuzumab

(E) Vinblastine

Item 90

A 59-year-old man is evaluated for a nonhealing painful tongue ulcer of 4 weeks' duration. The patient has smoked one pack of cigarettes per day for 40 years and drinks four to five beers daily. Medical history is otherwise unremarkable.

On physical examination, temperature is normal, blood pressure is 138/76 mm Hg, pulse rate is 72/min, and respiration rate is 17/min. Findings of the oral examination are shown.

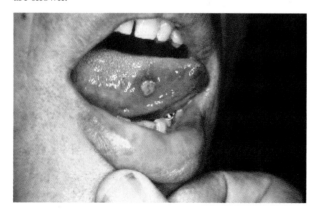

There are no other oral lesions. No cervical lymphadenopathy is noted. The lungs are clear.

Results of a complete blood count and a comprehensive metabolic panel are normal.

Which of the following is the most appropriate next step in management?

(A) Close surveillance

(B) Clotrimazole therapy

(C) Fine-needle aspiration biopsy of the lesion

(D) Triamcinolone therapy

Item 91

A 75-year-old woman with chronic lymphocytic leukemia who was previously asymptomatic on no therapy undergoes follow-up evaluation for community-acquired pneumonia for which she was hospitalized for 5 days and released 14 days ago. The patient completed a course of antibiotic therapy and currently feels well. She reports no fevers, chills, night sweats, weight loss, abdominal pain, or new lymphadenopathy, and her pulmonary symptoms have resolved. Medical history is significant for a previous episode of pneumonia for which she was hospitalized within the past year.

On physical examination, temperature is 36.7 °C (98.2 °F), blood pressure is 130/78 mm Hg, pulse rate is 72/min, and respiration rate is 14/min; BMI is 22. No palpable lymphadenopathy is noted. Cardiopulmonary examination is normal. Abdominal examination discloses splenomegaly.

Laboratory studies:

Hemoglobin	11 g/dL (110 g/L)
Leukocyte count	24,000/µL (24 × 10⁹/L), with 80% mature-appearing lymphocytes
Platelet count	120,000/µL (120 × 10⁹/L)
Absolute lymphocyte count	20,000/µL (20 × 10⁹/L)
IgG	500 mg/dL

Results of a posteroanterior/lateral radiograph of the chest taken during hospitalization show a resolving right lower lobe infiltrate.

Which of the following is the most appropriate next step in management?

(A) Intravenous immune globulin

(B) Prophylactic trimethoprim-sulfamethoxazole

(C) Splenectomy

(D) Repeat blood counts in 1 month

Item 92

A 60-year-old postmenopausal woman has a 2-week history of left-sided pelvic pain. She is otherwise asymptomatic. Medical and family histories are unremarkable, and she takes no medications.

On physical examination, temperature is 36.7 °C (98.0 °F), blood pressure is 130/80 mm Hg, pulse rate is 80/min, and respiration rate is 18/min. Pelvic examination discloses a 6-cm adnexal mass. The serum CA-125 level is 427 U/mL (427 kU/L); results of all other laboratory studies are normal. Ultrasonography of the abdomen and pelvis shows the pelvic mass. A CT scan of the abdomen and pelvis confirms the presence of the mass and no other masses in the abdomen.

Complete surgical resection is performed by a gynecologic oncologist. At surgery, the tumor is found to be limited to one ovary, and the capsule of the ovary is intact. There is no ascites.

Which of the following is the most appropriate postoperative management?

(A) Intraperitoneal carboplatin and paclitaxel
(B) Intravenous carboplatin and paclitaxel
(C) Oral etoposide
(D) Observation

Item 93

A 54-year-old postmenopausal woman is evaluated after she discovered a right axillary mass. She is otherwise healthy. She has never smoked cigarettes and drinks alcohol only socially. Family history is significant for her mother who developed breast cancer at age 62 years.

On physical examination, temperature is normal, blood pressure is 138/78 mm Hg, pulse rate is 64/min, and respiration rate is 16/min; BMI is 19. Thyroid examination is normal. A mobile, nontender 2-cm axillary lymph node mass is noted. There is no palpable breast mass or other lymphadenopathy. An excisional biopsy reveals adenocarcinoma. Results of mammography and breast MRI are normal. The complete blood count, metabolic panel, urinalysis, and chest radiograph are normal. Immunohistochemical staining results are positive for CK-7 and are negative for CK-20, estrogen receptor and progesterone receptor, and TTF-1 expression.

Which of the following is the most appropriate next step in management?

(A) Chest CT scan
(B) Panendoscopy of the aerodigestive tract
(C) Right mastectomy and axillary lymph node dissection
(D) Thyroid ultrasonography

Item 94

A 45-year-old woman has a 4-week history of nontender bilateral preauricular swelling. She also has a 10-year history of Sjögren syndrome characterized by nonerosive arthritis, xerostomia, keratoconjunctivitis sicca, and positive anti-Ro/SSA antibodies. History is negative for cigarette smoking, alcohol use, and head or neck radiation therapy. There are no other medical problems. Current medications are ibuprofen, oral pilocarpine, and cyclosporin ophthalmic drops.

On physical examination, vital signs are normal. The patient has dry mucous membranes and decreased saliva production. Bilateral 3-cm preauricular lymph nodes and multiple bilateral 2-cm cervical lymph nodes are palpated. The thyroid gland is normal to palpation. The remainder of the examination is normal.

An excisional lymph node biopsy is scheduled.

Which of the following is the most likely diagnosis?

(A) Lymphadenitis
(B) Lymphoma
(C) Metastatic thyroid cancer
(D) Plasmacytoma
(E) Squamous cell carcinoma

Item 95

A 20-year-old man is admitted to the hospital after a recent diagnosis of acute myeloid leukemia. He is scheduled to begin therapy with cytarabine and daunorubicin.

Pre-treatment laboratory studies:

Hemoglobin	6.0 g/dL (60 g/L)
Leukocyte count	80,000/μL (80 × 10⁹/L)
Platelet count	60,000/μL (60 × 10⁹/L)
Creatinine	1.5 mg/dL (114.5 μmol/L)
Lactate dehydrogenase	250 U/L
Calcium	9.1 mg/dL (2.3 mmol/L)
Sodium	145 meq/L (145 mmol/L)
Potassium	5.0 meq/L (5.0 mmol/L)
Chloride	104 meq/L (104 mmol/L)
Bicarbonate	24 meq/L (24 mmol/L)
Phosphorus	5.6 mg/dL (1.8 mmol/L)
Uric acid	8.8 mg/dL (0.5 mmol/L)

Which of the following is the most appropriate next step before initiation of induction chemotherapy?

(A) Administration of granulocyte-macrophage colony-stimulating factor
(B) Administration of vancomycin
(C) Aggressive intravenous fluid hydration and allopurinol administration
(D) Alkalinization of the urine

Item 96

A 55-year-old postmenopausal woman is evaluated 4 years after a diagnosis of ductal carcinoma in situ for which she underwent lumpectomy and completed 6 weeks of radiation therapy. She has also been taking tamoxifen.

Physical examination reveals a well-healed right lumpectomy scar. No masses in either breast are palpated, and no axillary or supraclavicular lymphadenopathy is noted. Abdominal examination, including pelvic evaluation, is normal.

For which of the following diseases is the patient at increased risk as a result of her tamoxifen therapy?

(A) Acute myeloid leukemia
(B) Colon cancer
(C) Endometrial cancer
(D) Ovarian cancer

Item 97

A 46-year-old woman is evaluated in the emergency department because of shortness of breath and chest pain, which were first noted on a flight from San Francisco to New York and have been increasing in intensity since she arrived in New York this afternoon; she denies calf pain. The patient was diagnosed with stage I breast cancer 1 year ago for which she was treated with lumpectomy, four cycles of doxorubicin and cyclophosphamide, and radiation therapy. The remainder of the medical history and family history are negative. She currently takes tamoxifen.

On physical examination, she appears uncomfortable and short of breath. Temperature is 36.7 °C (98.0 °F), blood pressure is 80/60 mm Hg, pulse rate is 120/min, and respiration rate is 28/min; BMI is 24. Oxygen saturation on ambient air is 90%. Estimated central venous pressure is 8 cm H_2O. Carotid upstrokes are normal.

Cardiopulmonary examination reveals regular tachycardia with soft heart sounds and no extra sounds or murmurs and clear lungs. There is no peripheral edema or calf pain.

Arterial blood gas studies (ambient air):

pH	7.45
PO_2	85 mm Hg (11.3 kPa)
PCO_2	35 mm Hg (4.7 kPa)
Bicarbonate	24 meq/L (24 mmol/L)

Tachycardia without other abnormalities is noted on electrocardiogram. A chest radiograph discloses clear lungs and normal heart size and vasculature.

Which of the following medical interventions is most likely responsible for this patient's current symptoms?

(A) Cyclophosphamide
(B) Doxorubicin
(C) Radiotherapy
(D) Surgical lumpectomy
(E) Tamoxifen

Item 98

A 65-year-old man is evaluated because of intermittent hematuria, dysuria, and fatigue that did not improve after empiric ciprofloxacin. He is a current smoker with a 60-pack-year smoking history.

Physical examination is normal. Urinalysis shows 50 to 100 erythrocytes/hpf and is negative for leukocyte esterase, nitrites, and protein. Ultrasound of the abdomen and pelvis is normal.

Which of the following is the most appropriate management?

(A) Course of trimethoprim-sulfamethoxazole
(B) Cystoscopy and biopsy
(C) Prothrombin time, activated partial thromboplastin time, and bleeding time
(D) Urine culture

Item 99

A 65-year-old woman is evaluated because of left jaw pain that has persisted for 3 weeks. The patient denies recent dental trauma but notes that she underwent a recent, left lower molar dental extraction 6 weeks ago. Medical history is significant for a 2-year history of estrogen receptor–positive and *HER2*-negative breast cancer metastatic to bone. A bone scan performed 1 month ago revealed no changes over the past 6 months.

Current medications are letrozole and zoledronic acid.

On physical examination, temperature is 38.2 °C (100.8 °F), blood pressure is 120/80 mm Hg, pulse rate is 84/min, and respiration rate is 12/min. There is swelling over her left mandible with tenderness and a decreased ability to open her mouth. Oral findings are shown.

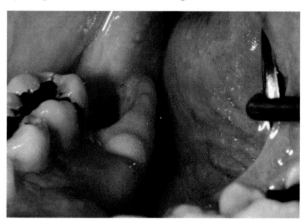

Which of the following is the most likely diagnosis?

(A) Letrozole-induced bone pain
(B) Metastatic breast cancer
(C) Osteonecrosis of the jaw
(D) Temporomandibular joint dislocation

Item 100

A 57-year-old woman has a 1-month history of increasing intermittent abdominal discomfort, constipation, and nausea. Two years ago, she underwent total abdominal hysterectomy with bilateral salpingo-oophorectomy followed by chemotherapy with six cycles of carboplatin and paclitaxel for stage IIIC serous papillary ovarian cancer. Chemotherapy was completed 18 months ago. Until now, there has been no evidence of disease recurrence. Medical history is otherwise unremarkable. Her only medications are a multivitamin, calcium and vitamin D supplements, and acetaminophen as needed for neuropathic pain.

On physical examination, temperature is normal, blood pressure is 134/85 mm Hg, pulse rate is 86/min, and respiration rate is 16/min; BMI is 28.5. The patient has gained 2.6 kg (6.0 lb) since her last office visit 3 months ago. There is no palpable lymphadenopathy. A healed midline abdominal scar is visible. The abdomen is soft and more distended than at her last examination. No dominant abdominal mass is noted, and there is no organomegaly. Pelvic examination is normal.

The complete blood count, serum creatinine level, and liver chemistry tests are normal. CA-125 concentration is 113 U/mL (113 kU/L) (normal range, 1.9-16.3 U/mL [1.9-16.3 kU/L]) compared with 102 U/mL (102 kU/L) 3 months ago.

CT scans of the chest, abdomen, and pelvis show studding of the peritoneal and bowel surfaces consistent with ovarian cancer recurrence. Paracentesis results of moderate ascites reveal malignant cells consistent with ovarian cancer.

There is no overt bowel obstruction, and the liver and lungs appear normal.

Which of the following is the most appropriate next step in managing this patient?

(A) Chemotherapy with a non–platinum-containing regimen
(B) Chemotherapy with a platinum-containing regimen
(C) Radiation therapy to the abdomen and pelvis
(D) Tumor debulking surgery

Answers and Critiques

Hematology Answers

Item 1   **Answer: C**

Educational Objective: Manage a patient with severe autoimmune hemolytic anemia who has indications for an incompatible transfusion.

This patient with symptomatic anemia has severe autoimmune hemolytic anemia secondary to chronic lymphocytic leukemia (CLL) confirmed by positive direct antiglobulin (Coombs) test results and the peripheral blood smear showing microspherocytes. In the absence of pregnancy and previous blood transfusions, the likelihood of alloimmunization to erythrocyte antigens is extremely low. Because of the broad specificity of autoantibodies in patients with autoimmune hemolytic anemia, most donor erythrocytes will be incompatible on cross-match. In this situation, transfusion of ABO-/Rh-specific, but otherwise incompatible, blood is necessary and can be life-saving. The transfused donor erythrocytes will survive as long as the patient's own erythrocytes and will provide oxygen-carrying capacity until definitive therapy, such as corticosteroids, becomes effective.

Erythropoietin is not indicated in patients with an appropriate reticulocyte response.

Splenectomy may be used to treat idiopathic autoimmune hemolytic anemia in a patient who does not respond to corticosteroid therapy. However, surgery is rarely indicated for patients with autoimmune hemolytic anemia secondary to CLL because therapy for the leukemia also treats the anemia. Transfusion of O-negative ("universal") blood is generally reserved for emergency situations in which the patient's ABO/Rh type is not known.

KEY POINT

- Because severe autoimmune hemolytic anemia can be life-threatening, an incompatible blood transfusion should not be withheld in a patient with this disorder.

Bibliography

Packman CH. Hemolytic anemia due to warm autoantibodies. Blood Rev. 2008;22(1):17-31. [PMID: 17904259]

Item 2   **Answer: A**

Educational Objective: Diagnose drug toxicity in a patient being treated for multiple myeloma.

Bortezomib, a novel proteosome inhibitor, is active against relapsed and refractory myeloma. Peripheral neuropathy is a common side effect of bortezomib therapy, occurring in approximately 30% of patients. The neuropathy is typically sensory and painful. Patients with preexisting neuropathy may experience increased symptoms during therapy with this agent. Reduction of the dosage may decrease symptoms, and some patients may have reversal of neuropathy after discontinuing bortezomib.

Diabetes mellitus most commonly causes a slowly progressive, distal, symmetric sensorimotor polyneuropathy. Autonomic dysfunction frequently is associated with diabetic neuropathy and is characterized by impotence, orthostatic hypotension, and gastroparesis. The acute onset of the neuropathy makes the diagnosis of diabetic neuropathy unlikely. However, patients with diabetes mellitus may be at increased risk for neurotoxicity from drugs for multiple myeloma, such as thalidomide and bortezomib. Although neuropathy can be a complication of myeloma, this symptom typically occurs on initial presentation and may improve with therapy for the myeloma and is usually not painful.

The POEMS syndrome is a rare plasma cell dyscrasia associated with polyneuropathy, organomegaly (hepatomegaly, splenomegaly, and lymphadenopathy), endocrinopathy (usually hypogonadism), monoclonal gammopathy, and skin manifestations (hyperpigmentation, hypertrichosis, acrocyanosis, plethora, hemangiomas, and/or telangiectasia). The patient's findings are incompatible with the POEMS syndrome.

KEY POINT

- Treatment of peripheral neuropathy due to bortezomib therapy requires discontinuation of therapy or dosage reduction.

Bibliography

Argyriou AA, Iconomou G, Kalofonos HP. Bortezomib-induced peripheral neuropathy in multiple myeloma: a comprehensive review of the literature. Blood. 2008;112(5):1593-1599. [PMID: 18574024]

Item 3   **Answer: A**

Educational Objective: Diagnose glucose 6-phosphate dehydrogenase deficiency.

Glucose 6-phosphate dehydrogenase (G6PD) deficiency is the most common disorder of erythrocyte metabolism. G6PD is necessary for generating adequate nicotinamide adenine dinucleotide phosphate-oxidase (NADPH) to prevent oxidant stress. G6PD is found on the X-chromosome, and deficiency, therefore, occurs rarely in women.

Several G6PD variants are detected electrophoretically, including G6PD B, the wild-type enzyme; and G6PD A−, which is responsible for oxidative hemolysis in aged erythrocyte cells. The acute onset of symptoms and findings in patients with this deficiency can be precipitated by drugs, infection, or diabetic ketoacidosis. In this patient, hemolysis was likely precipitated by diabetic ketoacidosis and trimethoprim-sulfamethoxazole.

At 2 to 4 days after introduction of the oxidative stress in patients with G6PD deficiency, there is the onset of jaundice and dark urine, with or without abdominal and back pain. The hemoglobin concentration decreases by 3 to 4 g/dL (30 to 40 g/L), and there is an appropriate increase in reticulocytes. The hemolysis spontaneously resolves in approximately 1 week as the older enzyme-depleted cells are replaced by new cells with sufficient G6PD to prevent further hemolysis. Additional laboratory findings in patients with G6PD deficiency include a negative direct and indirect anti-globulin (Coombs) test and the presence of "bite" or "blister" cells produced when accumulated oxidized hemoglobin remains adherent to the erythrocyte membrane with an adjacent membrane-bound clear zone. Such cells are visible on this patient's peripheral blood smear. Because reticulocytes can have normal G6PD levels in patients with the G6PD A– phenotype, measuring G6PD levels during an acute episode may produce a false-negative result.

Patients with warm antibody–mediated hemolysis have spherocytes on the peripheral blood smear as do patients with hereditary spherocytosis. The direct antiglobulin test is positive in patients with warm antibody–mediated hemolysis and negative in patients with hereditary spherocytosis. Patients with a microangiopathy have schistocytes on the peripheral blood smear and, typically, a low platelet count. Neither of these findings is present in the peripheral blood smear shown.

KEY POINT

- Because reticulocytes can have normal G6PD levels in patients with the G6PD A– phenotype, measuring G6PD levels during an acute episode may produce a false-negative result.

Bibliography

Mason PJ, Bautista JM, Gilsanz F. G6PD deficiency: the genotype-phenotype association. Blood Rev. 2007;21(5):267-283. [PMID: 17611006]

Item 4   Answer: C

Educational Objective: Treat a patient with polycythemia vera.

This patient has polycythemia vera, diagnosed by the elevated hematocrit level, decreased serum erythropoietin level, normal arterial oxygen saturation, and the presence of the *JAK2* mutation. Determination of the red blood cell mass is not needed when the hematocrit level is greater than 60% in men and 56% in women. Therapeutic phlebotomy should be instituted with the goal of lowering the hematocrit level to less than 45% for men and less than 42% for women. The major cause of death in untreated patients with polycythemia is thrombosis, which can be reduced by phlebotomy. Low-dose aspirin (70-100 mg) is also indicated for all patients unless there is a contraindication to

aspirin therapy or if the patient has symptoms of easy bruising and bleeding or an acquired platelet disorder, because some patients may develop a platelet dysfunction such as acquired von Willebrand disease. A meta-analysis of two randomized placebo-controlled trials concluded that low-dose aspirin was associated with a nonsignificant lower risk of fatal thrombotic events, and treatment did not increase the risk of major bleeding.

Therapeutic phlebotomy alone is sometimes insufficient treatment. Hydroxyurea is indicated for patients who cannot tolerate phlebotomy or do not respond to this procedure or who have marked thrombocytosis (thrombocyte count >1,500,000/µL [1500 × 10^9/L]). Anagrelide is used for treatment of essential thrombocytosis but may be helpful in treating patients with polycythemia vera in whom hydroxyurea is ineffective.

KEY POINT

- Initial treatment of polycythemia vera is therapeutic phlebotomy and low-dose aspirin.

Bibliography

Squizzato A, Romualdi E, Middeldorp S. Antiplatelet drugs for polycythaemia vera and essential thrombocythaemia. Cochrane Database Syst Rev. 2008;(2):CD006503. [PMID: 18425953]

Item 5   Answer: E

Educational Objective: Diagnose von Willebrand disease.

This patient has abnormal bleeding on tooth extraction, a history suggestive of a bleeding tendency, and a family history of a potential bleeding problem. His laboratory studies support both a qualitative platelet defect (prolonged bleeding time) and a mild coagulopathy (borderline elevated activated partial thromboplastin time [aPTT] and low factor VIII level). These findings are suggestive of the most common inherited hemostatic disorder, that of von Willebrand disease. von Willebrand disease is one of the few hemostatic disorders characterized by both a platelet and coagulation defect, due to a reduction or defect in von Willebrand factor (vWF), which supports platelet adhesion and also serves as a carrier protein for factor VIII. The diagnosis is confirmed by measuring the vWF antigen level and activity. Hemophilia A (factor VIII deficiency) is not associated with a prolonged bleeding time, nor would it be transmitted from father to son (X-linked inheritance).

The presence of a lupus inhibitor is generally associated with a thrombotic, not a bleeding, disorder; is an acquired disorder; does not prolong the bleeding time; and is not associated with decreased levels of factor VIII. Vitamin K deficiency can occur in patients receiving total parenteral nutrition or long-term antibiotics and in those who are malnourished, particularly in the setting of warfarin administration. This condition is characterized by a progressively prolonged prothrombin time (PT) and aPTT (with the PT proportionately more prolonged than the aPTT) and a normal thrombin time, findings not consistent with those in this patient. Factor XI deficiency might prolong the aPTT, but is not associated with a low factor VIII level or a prolonged bleeding time.

Bibliography

Kessler CM. Diagnosis and treatment of von Willebrand disease: new perspectives and nuances [erratum in Haemophilia. 2008;14(3): 669]. Haemophilia. 2007;13 Suppl 5:3-14. [PMID: 18078392]

Item 6   Answer: D

Educational Objective: Treat a patient with corticosteroid-refractory immune thrombocytopenic purpura.

Adult patients with immune thrombocytopenic purpura (ITP) often fail to have a sustained platelet response to corticosteroids and require other treatment. Splenectomy has been the traditional second-line therapy after corticosteroid failure, but in recent years, with the advent of other therapies, splenectomy is less-often performed, especially in older individuals who may have a higher surgical risk. Intravenous immune globulin or anti-D immunoglobulin (in Rh(+) patients with a spleen) is commonly used to immediately elevate the platelet count in patients with refractory ITP. Almost all patients who receive these treatments respond to varying degrees with an increase in platelet count to a safer level, but the rise is short-lived, lasting from a week to a few weeks, although occasionally longer. Repeated doses of these agents are effective. Such treatment, however, is not definitive, and other therapies, such as immunosuppressive agents, or, if necessary, splenectomy, should be re-considered.

High-dose cyclophosphamide or azathioprine may be used in treating refractory ITP, but an increased platelet count with these agents may not occur until after 4 months of treatment, which would not be helpful in immediately elevating this patient's severely low platelet count.

Platelet transfusions are contraindicated in patients with ITP except in the presence of life-threatening bleeding.

Danazol, an attenuated androgen, is helpful in treating some patients with ITP, but it is also a long-term treatment, with little ability to achieve an immediate increase in the platelet count.

Bibliography

Vesely SK, Perdue JJ, Rizvi MA, Terrell DR, George JN. Management of adult patients with persistent idiopathic thrombocytopenic purpura following splenectomy: a systematic review. Ann Intern Med. 2004;140(2):112-120. [PMID: 14734334]

Item 7   Answer: E

Educational Objective: Diagnose transfusion-related acute lung injury.

This patient has transfusion-related acute lung injury (TRALI), which occurs most frequently within 6 hours of transfusion of plasma-rich blood components. TRALI is an often severe reaction from donor antileukocyte antibodies that react with the patient's leukocytes. In TRALI, antibody-mediated activation of leukocytes causes leukocyte aggregates to become trapped in the pulmonary capillary bed, leading to neutrophil degranulation, alveolitis, or noncardiogenic pulmonary edema that often progresses to acute respiratory distress syndrome. TRALI is characterized by dyspnea, hypoxemia, and diffuse pulmonary infiltrates on radiography occurring within 6 hours of transfusion in the absence of circulatory overload. Plasma is the blood component most frequently responsible for TRALI, but packed erythrocytes, platelets, and even blood derivatives may also be implicated. Clinical improvement in TRALI begins in 2 to 3 days unlike in typical cases of acute respiratory distress syndrome. Management of TRALI involves stopping the transfusion and providing respiratory support and vasopressors for hypotension.

The absence of fever or a precipitating event and a normal level of consciousness make aspiration pneumonia unlikely. Anaphylaxis and pulmonary embolism cause respiratory distress without pulmonary infiltrates on a chest radiograph, and anaphylaxis is often associated with wheezing or stridor. Heart failure is effectively ruled out by the absence of an S_3 and jugular distention and a normal serum B-type-natriuretic peptide level.

Bibliography

Zhou L, Giacherio D, Cooling L, Davenport RD. Use of B-natriuretic peptide as a diagnostic marker in the differential diagnosis of transfusion-associated circulatory overload. Transfusion. 2005;45(7): 1056-1063. [PMID: 15987348]

Item 8   Answer: A

Educational Objective: Manage a patient with chronic myeloid leukemia.

This patient requires administration of imatinib. Chronic myeloid leukemia (CML) is the prototype of the myeloproliferative syndromes. It results from a balanced translocation between chromosomes 9 and 22 [t(9;22) the Philadelphia chromosome] creating a unique gene designated *BCR-ABL*, which codes a 210-kDa protein (p210) that functions as tyrosine kinase. The t(9;22) is not only diagnostic of CML, it is also the causative genetic event and a therapeutic target. The diagnosis of CML in this patient is based upon the presence of the *BCR/ABL* oncogene, peripheral blood smear findings showing increased granulocytes with a marked left shift and early erythrocyte precursors, and hypercellular bone marrow with marked myeloid proliferation. Patients with chronic-phase CML initially have less than 10% blasts in their bone marrow and peripheral blood. However, as the disease progresses, the blast count increases and is associated with an accelerated phase consisting of up to 20% blasts. A blast crisis may occur when the blast count is greater than 20%. Imatinib is a tyrosine kinase inhibitor that can lead to a complete cytogenetic remission in 70% of patients with CML and is most effective when used in the chronic phase of the disease. The optimal duration of therapy, long-term benefits, and toxicity of imatinib mesylate are under investigation. Imatinib has replaced hematopoietic stem cell transplantation (HSCT) as the initial treatment of patients with CML.

The best results for HSCT occur in patients with HLA-identical sibling donors. HSCT is curative for CML and was once the primary treatment option for patients with appropriately matched donors. However, HSCT is associated with significant morbidity and mortality and should be used only in very young patients with CML or in those who are resistant to the available tyrosine kinase inhibitors such as imatinib. Performing HLA typing in this patient and his sister to determine matching for HSCT is therefore not indicated at this time.

Leukapheresis is used to control the leukocytosis in patients with acute myeloid leukemia when the blast count is greater than 50,000/μL (50 × 10⁹/L). Patients with acute myeloid leukemia may have an elevated leukocyte count, but most leukocytes are circulating myeloblasts, and the blasts may contain Auer rods (clumped lysozymes that appear as azurophilic cytoplasmic rods). Auer rods are not present in patients with CML.

Because treatment of patients with CML is most effective when initiated in the chronic phase, close observation is inappropriate at this time.

KEY POINT
- Imatinib is a tyrosine kinase inhibitor that can lead to a complete cytogenetic remission in 70% of patients with chronic myeloid leukemia (CML); it is most effective when used in the chronic phase of CML.

Bibliography

Hughes T, Deininger M, Hochhaus A, et al. Monitoring CML patients responding to treatment with tyrosine kinase inhibitors - Review and recommendations for 'harmonizing' current methodology for detecting BCR-ABL transcripts and kinase domain mutations and for expressing results. Blood. 2006;108(1):28-37. [PMID: 16522812]

Item 9   Answer: C

Educational Objective: Manage a patient with transient risk factors for recurrent deep venous thrombosis.

In patients with venous thromboembolism (VTE) occurring secondary to transient risk factors such as in this patient, anticoagulation therapy should continue for 3 to 6 months, and in those with recurrent VTE, treatment should continue for more than 12 months. Although the appropriate duration of anticoagulation for idiopathic or recurrent VTE is not definitively known, extended-duration therapy is associated with significant benefit.

Treatment of 3 or 6 months' duration in patients with VTE secondary to transient risk is associated with similar risks for recurrent VTE. In one study in which patients with a second episode of VTE were enrolled exclusively, extended-duration (>12 months or indefinite) anticoagulant therapy was associated with fewer recurrences than was cessation of therapy after 6 months. For patients with idiopathic VTE (including those with recurrent VTE), extended-duration therapy was shown to decrease the relative risk for recurrence by 64% to 95%. Duration of therapy in the trials varied widely, from greater than 3 months, to 12 months, to up to 4 years. The results for extended-duration therapy reflect follow-up only to 4 years; the risk–benefit ratio is not known for longer durations. Clinicians should weigh the benefits, harms, and patient preferences in deciding on the duration of anticoagulation.

This patient has two transient risk factors contributing to her deep venous thrombosis (DVT), a long airplane flight predisposing to venous stasis and oral contraceptives. Thus, a course of therapy for 3 to 6 months would be appropriate; 6 weeks would be considered too short and 12 months unnecessarily long. Decreasing warfarin treatment to 4 or 6 weeks results in a doubling of the rate of recurrent VTE compared with 6 months. Lifelong anticoagulation is unnecessary in a patient with transient, reversible risk factors for DVT.

- A 3- to 6-month regimen is adequate anticoagulation in a patient with a deep venous thrombosis caused by reversible risk factors.

Bibliography
Segal JB, Streiff MB, Hoffman LV, Thornton K, Bass EB. Management of Venous Thromboembolism: A Systematic Review for a Practice Guideline [erratum in Ann Intern Med. 2007;146(5): 396]. Ann Intern Med. 2007;146(3):211-222. [PMID: 17261856]

Item 10   Answer: A

Educational Objective: Diagnose inflammatory anemia.

This patient has inflammatory anemia as characterized by a low serum iron concentration and low total iron-binding capacity (TIBC) with an elevated serum ferritin concentration. Although the initial presentation of inflammatory anemia is typically a normochromic normocytic anemia, over time, microcytosis can be observed. Inflammatory anemia is associated with increased levels of the peptide hepcidin, which is produced in the liver and causes decreased iron absorption from the gut and decreased iron release from macrophages. Hepcidin directly affects the iron transporter, ferroportin, and causes internalization of this ion channel. Hepcidin measurement is not available for clinical diagnostic use.

Hemoglobin C disease produces a mild hemolytic anemia in persons of African ancestry. Laboratory evaluation typically reveals normal iron studies. The peripheral blood smear shows prominent targeting in addition to microcytosis. This patient's abnormal iron studies and normal peripheral blood smear exclude hemoglobin C disease as the cause of his anemia.

Iron deficiency is characterized by a low serum iron concentration, an elevated TIBC, and a decreased serum ferritin concentration, a pattern different from that observed in this patient. Patients with inflammatory anemia and iron deficiency have a low mean corpuscular volume and low serum iron levels because both experience iron-limited erythropoiesis.

Patients with thalassemia would have an elevated serum lactate dehydrogenase level and reticulocyte count caused by hemolysis, values unlike those found in this patient.

- Inflammatory anemia is characterized by a low or normal serum iron level, a low total iron-binding capacity, and an elevated ferritin concentration.

Bibliography
Weiss G, Goodnough LT. Anemia of chronic disease. N Engl J Med. 2005;352(10):1011-1023. [PMID: 15758012]

Item 11   Answer: C

Educational Objective: Treat a patient with hyperviscosity syndrome and lymphoplasmacytic lymphoma (Waldenström macroglobulinemia).

Patients with lymphoplasmacytic lymphoma (Waldenström macroglobulinemia) have an elevated serum IgM concentration associated with lymphoplasmacytic infiltrates of the bone marrow, lymphadenopathy, anemia, neuropathy, organomegaly, IgM monoclonal gammopathy, and hyperviscosity syndrome. Symptoms of hyperviscosity syndrome include blurred vision, fatigue, mucosal bleeding, headache, heart failure, and altered mentation. Plasma exchange is indicated for managing acute symptoms in conjunction with administration of rituximab or fludarabine for treating the lymphoplasmacytic lymphoma.

Blood transfusion is contraindicated because it may increase serum viscosity even more and exacerbate hyperviscosity symptoms in patients with Waldenström macroglobulinemia.

Furosemide would be indicated in patients with heart failure; however, this patient has symptoms of hyperviscosity syndrome, and diuresis will not improve her symptoms.

Intravenous immune globulin can be used in the treatment of autoimmune hemolytic anemia; however, this patient does not have hemolytic anemia because the serum lactate dehydrogenase level is normal.

- Plasma exchange is appropriate for treating hyperviscosity syndrome, and rituximab or fludarabine is indicated for specific treatment of lymphoplasmacytic lymphoma (Waldenström macroglobulinemia).

Bibliography
Dimopoulos MA, Kyle RA, Anagnostopoulos A, Treon SP. Diagnosis and management of Waldenstrom's macroglobulinemia. J Clin Oncol. 2005;23(7):1564-1577. [PMID: 15735132]

Item 12   Answer: A

Educational Objective: Evaluate a patient with paroxysmal nocturnal hemoglobinuria.

The coexistence of pancytopenia, hemolytic anemia, and thrombosis should raise the suspicion for paroxysmal nocturnal hemoglobinuria (PNH). PNH is caused by loss of glycosylphosphatidylinositol (GPI)–linked proteins on the cell surface. Two such proteins, CD55 and CD59, help reduce erythrocyte sensitivity to complement. Deficiency of CD55 and CD59 can be detected by flow cytometry. Because of the unopposed actions of complement, patients with PNH have direct antiglobulin (Coombs)–negative hemolysis. Iron deficiency is also a common finding in patients with PNH owing to iron loss in the urine. PNH is associated with thrombosis, perhaps secondary to loss of naturally occurring anticoagulants that are linked to membranes by GPI anchors. Finally, this disorder is associated with aplasia, myelodysplasia, and, rarely, acute leukemia. Recently, eculizumab, a monoclonal antibody to C5, has been reported to offer a sustained response to patients with PNH.

This patient does not have a history suggestive of a congenital hemoglobin disorder necessitating hemoglobin electrophoresis. A hemoglobinopathy would not explain the low leukocyte count or thrombocytopenia in this patient. Erythrocyte osmotic fragility is used to assess hereditary spherocytosis, but that disorder would not explain this patient's pancytopenia nor the deep venous thrombosis (DVT).

Parvovirus B19 may cause anemia or, especially in immunocompromised patients, pancytopenia, but the reticulocyte count should be less than 2%, and there is no association with DVT.

KEY POINT

- Paroxysmal nocturnal hemoglobinuria is characterized by direct antiglobulin (Coombs)–negative hemolysis, pancytopenia, and thrombosis.

Bibliography

Hill A, Richards SJ, Hillmen P. Recent developments in the understanding and management of paroxysmal nocturnal haemoglobinuria. Br J Haematol. 2007;137(3):181-192. [PMID: 17408457]

Item 13   Answer: B

Educational Objective: Diagnose immune thrombocytopenic purpura.

This healthy young woman has petechiae caused by her very low platelet count with a subacute onset. Although most of her remaining laboratory studies are normal, her peripheral blood smear showing few, but large, platelets supports the presence of a young population of platelets, consistent with increased turnover. These findings are suggestive of immune thrombocytopenic purpura (ITP), and a bone marrow examination is not essential. Instead, a presumptive diagnosis of ITP should be established, and the patient should receive high-dose corticosteroids. Corticosteroids are generally indicated in patients with ITP who have symptomatic bleeding and platelet counts below 50,000/μL (50 × 10^9/L) or in those with severe thrombocytopenia and platelet counts below 15,000/μL (15 × 10^9/L).

Platelet transfusions would not be indicated in this patient unless serious, life-threatening bleeding was present. A bone marrow biopsy is not necessary in this setting given the absence of any other signs of a bone marrow stem cell disorder, such as leukopenia or the presence of nucleated erythrocytes, and early myeloid forms suggest a myelophthisic process as occurring in neoplastic and metastatic disease, lymphoma, granulomatous disease, and infections of the bone marrow. Observation alone would be inappropriate in this patient considering her very low platelet count

and the risk for bleeding. Splenectomy is not indicated as first-line therapy for ITP but may be considered when other less-invasive therapies have failed.

KEY POINT

- Corticosteroids are the first-line treatment for patients with immune thrombocytopenic purpura.

Bibliography

Cines DB, Bussel JB. How I treat idiopathic thrombocytopenic purpura (ITP). Blood. 2005;106(7):2244-2251. [PMID: 15941913]

Item 14   Answer: D

Educational Objective: Manage a patient with antiphospholipid antibodies after a first deep venous thrombosis.

A systematic review reported that the absolute risk of new venous thromboembolism (VTE) in patients with antiphospholipid antibodies is low (less than 1% per year). However, this risk may be increased to up to 10% per year in women with antiphospholipid antibodies or antiphospholipid antibody syndrome and recurrent fetal loss and more than 10% per year in patients with antiphospholipid antibodies and previous VTE who have discontinued anticoagulants within 6 months. Current recommendations are to treat these patients with anticoagulation indefinitely. The benefit of VTE prevention with long-term anticoagulation in these high-risk patients may outweigh the risk for bleeding complications. Randomized studies have now shown that most patients can be treated effectively with standard-intensity anticoagulation (target INR, 2.5). Selected patients with resistant disease or recurrence despite therapy should be treated at a higher intensity (target INR, 3.0). Positive results for anticardiolipin antibody or lupus inhibitor assay should be confirmed over time to ensure that they are not transient, which can occur after viral infections. Ideally, at least two positive laboratory tests (anticardiolipin antibody or lupus inhibitor assay) at least 12 weeks apart should be documented to confirm the presence of an antiphospholipid antibody syndrome before a patient is committed to lifelong anticoagulation.

KEY POINT

- Patients with an antiphospholipid antibody syndrome and deep venous thrombosis have a high risk for recurrence once anticoagulation therapy is discontinued and require anticoagulation therapy indefinitely.

Bibliography

Lim W, Crowther MA, Eikelboom JW. Management of antiphospholipid antibody syndrome: A systematic review. JAMA. 2006;295(9):1050-1057. [PMID: 16507806]

Item 15   Answer: C

Educational Objective: Treat a patient with the 5q- syndrome.

This patient should receive lenalidomide. Myelodysplastic syndromes (MDS) are clonal disorders of the hematopoietic stem cells that occur predominantly in patients older than 50 years and are characterized by ineffective hematopoiesis and peripheral cytopenia. Dysplasia of erythroid, granulocytic, or megakaryocytic lineages in a patient with a hypercellular bone marrow and low peripheral blood counts suggests MDS. Detection of clonal abnormalities commonly involving chromosomes 3, 5, 7, 8, and 17 supports the diagnosis. This patient has the 5q- syndrome (interstitial deletion of the long arm of chromosome 5), which is a subtype of MDS, characterized by an elevated platelet count and anemia. Most patients are elderly women who have an indolent course associated with transfusion-dependent anemia, a low incidence of neutropenia and thrombocytopenia, and a low rate of transformation to acute myeloid leukemia. This subtype of MDS responds favorably to lenalidomide, an analogue of thalidomide, which results in resolution of the anemia in two thirds of patients. Lenalidomide is U.S. Food and Drug Administration approved for patients with the 5q- syndrome, but they must register with the "Revassist" program, and they must complete an informed consent to ensure that they understand the need to minimize fetal exposure. Lenalidomide can cause neutropenia and infections, and blood counts must be monitored closely.

Patients with classic MDS treated with azacitidine have better outcomes than patients who receive supportive care only. In these patients, azacitidine therapy significantly delays leukemic transformation and significantly improves quality of life. Azacitidine is not as effective as lenalidomide for a patient with the 5q- syndrome. Danazol has been used to treat the anemia associated with MDS. However, danazol has a low response rate and many side effects (especially masculinizing effects in women) and is therefore not recommended as first-line therapy. In selected patients with MDS, co-administration of erythropoietin and granulocyte colony-stimulating factor has a synergistic effect in increasing hemoglobin levels and decreasing transfusion requirements, particularly in patients requiring less than 2 units of packed erythrocytes per month and in those with serum erythropoietin levels less than 500 U/L.

KEY POINT
- Patients with the 5q- syndrome have a subtype of myelodysplastic syndrome that responds to lenalidomide.

Bibliography
List A, Dewald G, Bennett J, et al; Myelodysplastic Syndrome-003 Study Investigators. Lenalidomide in the myelodysplastic syndrome with chromosome 5q deletion. N Engl J Med. 2006;355(14):1456-1465. [PMID: 17021321]

Item 16   Answer: B

Educational Objective: Manage a patient with factor XI deficiency prior to minor surgery.

This patient may proceed to surgery with no preoperative treatment. Hematologic problems commonly encountered perioperatively include coagulopathy, thrombocytopenia, and anemia. Patients with a negative history for bleeding and normal physical examination findings undergoing low-risk procedures do not need screening for coagulopathy. Although routine screening for a bleeding disorder is not indicated unless there is a personal or family history suggestive of a problem, it was performed in this patient. Unexpected findings are uncommon, and even when present in a patient without a history of abnormal bleeding, rarely result in a change in preoperative management. The relationship between an abnormal screening coagulation test and the risk of surgical bleeding is low in this group of patients. Because isolated factor XI deficiency, also called Rosenthal syndrome and hemophilia C, is seldom related to a bleeding tendency or is only a minimal bleeding risk at best, this patient who is undergoing minor surgery may proceed to surgery with no preoperative treatment; canceling surgery is also unnecessary.

Isolated factor XI deficiency is found most commonly in patients of Jewish ancestry from northern Europe (Ashkenazi ethnicity). Because factor VII in the extrinsic pathway can cross over and also activate factor IX in the intrinsic pathway, those factors higher up in the clotting cascade (factors XI and XII) are bypassed, resulting in relatively normal hemostasis.

KEY POINT
- Patients with isolated factor XI deficiency seldom have a bleeding tendency and do not require prophylactic treatment prior to surgery.

Bibliography
Franchini M, Veneri D, Lippi G. Inherited factor XI deficiency: a concise review. Hematology. 2006;11(5):307-309. [PMID: 17607578]

Item 17   Answer: D

Educational Objective: Manage a patient with a severe iron deficiency refractory to oral iron.

Because iron is absorbed in the proximal small bowel, patients with disorders of the small bowel such as malabsorption, or those with a history of surgical resection, frequently cannot absorb oral iron. Such patients can become profoundly iron deficient, as this patient has, unless parenteral iron therapy is initiated. Intravenous iron is an effective iron replacement therapy in patients who cannot absorb oral iron salts. After the initiation of iron therapy, reticulocytosis is seen within 4 days. Noticeable increases in hemoglobin are usually obtained within several weeks.

Older parenteral preparations, such as iron dextran, confer a much higher risk of anaphylaxis than that associated with newer preparations such as intravenous iron or ferric gluconate. In patients who have had resection of large portions of the proximal segment of the small bowel, doubling the oral dose of iron will not resolve the iron deficiency.

Similarly, although ascorbic acid can augment oral iron absorption, it does so poorly and increases the possibility of gastrointestinal side effects, and the combination of oral iron and ascorbic acid will not replace iron stores in a patient without an intact proximal small bowel.

Deferoxamine is an iron chelator used to treat iron overload and is not appropriate in this patient.

KEY POINT
- For patients unable to absorb oral iron, intravenous iron is a suitable parenteral replacement.

Bibliography
Silverstein SB, Rodgers GM. Parenteral Iron therapy options. Am J Hematol. 2004;76(1):74-78. [PMID: 15114602]

Item 18   Answer: A
Educational Objective: Diagnose renal cell carcinoma in a patient with erythrocytosis and elevated erythropoietin levels.

Patients with erythrocytosis and elevated erythropoietin levels may have a tumor providing an exogenous source of erythropoietin, pulmonary or cardiac disease, or a high-oxygen–affinity hemoglobin. In this patient who has a normal arterial oxygen saturation level and normal cardiopulmonary findings with no family history of erythrocytosis, an erythropoietin-producing tumor such as renal cell carcinoma is the most likely diagnosis. Therefore, an ultrasound of the abdomen would be the most reasonable next diagnostic test. Only 1% to 5% of patients with renal cell carcinoma have erythrocytosis; approximately 20% to 80% of patients with renal cell carcinoma have anemia.

Because this patient is not cyanotic, has a normal arterial oxygen saturation level, and has normal physical examination findings, abnormalities of the cardiac and pulmonary systems are not likely. As such, an echocardiogram would not be helpful.

Patients with myeloproliferative disorders, such as polycythemia vera, have characteristically low, not elevated, erythropoietin levels. Therefore, a myeloproliferative disorder is unlikely in this patient, and a *JAK2* mutation analysis would be unnecessary.

Although sometimes advocated in the workup of polycythemia vera, the erythrocyte mass study in a patient with a hemoglobin concentration of 20 g/dL (200 g/L) is not likely to provide useful information. With an elevated hemoglobin concentration of this magnitude, the erythrocyte mass will invariably be elevated in this patient. In addition, this study is difficult to obtain, expensive to perform, and the results may be inaccurate in inexperienced hands.

KEY POINT
- Patients with erythrocytosis and elevated erythropoietin levels may have a tumor providing an exogenous source of erythropoietin, pulmonary or cardiac disease, or a high-oxygen–affinity hemoglobin.

Bibliography
Hodges VM, Rainey S, Lappin TR, Maxwell AP. Pathophysiology of anemia and erythrocytosis. Crit Rev Oncol Hematol. 2007;64(2): 139-158. [PMID: 17656101]

Item 19   Answer: D
Educational Objective: Provide stroke prophylaxis in a patient with sickle cell anemia and a history of stroke.

The pathophysiology of stroke in patients with sickle cell disease is complex, involving adherent erythrocyte membranes, constricted arterioles, nitric oxide depletion, and other factors. Strokes recur in up to 70% of patients with sickle cell disease following an initial stroke if left untreated. Randomized trials have confirmed the ability of monthly erythrocyte transfusions (hypertransfusions) of two units per month in adults to decrease stroke recurrence by 50% in patients with sickle cell disease. In fact, in children at risk for stroke based on abnormal cranial Doppler flow measurements, such hypertransfusion therapy is an effective prophylactic treatment. Furthermore, increased stroke risk returns to baseline in children in whom transfusions are stopped once initiated.

Dipyridamole, clopidogrel, and angiotensin-converting enzyme inhibitors have a role in stroke prevention in patients with atherosclerotic disease; however, their role in patients with sickle cell disease remains undefined. Hydroxyurea would be continued, although its role in stroke prevention is unclear.

KEY POINT
- Hypertransfusion can reduce the risk of stroke recurrence in patients with sickle cell disease by 50%.

Bibliography
Wang WC. The pathophysiology, prevention and treatment of stroke in sickle cell disease. Curr Opin Hematol. 2007;14(3):191-197. [PMID: 17414206]

Item 20   Answer: B
Educational Objective: Manage preoperative anticoagulation needs in a patient with a high risk for thrombosis.

Patients with a mechanical valve in the mitral position have a high risk for thrombosis when they are not taking anticoagulants, even for short periods. Other high-risk conditions include high-risk atrial fibrillation (for example, valvular atrial fibrillation, previous stroke, or transient ischemic attack), and a recent history (<3 months) of venous thromboembolism. This patient is scheduled to have a polypectomy, a procedure associated with a bleeding risk, especially in the setting of anticoagulation. Consequently, stopping oral anticoagulation in this patient is appropriate; however, the use of a short-acting anticoagulant, such as unfractionated heparin or low-molecular-weight heparin (LMWH), is required to provide additional short-term protection while he is not taking warfarin. This process, called "bridging," is a common procedure in patients who take warfarin and require that it be temporarily interrupted for an invasive procedure. Warfarin is usually stopped 5 days preoperatively to allow the INR to normalize. Heparin is then initiated approximately 3 days before the procedure as the INR decreases. Although unfractionated heparin can be used for this purpose, use of this agent requires hospitalization for intravenous administration and monitoring, whereas LMWH can be administered at home, twice daily; does not need monitoring; and is recommended. The second dose of LMWH the evening before the procedure is omitted, and then LMWH is resumed, with warfarin, 12 to 24 hours postoperatively, as long as hemostasis is secured. In some cases, the LMWH may be postponed for 36 to 48 hours depending on the bleeding risk. When the INR reaches a therapeutic level several days later, the LMWH can be discontinued. This process can be managed by the patient or a caregiver on an outpatient basis.

If the bleeding risk during a procedure is extremely low, such as in a dental procedure, then warfarin does not need to be discontinued. Depending on the risk for thrombosis, the warfarin may be discontinued without bridging medication (for example, in the case of a patient with a history of deep venous thrombosis that occurred 3 months ago). In some cases, the risk of thrombosis from the procedure is considered to be low such that postoperative bridging with LMWH can be given without preoperative bridging, or low-dose LMWH can be used for bridging. Such bridging decisions require a careful assessment of the risk of thromboembolism if warfarin is discontinued versus the risk of bleeding if warfarin is continued.

KEY POINT

• In patients at high risk for thromboembolism who must have a temporary interruption of warfarin therapy for a procedure, bridging anticoagulation with low-molecular-weight heparin is recommended before and after the procedure.

Bibliography

Douketis JD, Berger PB, Dunn AS, et al; American College of Chest Physicians. The perioperative management of antithrombotic therapy: ACCP Evidence–based clinical practice guidelines. Chest. 2008;133(6 Suppl):299S-339S. [PMID: 18574269]

Item 21   Answer: D

Educational Objective: Treat a patient with essential thrombocythemia who is to undergo surgery.

This patient has essential thrombocythemia characterized by menorrhagia, epistaxis, easy bruising, and marked thrombocytosis with abnormal platelet aggregation studies. Patients with essential thrombocythemia may develop both thrombotic and hemorrhagic complications, especially when the platelet count is greater than 1 million/μL (1000 × 10^9/L). The platelet count must be lowered quickly in patients with life-threatening symptoms, such as transient ischemic attack, stroke, myocardial infarction, or gastrointestinal bleeding, and prior to surgery. The postoperative period is a time of great risk for developing thrombotic and hemorrhagic complications. When hemorrhages occur, they are mostly mucosal, and significant gastrointestinal bleeding may develop. This patient's platelet count should therefore be lowered preoperatively, and platelet apheresis will do this quickly. However, because significant rebound thrombocytosis may develop, additional myelosuppression with hydroxyurea is needed postoperatively.

Hydroxyurea alone may be used to treat essential thrombocythemia but should be started well in advance of surgery so that the platelet count can be lowered preoperatively. Although anagrelide may also be used, it does not act quickly enough to provide protection if given only 2 days preoperatively. The risk for acute leukemia after long-term use of hydroxyurea is 3% to 4% in essential thrombocythemia, although the exact role of hydroxyurea in leukemogenesis is not clear. Anagrelide therapy has been associated with higher risk of arterial thrombosis, bleeding, and fibrotic transformation than hydroxyurea in patients with essential thrombocythemia. Aspirin is contraindicated in this patient with abnormal platelet function but would be added to her therapy if the platelet count were normal.

KEY POINT

• Platelet apheresis can quickly lower the platelet count in patients with essential thrombocythemia and life-threatening symptoms but must be followed by additional myelosuppressive therapy to prevent rebound thrombocytosis.

Bibliography

Schafer AI. Thrombocytosis. N Engl J Med. 2004;350(12):1211-1219. [PMID: 15028825]

Item 22   Answer: D

Educational Objective: Evaluate a patient with idiopathic pulmonary embolism and family history of venous thromboembolism.

This patient with an idiopathic pulmonary embolism (PE) and a family history of venous thromboembolism has a high likelihood of having an underlying thrombophilic condition. Screening decisions in patients with possible thrombophilic disorders are based on whether they are considered to be strongly or weakly thrombophilic. Patients who are considered strongly thrombophilic 1) will have had their first idiopathic venous thrombosis before 50 years of age; *or* 2) have a history of recurrent thrombotic episodes; *or* 3) have first-degree relative(s) in whom a documented thromboembolism has occurred before the age of 50 years. This patient meets not one but two of these criteria with her family history and recent pulmonary embolism; therefore, she should undergo testing for activated protein C resistance, the prothrombin gene mutation, antiphospholipid antibodies, factor V Leiden, antithrombin deficiency, protein C deficiency, protein S deficiency, and the lupus inhibitor.

Screening for thrombophilia should not be done during anticoagulant therapy because both heparin and warfarin will influence the results of certain tests. Neither should it be done during the acute presenting episode before anticoagulants are initiated because the thrombosis itself may influence the results of certain tests. Thus, thrombophilia testing is best done at least a couple weeks after a course of therapy is completed. If D-dimer testing is to be performed as part of the risk assessment for recurrent deep venous thrombosis, testing should be done no earlier than 4 weeks after cessation of therapy.

Polycythemia vera and essential thrombocythemia predispose patients to venous and arterial thrombotic events, particularly when the red blood cell mass or platelet count is not controlled. Although the *JAK2* mutation is found in almost all patients who have polycythemia vera and in approximately 50% of patients with essential thrombocythemia, routine screening for this mutation is not recommended except in patients with the Budd-Chiari syndrome or portal vein thrombosis in whom a myeloproliferative disease is suspected. Because this patient has a normal complete blood count and her thrombotic disorder was a PE, screening for the *JAK2* mutation would be inappropriate.

Performing no further testing in this patient considering her recent idiopathic PE and family history of thrombotic issues would be inappropriate because the risk of recurrent venous thromboembolism cannot be estimated without screening for inherited thrombophilia.

Certain thrombophilic disorders are associated with a high risk for recurrence, and patients with these disorders are candidates for long-term, if not lifelong, therapy. These include individuals with antithrombin, protein C, or protein S deficiency, and those who are homozygous for factor V Leiden or the prothrombin gene mutation or who are doubly heterozygous for each.

KEY POINT

- **Thrombophilic screening should not be done at the onset of a thrombotic event or during anticoagulant therapy but should be performed 2 weeks after completion of therapy.**

Bibliography

Bauer KA. The thrombophilias: Well-defined risk factors with uncertain therapeutic implications. Ann Intern Med. 2001;135(5):367-373. [PMID: 11529700]

Item 23   Answer: D

Educational Objective: Manage a patient with thrombotic thrombocytopenic purpura.

This patient has evidence of microangiopathic hemolytic anemia, thrombocytopenia with normal coagulation, and central nervous system symptoms, the principal triad of thrombotic thrombocytopenic purpura (TTP); renal failure and fever compose the pentad of symptoms. Plasma exchange is the principal treatment modality for TTP and should be initiated as soon as possible to decrease patient morbidity. Plasma exchange reverses the platelet consumption that is responsible for the thrombus formation causing the findings associated with TTP. It is acceptable to initiate plasma exchange even in circumstances when the diagnosis is in question, only to be stopped when an alternative diagnosis is established.

Intravenous immune globulin is useful in treating patients with immune thrombocytopenic purpura (ITP) but not TTP. The presence of severe microangiopathic hemolytic anemia is inconsistent with ITP and, therefore, precludes the use of intravenous immune globulin in this patient.

A direct antiglobulin (Coombs) test would be appropriate for patients with suspected immune hemolytic anemia, but this is a case of microangiopathic hemolytic anemia as evidenced by schistocytes on the peripheral blood smear.

An activated partial thromboplastin time (aPTT) mixing study is not indicated in this patient because her aPTT is normal.

Platelet antibody assays are generally not very sensitive or specific in patients with thrombocytopenia and would not be helpful in this case. A positive test result would not explain the presence of schistocytes on the peripheral blood smear.

KEY POINT

- **Microangiopathic hemolytic anemia, thrombocytopenia with normal coagulation, and central nervous system symptoms are the principal triad of thrombotic thrombocytopenic purpura; renal failure and fever compose the pentad of symptoms.**

Bibliography

George JN. Clinical practice. Thrombotic thrombocytopenic purpura. N Engl J Med. 2006;354(18):1927-1935. [PMID: 16672704]

Item 24   Answer: B

Educational Objective: Diagnose Sβ+ thalassemia.

Hemoglobin electrophoresis is a method for identifying hemoglobin subcomponents by separating out individual hemoglobin species in an electric field. This patient has Sβ+ thalassemia, characterized by a hemoglobin S level that is greater than 60%, with an elevated hemoglobin A_2 level and mild microcytosis. These patients have painful crises, but to a lesser extent than patients homozygous for hemoglobin S. Patients with Sβ+ thalassemia have target cells and few or no sickled erythrocytes on the peripheral blood smear. Patients with sickle cell trait (AS), who are often confused with patients with Sβ+ thalassemia, have a hemoglobin S level that is less than 50% and a hemoglobin A level that is correspondingly greater than 50%. Patients with the sickle cell trait also have normal-sized erythrocytes. Patients with hemoglobin SC disease have painful crises in addition to an approximately 50:50 ratio of hemoglobin S to hemoglobin C on electrophoresis. Patients with hemoglobin SC disease also typically have hepatosplenomegaly. Sickled erythrocytes, reticulocytosis, and Howell-Jolly bodies are found on the peripheral blood smear in affected patients. Patients heterozygous for hemoglobin S with hereditary persistence of fetal hemoglobin have less than 70% hemoglobin S and greater than 30% hemoglobin F on electrophoresis.

KEY POINT

- Sβ+ thalassemia is characterized by a hemoglobin S level greater than 60%, with an elevated hemoglobin A_2 level and mild microcytosis.

Bibliography

Rund D, Rachmilewitz E. Beta-thalassemia. N Engl J Med. 2005;353(11):1135-1146. [PMID: 16162884]

Item 25   Answer: C

Educational Objective: Treat pure red cell aplasia due to parvovirus B19 infection.

This patient with HIV infection has pure red cell aplasia secondary to parvovirus B19 infection. Immunocompromised patients often lack the characteristic rash and arthralgia observed in immunocompetent patients. The diagnosis is suggested by the presence of giant pronormoblasts in the bone marrow and confirmed by the presence of viral DNA in the serum and bone marrow. Patients with HIV infection may not be able to mount an appropriate antibody response to parvovirus B19 and subsequently develop pure red cell aplasia due to the destruction of erythroid precursors. Once the diagnosis is made, treatment includes erythrocyte transfusions and pooled intravenous immune globulin to infuse antibodies against parvovirus.

Antithymocyte globulin and cyclosporine are effective for treating autoimmune aplastic anemia, characterized by an aplastic or hypoplastic bone marrow, without giant pronormoblasts. This patient's anemia is characterized by a hypocellular bone marrow, giant pronormoblasts, and evidence of parvovirus infection, making aplastic anemia an unlikely diagnosis. Cytarabine and anthracyclines are chemotherapeutic agents that are used to treat acute myeloblastic leukemia (AML). The diagnosis is of AML is suggested by an elevated leukocyte count, anemia, thrombocytopenia, and blasts on the peripheral blood smear. These findings are absent, making AML an unlikely diagnosis. Recombinant erythropoietin is not indicated because this patient already has a very high baseline serum erythropoietin level, and more erythropoietin is unlikely to improve his anemia and will not treat the underlying infectious disease.

KEY POINT

- Treatment of pure red cell aplasia in patients with parvovirus B19 infection consists of erythrocyte transfusion and intravenous immune globulin.

Bibliography

Claster S. Biology of anemia, differential diagnosis, and treatment options in human immunodeficiency virus infection. J Infect Dis. 2002;185 Suppl 2:S105-9. [PMID: 12001030]

Item 26   Answer: B

Educational Objective: Manage anticoagulation therapy in a patient with an idiopathic deep venous thrombosis.

Patients who experience an idiopathic deep venous thrombosis (DVT) have a relatively high rate of recurrence (approximately 8% to 10% per year over the next several years) if anticoagulation is stopped at 6 months. Some experts recommend long-term or lifelong treatment. Because oral anticoagulant therapy confers a risk for major bleeding, a risk-benefit assessment must be performed when deciding whether to continue or discontinue anticoagulation therapy. One option in determining the risk for recurrent venous thrombosis in high-risk individuals is to measure the D-dimer concentration after 6 months of anticoagulation therapy. Patients at high risk may include those with idiopathic DVT occurring at a young age, in unusual locations, or with a strong family history. An elevated D-dimer level, obtained while the patient has ceased taking therapy for 1 month, is associated with an increased recurrence risk compared with a normal D-dimer level. Because this idiopathic DVT occurred in a young individual, the likelihood of an underlying thrombophilic condition (either inherited or acquired) is possible, and thrombophilic testing may also be indicated. Identifying selected thrombophilic conditions may help further in determining the duration of anticoagulant therapy.

Continuing warfarin therapy without first measuring the D-dimer level to determine the patient's risk for recurrence does not provide the needed data for informed decision-making in this case.

Measuring the C-reactive protein level, a marker of inflammation, does not reliably predict recurrence rates for DVT.

Evidence drawn from a meta-analysis suggests that it is unlikely that the methylenetetrahydrofolate reductase (MTHFR) genotype is a predictor independent of homocysteine for venous or arterial disease, and screening for MTHFR in patients with arterial or venous thrombosis is not recommended. Furthermore, there is no evidence that patients with elevated homocysteine levels require additional warfarin therapy, and elevated homocysteine is not a predictor of risk for DVT recurrence.

KEY POINT

- Patients with idiopathic deep venous thrombosis and an elevated D-dimer level measured 1 month after cessation of a 6-month anticoagulation regimen have an increased recurrence risk compared with patients in whom D-dimer levels are normal.

Bibliography

Palareti G, Cosmi B, Legnani C, et al; PROLONG Investigators. D-dimer testing to determine the duration of anticoagulation therapy [erratum in N Engl J Med. 2006;355(26):2797]. N Engl J Med. 2006;355(17):1780-1789. [PMID: 17065639]

Item 27   Answer: C
Educational Objective: Diagnose myelofibrosis.

Myeloproliferative syndromes are clonal stem cell disorders characterized by chronic unregulated hyperproliferation of the myeloid elements in the bone marrow (granulocytes, erythrocytes, platelets, and stromal cells). This patient has myelofibrosis, one of the four entities that constitute the myeloproliferative syndrome. Myelofibrosis causes clonal proliferation of abnormal stromal cells that release fibrosis-promoting cytokines in the bone marrow. His peripheral blood smear shows a classic leukoerythroblastic picture of immature granulocytes (a metamyelocyte) and early erythrocyte forms (nucleated erythrocytes) as well as dysmorphic erythrocytes (tear-drop cells). Splenomegaly and hepatomegaly result from extramedullary hematopoiesis, and patients can develop portal hypertension. Bone marrow hypercellularity is the hallmark of this disease and often results in dry bone marrow aspiration. This patient's bone marrow biopsy reveals typical findings of myelodysplasia, including a hypercellular marrow with dysmorphic megakaryocytes and no evidence of increased blast forms, resulting in inadequate hematopoiesis. Median survival is 3 to 5 years, and death commonly results from marrow

failure, transformation to acute leukemia, or complications of portal hypertension.

Patients with chronic myeloid leukemia characteristically have an elevated leukocyte count, a low platelet count, and splenomegaly, but the leukocyte count is often higher than this patient's count, and the peripheral blood smear shows the characteristic full array of maturing granulocytes. Bone marrow is hypercellular with marked myeloid hyperplasia and minimal fibrosis, and cytogenetic analysis shows the Philadelphia chromosome.

Aplastic anemia is a disorder in which myeloid progenitor cells and stem cells are severely diminished or absent in the bone marrow because of an intrinsic defect of the stem cells or immune-mediated stem cell destruction, which leads to transfusion-dependent anemia, thrombocytopenia, and severe neutropenia. The bone marrow is typically aplastic or hypoplastic, without evidence of infiltrating malignant cells, and there is no evidence of hepatomegaly or splenomegaly.

Acquired chronic pure red cell aplasia is characterized by the absence or marked decrease of erythrocyte production, probably as the result of immune-mediated destruction of erythroid progenitors. Affected patients typically have severe normochromic and normocytic or macrocytic anemia as well as reticulocytopenia with normal leukocyte and platelet counts. Nucleated and dysmorphic erythrocytes are not present in the peripheral blood smear, and the bone marrow shows profound erythroid hypoplasia.

KEY POINT

- Myelofibrosis is characterized by splenomegaly, normocytic anemia, circulating erythroblasts and myeloid precursors, teardrop cells, and bone marrow fibrosis.

Bibliography

Tefferi A. Myelofibrosis with myeloid metaplasia. N Engl J Med. 2000;342(17):1255-1265. [PMID: 10781623]

Item 28   Answer: A
Educational Objective: Diagnose acute lymphoblastic leukemia.

This patient has acute lymphoblastic leukemia (ALL), precursor T-cell subtype (as determined by immunophenotyping and the presence of terminal deoxynucleotidyl transferase [TdT]). ALL typically develops in young men in their teens and twenties who present with leukocytosis, lymphadenopathy, organomegaly, and bone marrow that is infiltrated with lymphoblasts. Patients often have mediastinal masses, which is a favorable prognostic sign. Adult patients with T-cell lineage ALL have a better prognosis than those with B-cell lineage ALL, and the absence of the Philadelphia chromosome (absence of the *BCR/ABL* translocation) is a good prognostic sign.

Patients with acute myeloid leukemia usually do not have lymphadenopathy or organomegaly, and histochemical studies show positive staining for myeloperoxidase. Although patients with chronic lymphocytic leukemia may have lymphadenopathy and organomegaly, they do not have bone marrow blasts. In addition, chronic lymphocytic leukemia is typically a B-cell disorder. Although the presence of lymphadenopathy in this patient does suggest a possible lymphoma, the presence of leukocytosis and the infiltration of the bone marrow with blasts and the types of immunophenotypic markers that are present are inconsistent with a diagnosis of Hodgkin lymphoma.

KEY POINT

- **T-cell acute lymphoblastic leukemia is frequently diagnosed in young men with lymphadenopathy and organomegaly.**

Bibliography

Jabbour EJ, Faderl S, Kantarjian HM. Adult acute lymphoblastic leukemia. Mayo Clin Proc. 2005;80(11):1517-1527. [PMID: 16295033]

Item 29   Answer: D
Educational Objective: Diagnose multiple myeloma in a patient with hypercalcemia.

This patient has hypercalcemia, diffuse osteopenia, anemia, leukopenia, renal insufficiency, and a history of encapsulated organism–related pneumonia, which is a characteristic presentation of multiple myeloma. The diagnosis is supported by the bone marrow aspirate, which shows clusters of plasma cells. These cells can easily be distinguished from megaloblastoid erythrocytes by their dispersed chromatin pattern and perinuclear halo (Golgi apparatus).

Acute myeloid leukemia rarely causes hypercalcemia. In addition, more severe bone marrow failure and a decreased platelet count would be likely, and the bone marrow aspirate would not show leukemic blasts. Chronic lymphocytic leukemia (CLL) may rarely cause hypercalcemia along with renal insufficiency; an elevated leukocyte count is typical. Moreover, the morphologic findings of the bone marrow aspirate in this patient rule out a diagnosis of CLL.

Metastatic small cell lung cancer to the bone marrow may cause cytopenia. The peripheral blood smear would show leukoerythroblastic features with tear drop erythrocytes and immature myeloid and erythroid cells. Furthermore, the morphologic findings of the bone marrow aspirate in this patient, which shows a proliferation of plasma cells, is inconsistent with metastasis from any other cancer.

KEY POINT

- **Hypercalcemia is a common complication of multiple myeloma.**

Bibliography

Kyle RA, Rajkumar SV. Multiple myeloma [erratum in N Engl J Med. 2005;352(11):1163]. N Engl J Med. 2004;351(18):1860-1873. [PMID: 15509819]

Item 30   Answer: C
Educational Objective: Diagnose pulmonary hypertension in a patient with sickle cell anemia.

Pulmonary hypertension is a newly recognized cause of morbidity and mortality in patients with homozygous sickle cell (SS) disease. In a recent cross-sectional study on 40 adult patients with sickle cell anemia, pulmonary hypertension was present in two thirds of the patients and was minimal to moderate as assessed by Doppler techniques. Other studies suggest a prevalence of 20% to 40%. Patients with SS disease and pulmonary hypertension tend to have lower hemoglobin levels and higher levels of lactate dehydrogenase and bilirubin than patients with SS disease who do not have pulmonary hypertension. Furthermore, retinopathy and lower extremity ulcers are more common in patients with SS disease and pulmonary hypertension than in patients with SS disease and normal pulmonary artery pressures. The presentation of pulmonary hypertension is characterized by right-sided heart failure. In addition, the echocardiographic results described for this patient are consistent with those of patients with pulmonary hypertension.

Constrictive pericarditis is characterized by a thickened, fibrotic, and adherent pericardium that restrains ventricular diastolic expansion, leading to impaired filling. Patients with this disorder have dyspnea, fatigue, jugular venous distention, peripheral edema, hepatomegaly, and ascites. Pulmonary congestion is absent, and a pericardial knock may be auscultated. Systemic venous pressure may increase with inspiration (Kussmaul sign). Echocardiography can confirm the pathophysiology of constrictive pericarditis and shows: (1) accentuated transmitral or tricuspid early filling velocity with a rapid decrease in early filling velocities, (2) accentuated phasic changes in filling with respiration, and (3) abnormal diastolic septal motion. None of these findings were present in this patient.

Giant cell myocarditis is a rare disease of uncertain etiology that presents with cardiogenic failure, marked biventricular enlargement, and refractory ventricular arrhythmias in young to middle-aged adults. This patient's clinical presentation, physical examination, and echocardiographic results are not compatible with this diagnosis.

Most patients with hypertrophic cardiomyopathy are relatively asymptomatic; however, some may develop symptoms of pulmonary congestion (exertional dyspnea, orthopnea, paroxysmal nocturnal dyspnea) as well as chest pain, fatigue, palpitations, dizziness, and syncope. In affected patients, physical examination in the presence of left ventricular outflow obstruction shows a variable and dynamic systolic murmur that is increased by the Valsalva maneuver and standing, and is diminished by hand-gripping, leg elevation, and squatting. There is no change in the murmur with respiration. Echocardiography in patients with hypertrophic cardiomyopathy delineates the pattern of the left ventricular or septal hypertrophy, quantifies the severity of left ventricular obstruction, and confirms the presence of diastolic filling abnormalities.

> **KEY POINT**
> - Pulmonary hypertension is a common cause of morbidity and mortality in patients with sickle cell disease.

Bibliography

Gladwin MT, Sachdev V, Jison ML, et al. Pulmonary hypertension as a risk factor for death in patients with sickle cell disease. N Engl J Med. 2004;350(9):886-895. [PMID: 14985486]

Item 31   Answer: A
Educational Objective: Recognize the expected increment in platelets following platelet transfusion.

The dosage of platelets should be calculated for each patient on the basis of the desired increment in platelet count and the size of the patient. A commonly used adult transfusion dose is a pool of four to five concentrates ("five pack"). Platelets can also be prepared from a single donor using apheresis separation, collecting enough for a transfusion without the need to pool products. A platelet count of 50,000/µL (50 × 10^9/L) is considered adequate for patients undergoing most surgical procedures (except central nervous system procedures). One bag of apheresis platelets is appropriate for this patient, because it provides a platelet dose equivalent to four to six units of platelet concentrate and increases the platelet count of an average-sized adult by approximately 25,000/µL (25 × 10^9/L). The posttransfusion platelet increment would therefore be approximately 50,000/µL (50 × 10^9/L) in the absence of fever, bleeding, or splenomegaly.

Transfusing two bags of apheresis platelets is excessive. Fresh frozen plasma (FFP) is separated from blood and frozen within 6 hours to preserve all labile proteins. The chief indication for use of FFP is to replace coagulation factors. Transfusion of FFP is inappropriate in a patient with thrombocytopenia. A unit of platelets is derived from the platelet-rich plasma obtained from a unit of whole blood, which is then concentrated to a volume of approximately 50 mL. One unit of platelet concentrate is inadequate for an adult.

> **KEY POINT**
> - For most adults, one bag of apheresis platelets increases the platelet count by approximately 25,000/µL (25 × 10^9/L).

Bibliography

Stroncek DF, Rebulla P. Platelet transfusions. Lancet. 2007;370 (9585):427-438. [PMID: 17679020]

Item 32   Answer: D
Educational Objective: Diagnose secondary polycythemia due to sleep apnea.

This obese man most likely has sleep apnea with secondary polycythemia. Excessive daytime sleepiness is the hallmark of sleep apnea. Other clinical manifestations that should alert the clinician to the presence of sleep apnea include morning headaches, nocturia, and alterations in mood. Hypoxia is the main inducer of erythropoietin production by the proximal nephrons, and an elevated erythropoietin level strongly supports a diagnosis of secondary polycythemia. Some patients with cardiopulmonary disease or sleep apnea will not show reduced oxygen saturation at rest or during the daytime. In these cases, pulse oximetry should be obtained after exertion, and, depending on the clinical history, sleep studies may be indicated to confirm the diagnosis of sleep apnea and to detect nocturnal oxygen desaturation. In patients with sleep apnea, the secondary polycythemia will most likely resolve once the sleep apnea is corrected.

Relative polycythemia often accompanies plasma volume contraction as a result of excessive sweating, diarrhea, vomiting, capillary leak syndrome, and, occasionally, diuretic use. The hematocrit or hemoglobin appears increased because of a reduction in plasma volume. There is nothing in the history to suggest the presence of relative polycythemia, and relative polycythemia cannot explain the increase in this patient's erythropoietin level.

Polycythemia vera is characterized by an increased erythrocyte mass and may be accompanied by mild elevation in leukocyte and platelet counts. Hematocrit values greater than 60% for men and 56% for women in the absence of secondary causes of erythrocytosis and the presence of splenomegaly establish the diagnosis of polycythemia vera. A *JAK2* mutation is detected in 65% to 95% of patients with polycythemia vera, and a polymerase chain reaction assay for this mutation can aid in establishing the differential from secondary causes of erythrocytosis. The patient's strongly suggestive history of sleep apnea and absence of leukocytosis and thrombocythemia, elevated erythropoietin level, and absence of *JAK2* mutation argue strongly against the diagnosis of polycythemia vera.

Congenital polycythemia due to a high-oxygen-affinity hemoglobin is suspected when polycythemia is discovered during childhood or when it is associated with a positive family history of polycythemia. In these cases, the serum erythropoietin level is normal. This patient lacks an appropriate childhood or family history, and his elevated erythropoietin level is also incompatible with a high-oxygen-affinity hemoglobin.

> **KEY POINT**
> - Polycythemia associated with an increased serum erythropoietin level helps exclude polycythemia vera and suggests a diagnosis of secondary erythrocytosis.

Bibliography

Spivak JL. Polycythemia vera: Myths, mechanisms, and management. Blood. 2002;100(13):4272-4290. [PMID: 12393615]

Item 33   Answer: B

Educational Objective: Evaluate a patient with a prolonged activated partial thromboplastin time.

This patient has a prolonged activated partial thromboplastin time (aPTT). The first diagnostic step in determining the cause of an abnormal aPTT or prothrombin time (PT) is to perform an inhibitor mixing study. In a mixing study, the patient's plasma is mixed in a 1:1 ratio with normal pooled plasma, and the clotting tests with abnormal results are repeated. A mixing study that corrects to normal indicates a factor clotting deficiency, whereas one that does not correct (or only poorly corrects) indicates the presence of a clotting inhibitor or antibody. Once the results of the inhibitor mixing study are established, other assays to identify the deficient clotting factor or the type of clotting inhibitor can be done.

Although this patient might have von Willebrand's disease, hemophilia A, or the antiphospholipid antibody syndrome with a mild factor VIII deficiency causing an elevated aPTT, understanding the mechanism responsible for the elevated aPTT is necessary before performing tests to rule out these diagnoses.

KEY POINT

- Performing an inhibitor mixing study is the first step in identifying the cause of an abnormal activated partial thromboplastin time or prothrombin time.

Bibliography

Kamal AH, Tefferi A, Pruthi RK. How to interpret and pursue an abnormal prothrombin time, activated partial thromboplastin time, and bleeding time in adults. Mayo Clin Proc. 2007;82(7):864-873. [PMID: 17605969]

Item 34   Answer: C

Educational Objective: Manage a patient with acute promyelocytic leukemia.

This patient has acute myeloid leukemia, promyelocytic subtype (subtype M3), based on the number of myeloblasts and promyelocytes in the bone marrow and confirmed by the presence of t(15;17). The 15;17 translocation results in a unique fusion gene, PML/RARα, which has been implicated in leukemogenesis. Patients with acute promyelocytic leukemia often present with pancytopenia and symptoms referable to the anemia, neutropenia, and thrombocytopenia, or they may be asymptomatic, like this patient. Patients with acute promyelocytic leukemia have an excellent response to chemotherapy plus a differentiating agent that interferes with PML/RARα protein function, such as

all-*trans*-retinoic acid or arsenic trioxide. Response rates approach 85% to 95% for patients on this regimen.

Since this patient is not febrile, broad-spectrum antibiotics are not needed despite the low leukocyte count. Chemotherapy alone is insufficient treatment because randomized clinical trials have shown the superiority of combining differentiating agents such as all-*trans*-retinoic acid and chemotherapy as induction therapy. Given the excellent results with current combined regimens, bone marrow transplantation is generally not considered a postremission treatment option in the first complete remission. Therefore, HLA typing for hematopoietic stem cell transplantation is not indicated at this time.

KEY POINT

- Acute promyelocytic leukemia is treated with chemotherapy plus a differentiating agent such as all-*trans*-retinoic acid or arsenic trioxide.

Bibliography

Advani SH, Nair R, Bapna A, et al. Acute promyelocytic leukemia: All-*trans* retinoic acid (ATRA) along with chemotherapy is superior to ATRA alone. Am J Hematol. 1999;60(2);87-93. [PMID: 9929098]

Item 35   Answer: C

Educational Objective: Treat a patient with thrombophilia and the antiphospholipid antibody syndrome during pregnancy.

There is considerable evidence showing the association between thrombophilia and recurrent pregnancy loss, especially in women with the antiphospholipid antibody syndrome. Studies have shown that aspirin alone does not reduce the rate of pregnancy loss in such patients, but the combination of unfractionated heparin and low-dose aspirin has been shown to do so. Current guidelines recommend low- or intermediate-dose unfractionated heparin or prophylactic-dose low-molecular-weight heparin (LMWH), both with low-dose aspirin, as the treatment of choice in pregnant patients with thrombophilia and the antiphospholipid antibody syndrome.

Head-to-head studies of unfractionated heparin and LMWH have not been done. Because LMWH is less likely than unfractionated heparin to cause heparin-induced thrombocytopenia, it tends to be preferred over unfractionated heparin. Vitamin K antagonists, such as warfarin, are generally not recommended for use in pregnant patients because of their teratogenic potential except possibly in the setting of mechanical heart valves.

KEY POINT

- Heparin plus aspirin is required to reduce the risk of pregnancy loss in women with the antiphospholipid antibody syndrome.

Bibliography

Bates SM, Greer IA, Pabinger I, Sofaer S, Hirsh J. American College of Chest Physicians. Venous thromboembolism, thrombophilia, antithrombotic therapy, and Pregnancy: American College of Chest Physicians Evidence-Based Clinical Practice Guidelines (8th Edition). Chest 2008;133(6 Suppl):844S-886S. [PMID: 18574280]

Item 36   Answer: A

Educational Objective: Diagnose cyclosporine-induced hemolytic uremic syndrome.

This patient's peripheral blood smear shows schistocytes and is absent platelets, findings characteristic of microangiopathic hemolytic anemia (MAHA). The negative direct and indirect antiglobulin (Coombs) tests rule out autoimmune hemolytic anemia in this patient. In addition, the patient's laboratory results are consistent with hemolysis (elevated lactate dehydrogenase level) and include an elevated creatinine concentration. An elevated creatinine concentration is consistent with cyclosporine toxicity or renal graft failure. In this patient, cyclosporine should be stopped and alternative methods of immunosuppression should be initiated. Plasma exchange is used in patients with thrombotic thrombocytopenic purpura and hemolytic-uremic syndrome (HUS), but its use in the management of patients with cyclosporine-induced HUS is controversial.

Mycophenolate and trimethoprim-sulfamethoxazole can both cause bone marrow suppression, but neither is associated with MAHA.

Prednisone does not lead to hemolytic anemia.

> **KEY POINT**
> - Calcineurin inhibitors such as cyclosporine and tacrolimus can cause microangiopathic hemolytic anemia and acute kidney injury.

Bibliography

Qu L, Kiss JE. Thrombotic microangiopathy in transplantation and malignancy. Semin Thromb Hemost. 2005;31(6):691-699. [PMID: 16388420]

Item 37   Answer: D

Educational Objective: Diagnose vitamin K deficiency in a malnourished patient treated with antibiotics.

Clotting factors II, VII, IX, and X, as well as protein C and protein S, require vitamin K–dependent gamma carboxylation for full activity. Dietary vitamin K is obtained primarily from the intake of dark green vegetables and is modified by gut flora to the active form. Interruption of bile flow prevents absorption of vitamin K. Antibiotic-related elimination of enteric bacteria limits intestinal sources of vitamin K, whereas warfarin directly antagonizes vitamin K activity. The prothrombin time (PT) is the first clotting time to become prolonged, but the activated partial thromboplastin time (aPTT) will also lengthen with further factor deficiencies. Therefore, a progressively

prolonged PT (with the PT proportionately more prolonged than the aPTT) and a normal thrombin time in a malnourished patient receiving antibiotics should raise the suspicion for vitamin K deficiency. In adults with normal hepatic function, oral or subcutaneous vitamin K usually corrects the clotting times within 24 hours; intravenous vitamin K confers an increased risk for anaphylaxis. Fresh frozen plasma is used when urgent correction is required.

In this patient, the normal thrombin time and platelet count and elevated fibrinogen level are not suggestive of a diagnosis of disseminated intravascular coagulation (DIC) or liver disease. DIC would be a consideration in patients with a constellation of findings, including elevated levels of fibrin degradation products and/or fibrinogen D-dimer, sometimes accompanied by a prolonged PT, a decreased fibrinogen level, and thrombocytopenia.

Antibodies directed against clotting factors are rare but can result in potentially lethal, acquired bleeding disorders. Most such antibodies are considered idiopathic, but they may develop because of drugs or as part of an underlying illness, such as malignancy or autoimmune disorders (for example, systemic lupus erythematosus or rheumatoid arthritis). Diagnosis is made by identification of a protracted clotting time that does not correct with a mixing study. Quantifying the inhibitor by obtaining an inhibitor titer helps determine treatment options. Causes of such acquired bleeding disorders include the use of fibrin sealants during procedures, the presence of antiphospholipid antibodies, and the use of antibiotics. Because the PT/INR mixing study corrects to normal, a lupus inhibitor is excluded in this patient. In addition, low-dose heparin has no effect on INR and should not result in the clinical bleeding present in this patient. Finally, positive D-dimer results are to be expected in any hospitalized, ill patient with ongoing inflammation, and in the absence of any other findings, have no diagnostic significance.

> **KEY POINT**
> - A progressively prolonged prothrombin time (PT) and activated partial thromboplastin time (aPTT) (with the PT proportionately more prolonged than the aPTT) with a normal thrombin time in a malnourished patient who has received antibiotics is suggestive of vitamin K deficiency.

Bibliography

Crowther MA, McDonald E, Johnston M, Cook D. Vitamin K deficiency and D-dimer levels in the intensive care unit: a prospective cohort study. Blood Coagul Fibrinolysis. 2003;13(1):49-52. [PMID: 11994567]

Item 38   Answer: C

Educational Objective: Diagnose subclinical cobalamin deficiency.

Levels of methylmalonic acid and homocysteine become elevated in patients with vitamin B$_{12}$ deficiency before serum vitamin B$_{12}$ levels decrease below the normal range (200-800 pg/mL [148-590 pmol/L]). In contrast, only homocysteine is elevated in folate deficiency. Subclinical vitamin B$_{12}$ deficiency in patients with subtle signs and symptoms of vitamin B$_{12}$ deficiency, as in this case, can be detected by identification of elevated methylmalonic acid levels. This is particularly true for patients whose vitamin B$_{12}$ levels are in the "low-normal" range. Additionally, pancytopenia can occur in vitamin B$_{12}$-deficient patients. Interestingly, metformin has been recently associated with vitamin B$_{12}$ deficiency, although malabsorption, independent of pernicious anemia, is the most likely cause of vitamin B$_{12}$ deficiency in an older patient.

Although bone marrow biopsy can be suggestive of vitamin B$_{12}$ deficiency, it is not a specific test for confirming this disorder because there are other potential causes of megaloblastic marrow, including myelodysplasia.

Erythrocyte folate levels have been touted as a better indication of folate stores than are serum folate levels but are subject to problems of defining normal values and may not be that helpful clinically. Erythrocyte folate levels can also be depressed in patients with vitamin B$_{12}$ deficiency. Additionally, folate deficiency would not cause the neurologic symptoms present in this patient.

Parietal cell antibodies are elevated in patients with pernicious anemia but may not be elevated in patients whose vitamin B$_{12}$ deficiency is due to malabsorption, which is a very common cause of deficiency in the elderly.

KEY POINT

• Methylmalonic acid levels become elevated before cobalamin levels decrease below the normal range in patients with vitamin B$_{12}$ deficiency.

Bibliography
Hvas AM, Nexo E. Diagnosis and treatment of vitamin B12 deficiency—an update. Haematologica. 2006;91(11):1506-12. [PMID: 17043022]

Item 39   Answer: C
Educational Objective: Diagnose a delayed hemolytic transfusion reaction.

A delayed hemolytic transfusion reaction is an anamnestic antibody response to previous erythrocyte antigen sensitization that typically occurs 7 to 14 days after the index transfusion. The primary alloimmunization event is generally a remote transfusion or pregnancy. At the time of the index transfusion, the antibody level has declined below the detectable threshold that can be determined by routine blood bank screening. For patients who have received multiple transfusions at another facility, obtaining a transfusion history from the previous blood bank may be very helpful. A delayed hemolytic transfusion reaction is associated with jaundice, low-grade fever, and an otherwise unexplained decrease in the hemoglobin concentration. Laboratory

testing in these patients shows indirect hyperbilirubinemia and positive results on direct and indirect antiglobulin (Coombs) tests.

Patients with sickle cell disease may have pain typical of a vaso-occlusive crisis, but they would not have positive direct antiglobulin test results or the appearance of a new alloantibody on antibody testing. Furthermore, a vaso-occlusive crisis would not explain the sudden decrease in this patient's hemoglobin concentration.

Patients with aplastic anemia have pancytopenia and a low reticulocyte count, findings not present in this patient.

Autoimmune hemolytic anemia is less likely because a specific erythrocyte alloantibody has been identified in this patient. Occasionally, an autoantibody develops concomitantly with development of one or more alloantibodies. This finding is not specific for patients with sickle cell disease. However, bystander hemolysis in the absence of detectable auto- or alloantibodies (sometimes referred to as the hyperhemolysis syndrome) is well documented in patients with sickle cell disease.

KEY POINTS

• A delayed hemolytic transfusion reaction is an anamnestic antibody response to previous erythrocyte antigen sensitization that occurs 7 to 14 days after an index transfusion.
• In patients with sickle cell disease, a delayed hemolytic transfusion reaction may mimic a vaso-occlusive crisis.

Bibliography
Telen MJ. Principles and problems of transfusion in sickle cell disease. Semin Hematol. 2001;38(4):315-323. [PMID: 11605166]

Item 40   Answer: B
Educational Objective: Diagnose acute myeloid leukemia.

Myelodysplastic syndromes are clonal disorders of the hematopoietic stem cells in patients older than 50 years and are characterized by ineffective hematopoiesis and peripheral cytopenia. Although the natural history of distinct subtypes of myelodysplasia ranges from indolent chronic anemia to rapid death from progression to acute leukemia, most patients eventually progress to leukemic syndromes or die from complications of bone marrow failure. This patient has acute myeloid leukemia, as indicated by the peripheral blood smear that shows a myeloblast with Auer rods. Auer rods are clumps of azurophilic, needle-shaped crystals made from primary cytoplasmic granules. They occur most often in patients with acute myeloid leukemia and rarely in patients with myelodysplasia. Fever in patients with AML is almost always related to infection, and this patient must be quickly and thoroughly evaluated for a source of infection and treated empirically with broad-spectrum antibiotics.

Auer rods do not occur in patients with acute lymphoblastic leukemia. Patients with acute promyelocytic leukemia may have circulating blasts, but the predominant cell is a large immature granulocyte with multiple granules overlying the cytoplasm and nucleus. Patients with chronic myeloid leukemia may have circulating blasts but will also have more mature granulocytes and will not have Auer rods.

KEY POINT

- A peripheral blood smear showing myeloblasts that contain Auer rods is diagnostic of acute myeloid leukemia.

Bibliography

Nimer SD. Myelodysplastic syndromes. Blood. 2008;111(10):4841-4851. [PMID: 18467609]

Item 41　　Answer:　E

Educational Objective: Treat sickle cell disease in a pregnant patient.

Although the RNA-reductase inhibitor hydroxyurea has been shown to decrease the incidence of painful crises and improve mortality in patients with sickle cell disease, it is contraindicated in pregnancy because of its documented teratogenicity, and, as such, is classified as a class D drug in pregnancy.

Oxycodone and acetaminophen are classified as Food and Drug Administration (FDA) pregnancy risk category B drugs. The pregnancy risk factor increases to FDA risk category D if oxycodone is used for prolonged periods during pregnancy or in high doses close to term. Acetaminophen and oxycodone can be used with caution in pregnancy to manage less severe episodes of pain that do not require hospitalization if the benefits of administration outweigh any potential risks.

The influenza vaccine is offered annually to individuals at risk for complications from the flu, including patients older than 65 years, those with chronic disease, those who are immunocompromised, and pregnant women whose last two trimesters coincide with the influenza season (late December through mid-March). The main vaccine used in the United States is a trivalent inactivated virus, but an intranasally administered vaccine from a trivalent live-attenuated virus is also available for patients aged 5 to 49 years. The live vaccine is contraindicated in immunocompromised persons and pregnant women. Folic acid is important in pregnancy owing to requirements of the developing fetus and is also important in patients with hemolytic anemias who also have increased folate requirements. Folate is a pregnancy class A drug.

KEY POINT

- Hydroxyurea is contraindicated in pregnancy.

Bibliography

Dauphin-McKenzie N, Giles JM, Jacques E, Harrington T. Sickle cell anemia in the female patient. Obstet Gynecol Surv. 2006;61(5): 343-352. [PMID: 16635275]

Item 42　　Answer:　C

Educational Objective: Treat a patient with delayed heparin-induced thrombocytopenia and thrombosis.

This patient's deep venous thrombosis (DVT), recent hospitalization, and thrombocytopenia are clues possibly suggestive of delayed-onset, heparin-induced thrombocytopenia (HIT), and cessation of heparin, initiation of a direct thrombin inhibitor, and requesting a heparin platelet factor-4 antibody assay are appropriate. Heparin-induced thrombocytopenia and thrombosis (HITT) can occur in a delayed fashion, often within 3 months of heparin exposure. The patient was hospitalized 4 weeks earlier for an acute myocardial infarction, underwent cardiac catheterization, and received low-molecular-weight heparin. HIT may have been present at the time of discharge, but was unrecognized. Her current findings include a DVT and thrombocytopenia, which may be related to the DVT or to a potential case of delayed-onset HIT. The clinical suspicion of delayed-onset HIT is heightened by an abrupt decrease in the platelet count to $27,000/\mu L$ ($27 \times 10^9/L$) 12 hours after initiation of heparin treatment.

Platelet transfusions are contraindicated in patients in whom thrombocytopenia is caused by a consumptive process unless there is life-threatening bleeding. Corticosteroids would only be appropriate if the thrombocytopenia were thought to be typical for immune thrombocytopenic purpura, which it is not, especially considering the patient's associated thrombosis. Warfarin should not be initiated in the absence of a concurrently administered parenteral anticoagulant, because warfarin alone can potentiate a hypercoagulable state early in treatment.

KEY POINT

- Heparin-induced thrombocytopenia and thrombosis can occur in a delayed fashion, often within 3 months of heparin exposure and requires heparin cessation and initiation of a direct thrombin inhibitor.

Bibliography

Rice L, Attisha WK, Drexler A, Francis JL. Delayed-onset heparin-induced thrombocytopenia. Ann Intern Med. 2002;136(3):210-215. [PMID: 11827497]

Item 43　　Answer:　B

Educational Objective: Manage immune thrombocytopenic purpura in a pregnant patient.

Because the patient has no signs or symptoms of other causes of thrombocytopenia, including an otherwise-normal complete blood count, differential, and peripheral blood smear, it is therefore reasonable to assume a diagnosis of immune thrombocytopenic purpura (ITP), which was probably present before her pregnancy (platelet count of 102,000/µL [102×10^9/L]) but was never diagnosed. ITP often becomes apparent during the first trimester, and affected patients may have a history of thrombocytopenia or other autoimmune manifestations. ITP in patients with this level of platelets requires observation only. Treatment would be indicated only if her platelet count were to decrease well below 50,000/µL (50×10^9/L) on a sustained basis. Treatment of ITP in pregnancy, when required, is similar to that in nonpregnant patients, consisting of corticosteroid therapy or intravenous immune globulin to achieve an increase in the platelet count.

The incidence of thrombotic thrombocytopenic purpura (TTP) appears to be increased during pregnancy. Although some series suggest that most cases develop in the late second trimester, recent reports suggest that the disorder may also occur commonly near term. The manifestations of TTP in pregnant women are identical to those in nonpregnant women, consisting of microangiopathic hemolytic anemia and thrombocytopenia and may be associated with fever, renal injury, and neurologic abnormalities. The treatment of choice is immediate plasma exchanges. The course of TTP is not affected by pregnancy termination.

Platelet transfusion in patients with thrombocytopenia is generally reserved for patients with severe thrombocytopenia who have major bleeding. It should be considered as a temporizing measure to bridge the interval necessary for more durable treatments to take effect.

KEY POINT

- Immune thrombocytopenic purpura in pregnancy generally requires no therapy unless the platelet count is well below 50,000/µL (50×10^9/L) on a sustained basis.

Bibliography

Karim R, Sacher RA. Thrombocytopenia in pregnancy. Current Hematol Reports. 2004;3(2):128-133. [PMID: 14965489]

Item 44   Answer: B

Educational Objective: Diagnose warm antibody–mediated hemolytic anemia.

The hemolytic anemias are characterized by increased destruction of erythrocytes associated with a marrow response (reticulocytosis). Elevated levels of unconjugated bilirubin, lactate dehydrogenase, and uric acid, and depressed levels of haptoglobin are characteristic of hemolysis. Warm antibody–mediated hemolytic anemia is characterized by a positive direct antiglobulin (Coombs) test and the presence of spherocytes on the peripheral blood smear. Autoimmune hemolytic anemia (AIHA) may be idiopathic

or result from drugs, lymphoproliferative disorders, collagen vascular diseases, or malignancies. The disorder occurs when IgG, IgM, or, rarely IgA, autoantibodies bind to erythrocyte antigens. The most common type of AIHA is warm antibody–mediated. In this condition, IgG antibodies bind to Rh-type antigens on the erythrocyte surface at 37.0 °C (98.6 °F) . Although these antibodies may fix complement, they more commonly bind to the cell surface and facilitate Fc-receptor–mediated erythrocyte destruction by splenic macrophages. Warm antibodies are diagnosed by the direct antiglobulin test, which detects IgG or complement on the cell surface.

Microangiopathic hemolytic anemia is a nonimmune hemolytic anemia. Like other hemolytic anemias, it is characterized by reticulocytosis, elevated levels of unconjugated bilirubin, lactate dehydrogenase, and depressed levels of haptoglobin. Microangiopathic hemolysis may be associated with thrombocytopenia. Another distinguishing characteristic of microangiopathic hemolytic anemia is the presence of schistocytes on the peripheral blood smear.

α-Thalassemia is a congenital hemolytic anemia. Patients with a two-α-gene defect have target cells and an absence of spherocytes on the peripheral blood smear and will not have a positive direct antiglobulin test. Patients homozygous for hemoglobin C typically show polymerized hemoglobin C in erythrocytes on the peripheral blood smear and a less-severe degree of hemolysis than that observed in this case. Target cells, not spherocytes, are also visible on the peripheral blood smear, and the direct antiglobulin test results are negative in patients homozygous for hemoglobin C.

KEY POINT

- Warm antibody–mediated hemolytic anemia is characterized by spherocytes on the peripheral blood smear and is a common complication of lymphoid malignancies.

Bibliography

Hauswirth AW, Skrabs C, Schutzinger C, Gaiger A, Lechner K, Jager U. Autoimmune hemolytic anemias, Evans' syndromes, and pure red cell aplasia in non-Hodgkin lymphomas. Leuk Lymphoma. 2007;48(6):1139-1149. [PMID: 17577777]

Item 45   Answer: B

Educational Objective: Evaluate a patient in whom there is a low suspicion for deep venous thrombosis.

A patient in whom deep venous thrombosis (DVT) is suspected must undergo objective testing to exclude the diagnosis. Several imaging procedures can exclude DVT, but the diagnostic goal is to use the most efficient, least-invasive, and least-expensive method with the fewest side effects. A D-dimer assay is a simple, relatively noninvasive test that has been shown to have a high negative predictive value, especially if the suspicion for DVT is low. The Wells criteria have been established to help the clinician assess the likelihood of DVT, and studies have shown that with a low clinical suspicion (as in this patient) and a negative D-dimer assay, the presence of DVT can be reliably excluded without the need for more invasive or complex imaging.

In the Wells criteria, the following clinical variables each earn 1 point: active cancer; paralysis or recent plaster cast; recent immobilization or major surgery; tenderness along the deep veins; swelling of the entire leg; greater than a 3-cm difference in calf circumference compared with the other leg; pitting edema; and collateral superficial veins. The clinical suspicion that an alternative diagnosis is likely earns -2 points. Based on this system, the pretest probability of DVT is considered high in patients with scores of greater than or equal to 3, moderate in patients with scores of 1 to 2, and low in patients with scores less than or equal to 0. This patient's Wells score is -2, and the likelihood for DVT is therefore low. This patient's fever, circumscribed area of warmth, and tenderness localized to the posterior calf could represent cellulitis, a reasonable alternative to the diagnosis of venous thrombosis.

If the D-dimer assay is positive or the clinical suspicion is moderate to high for the presence of a DVT, an objective imaging study, such as ultrasonography, must be performed. Ultrasonography is highly sensitive and specific for detection of proximal (popliteal or above) DVT. However, ultrasonography has low sensitivity for identifying thrombi limited to the calf veins. About 1% to 2% of patients with a normal initial ultrasound have calf vein thrombosis that is destined to extend into the proximal veins, generally within 5 to 8 days.

Venography, the traditional gold standard for diagnosis of DVT, is rarely performed today because of its invasiveness, discomfort, costs, and complexity.

Neither an MRI nor CT of the leg has been substantially validated as a reliable diagnostic test for DVT.

KEY POINT

- Negative D-dimer assay results and a low Wells criteria score reliably exclude a diagnosis of deep venous thrombosis and preclude the need for more invasive testing or complex imaging.

Bibliography

Wells PS, Anderson DR, Bormanis J, et al. Value of assessment of pretest probability of deep-vein thrombosis in clinical management. Lancet. 1997;350(9094):1795-8. [PMID: 9428249]

Item 46   Answer: B
Educational Objective: Diagnose aplastic anemia.

This patient has aplastic anemia. Patients with this disorder have pancytopenia and a hypoplastic bone marrow (<20 cellularity) with normal maturation of all cell lines. Aplastic anemia is a fatal disorder in which myeloid progenitor cells and stem cells are severely diminished or absent in the bone marrow because of an intrinsic defect of the stem cells or

immune-mediated stem cell destruction, which leads to transfusion-dependent anemia, thrombocytopenia, and severe neutropenia. In approximately 50% of cases of aplastic anemia, there is no obvious cause, whereas chemicals, drugs, viral infections, collagen vascular diseases, and thymoma can be implicated in the remaining cases. Interferon-activated T lymphocytes are implicated in autoimmune destruction of stem cells in a significant proportion of patients with the idiopathic or the acquired form of the disease; this fact explains why immunosuppressive therapy is effective in some patients. Initial management involves withdrawal of any potentially causative agents and a CT scan of the chest to rule out an associated thymoma.

Patients with acute myeloid leukemia may have pancytopenia, but bone marrow examination shows infiltration with CD34 blasts, and circulating myeloblasts are likely to be present on the peripheral blood smear.

Patients with immune thrombocytopenic purpura (ITP) have petechiae and ecchymoses but do not have a decreased leukocyte count. Although patients with ITP and an associated autoimmune hemolytic anemia may have a low hemoglobin level, this patient's direct antiglobulin (Coombs) test was negative, and she had a low reticulocyte count. In addition, her bone marrow did not show the increased number of megakaryocytes characteristic of ITP. Finally, some patients with ITP may have anemia secondary to bleeding; however, this patient does not have a clinical history of bleeding, and her iron stores are normal, suggesting that hemorrhage is not the cause of her anemia.

Although pancytopenia may be present in patients with a myelodysplastic syndrome, bone marrow examination typically shows hypercellular marrow. In addition, the diagnosis of a myelodysplastic syndrome requires the presence of dysplasia in at least two cell lines, which is not present in this patient.

KEY POINT

- Patients with aplastic anemia have pancytopenia, a low reticulocyte count, and hypoplastic bone marrow.

Bibliography

Young NS, Calado RT, Scheinberg P. Current concepts in the pathophysiology and treatment of aplastic anemia. Blood. 2006;108(8): 2509-2519. [PMID: 16778145]

Item 47   Answer: A
Educational Objective: Treat a patient with an idiopathic deep venous thrombosis.

The appropriate treatment for a patient with noncancer-related deep venous thrombosis (DVT) that is idiopathic or associated with a transient risk factor is an initial short course of an immediate-acting anticoagulant such as unfractionated heparin, low-molecular-weight heparin, (LMWH), or fondaparinux for at least 5 days. Warfarin should be started at approximately the same time that heparin is administered, and the two drugs should be overlapped until the INR reaches a therapeutic range (≥2) measured on two occasions approximately 24 hours apart. This timing allows for further reduction of prothrombin, the vitamin K–dependent factor with the longest half-life (approximately 60 h), which is responsible for much of the antithrombotic effect of warfarin. Usually, 5 to 7 days of therapy are required to achieve this therapeutic level. The initial recommended daily warfarin dose is 5 mg, although, occasionally, 7.5 to 10 mg may be used. Lower doses (2.5 mg) are recommended in the elderly, especially in the setting of malnourishment, liver disease, or after major surgery.

KEY POINT

- Treatment of idiopathic or transient risk-related deep venous thrombosis consists of an immediate-acting anticoagulant such as unfractionated heparin, low-molecular-weight heparin, or fondaparinux for at least 5 days.

Bibliography

Crowther MA, Ginsberg JB, Kearon C, et al. A randomized trial comparing 5 mg and 10 mg warfarin loading doses. Arch Intern Med. 1999;159(1):46–48. [PMID: 9892329]

Item 48   Answer: D

Educational Objective: Diagnose and manage a patient with monoclonal gammopathy of undetermined significance.

This patient has monoclonal gammopathy of undetermined significance (MGUS) characterized by the presence of a low serum monoclonal protein (M-protein) concentration (≤3.0 g/dL [30 g/L]), less than 10% plasma cells in the bone marrow, and the absence of lytic bone lesions, anemia, hypercalcemia, and renal insufficiency associated with a plasma cell proliferative process or related B-cell lymphoproliferative disorder. The incidence of MGUS increases with age, and more than 5% of persons over 80 years of age may be affected. No specific treatment is required except for close follow-up to identify progression to myeloma or other disorders and periodic measurement of serum M-protein levels. The risk of progression correlates best with the concentration of M protein.

This patient does not require further staging with positron emission tomography. Bisphosphonate treatment is not indicated in the absence of lytic bone lesions.

This patient does not meet the criteria for multiple myeloma and therefore should not receive thalidomide and dexamethasone, which are agents used in the treatment of this disease.

KEY POINT

- Monoclonal gammopathy of undetermined significance is characterized by a serum monoclonal protein level less than 3.0 g/dL (30 g/L) without the overt clinical features of myeloma and less than 10% plasma cells in the bone marrow; routine follow-up to identify progression to a more serious disorder is indicated.

Bibliography

Blade J. Clinical practice. Monoclonal gammopathy of undetermined significance. N Engl J Med. 2006;355(26):2765-2770. [PMID: 17192542]

Item 49   Answer: C

Educational Objective: Diagnose folate deficiency in a patient with sickle cell anemia.

Patients with hemolytic anemia such as that in sickle cell disease have an increased requirement for folate because of excessive cell turnover. This is also true for patients with desquamative skin disorders. In this case, the patient probably has not been taking supplemental folate, perhaps because of oversight or due to difficulties with medical adherence in the setting of a previous stroke. The diagnosis can be confirmed with a serum folate measurement. The appropriate treatment for patients with folate deficiency is oral folic acid, 1 to 5 mg/d, for a duration of 1 to 4 months or until the patient achieves complete hematologic recovery. Following repletion, maintenance therapy with folate should continue indefinitely with 1 mg/d. Folate deficiency does not cause neurologic sequelae but is associated with anemia characterized by an elevated mean corpuscular volume (MCV) as is demonstrated in this patient. Importantly, patients taking hydroxyurea may also have an elevated MCV that can confuse the diagnosis.

Hyperhemolysis in sickle cell disease is characterized by an increased reticulocyte count, which is not present in this patient. Anemia of chronic disease is typified by a normal or decreased MCV, not an increased MCV as found in this case. Patients can have coexisting cobalamin deficiency with sickle cell disease, although this is not as likely a diagnosis as folate deficiency because cobalamin deficiency takes years to develop and hemolysis leads to increased folate requirements. Additionally, cobalamin deficiency that causes anemia may also be associated with loss of vibratory sense, which was absent in this patient's neurologic examination findings. However, the anemia of cobalamin deficiency can be reversed with folate therapy, necessitating establishment of a firm diagnosis before folate therapy is begun.

KEY POINT

- Patients with hemolytic anemia have increased folate requirements.

Bibliography

Lottenberg R, Haskell KL. An evidence-based approach to the treatment of adults with sickle cell disease. Hematology Am Soc Hematol Educ Program. 2005;58-65. [PMID: 16304360]

Item 50   Answer: A

Educational Objective: Manage a patient with multiple myeloma.

Thalidomide plus dexamethasone is standard first-line chemotherapy for patients younger than 65 years who are candidates for autologous stem cell transplantation. The overall response rate to this chemotherapy is approximately 65% to 75%. In patients who do have a favorable hematologic response to initial therapy, several randomized clinical trials have shown improvement in both overall and disease-free survival if these patients are subsequently treated with autologous stem cell transplantation. Patients who have no contraindications to intensive therapy with thalidomide and dexamethasone and autologous stem cell transplantation should therefore be offered this treatment as the best option to improve overall and disease-free survival.

Continuation of thalidomide with or without dexamethasone cannot be recommended, although clinical trials are evaluating the effectiveness of this agent as maintenance therapy after stem cell transplantation. Thalidomide has not been studied in this setting and is not approved for this indication. Furthermore, it is unknown whether thalidomide confers a survival advantage compared with autologous stem cell transplantation for patients with advanced multiple myeloma who have responded to initial therapy. Although parenteral bisphosphonates may reduce or prevent skeletal complications in patients with multiple myeloma, they do not improve disease-free survival.

Oral melphalan should not be used in patients who are potential candidates for stem cell transplantation because this treatment can impair the future collection of peripheral stem cells necessary for stem cell transplantation.

KEY POINT

- **Autologous stem cell transplantation following high-dose chemotherapy can improve overall and disease-free survival in patients with multiple myeloma.**

Bibliography

Child JA, Morgan GJ, Davies FE, et al; Medical Research Council Adult Leukaemia Working Party. High-dose chemotherapy with hematopoietic stem-cell rescue for multiple myeloma. N Engl J Med. 2003;348(19):1875-1883. [PMID: 12736280]

Item 51   Answer: B

Educational Objective: Recognize the indications for transfusion of leukoreduced and irradiated blood components.

This immunocompromised patient is at risk for a febrile reaction (because of previous transfusions) and cytomegalovirus infection (because of posttransplantation immunosuppression). Leukoreduction removes leukocytes by filtration and reduces the incidence of both of these transfusion-related complications. In addition, γ irradiation of cellular blood components (packed erythrocytes and platelets) is required in immunocompromised patients to prevent transfusion-associated graft-versus-host disease. Patients with anemia (hemoglobin less than 11 g/dL [110 g/L]) are not good candidates for autologous blood donation. Washing removes plasma from blood components and is indicated only for patients who have had documented recurrent allergic reactions.

KEY POINT

- **Irradiated blood components are indicated to prevent transfusion-associated graft-versus-host disease in at-risk patients.**

Bibliography

Klein HG, Spahn DR, Carson JL. Red blood cell transfusion in clinical practice. Lancet. 2007;370(9585):415-426. [PMID: 17679019]

Item 52   Answer: D

Educational Objective: Treat resistant immune (idiopathic) thrombocytopenic purpura.

This patient has chronic refractory immune (idiopathic) thrombocytopenic purpura (ITP). Romiplostim and eltrombopag are new thrombopoietin receptor agonists recently approved by the U.S. Food and Drug Administration for treatment of refractory ITP. Clinical studies of recombinant human thrombopoietin resulted in antibody formation to thrombopoietin and thrombocytopenia in normal subjects. Because of this, recombinant thrombopoietin is not useful in ITP or other clinical disorders. Romiplostim is given parenterally, once weekly; and eltrombopag is given orally, daily. Neither have sequence homology with thrombopoietin, and it is unlikely to cause antibody formation against the growth hormone. Romiplostim is effective in both splenectomized and nonsplenectomized patients and both agents allow corticosteroids or other therapies to be tapered during treatment. Serious adverse events are uncommon with either agent. There have been episodes of thrombosis and increased bone marrow reticulin reported.

Pulse administration of dexamethasone is an initial treatment option for patients with ITP, but this patient has not improved following treatment with prednisone and is very unlikely to respond to administration of another corticosteroid.

Plasmapheresis is not effective in removing the autoantibodies in patients with ITP, because these are usually IgG antibodies that are found in both the intravascular and the extravascular compartments. The IgG that is removed from the intravascular compartment is therefore rapidly replaced after equilibration within the extravascular space.

- Romiplostim and eltrombopag are recently approved thrombopoietin receptor agonists that are effective in the treatment of chronic immune (idiopathic) thrombocytopenic purpura.

Bibliography

Kuter DJ, Bussel JB, Lyons RM, et al. Efficacy of romiplostim in patients with chronic immune thrombocytopenic purpura: a double-blind randomised controlled trial. Lancet. 2008;371(9610): 395-403. [PMID: 18242413]

Item 53   Answer: A

Educational Objective: Diagnose AL amyloidosis.

AL amyloidosis should be suspected in patients with nephrotic-range proteinuria, acquired factor X deficiency leading to an elevated INR, postural hypotension caused by autonomic neuropathy, and macroglossia causing indented tooth marks on the lateral borders of tongue. These findings are usually associated with a low-grade plasma cell dyscrasia without large M proteins detected on serum and urine protein electrophoresis. The diagnosis can be confirmed by organ biopsy showing amyloid deposits. Fat pad aspiration, the results of which are positive in approximately 80% of patients, is a less-invasive means of establishing the diagnosis.

POEMS syndrome is characterized by this constellation of findings: *p*olyneuropathy, *o*rganomegaly, *e*ndocrinopathy, *m*onoclonal protein (usually < 2.0 g/dL [20 g/L]), and *s*kin changes. Additional features are sclerotic bony lesions. Because this patient does not have organomegaly or polyneuropathy, this diagnosis is ruled out.

Monoclonal gammopathy of undetermined significance (MGUS) is characterized by a serum monoclonal protein level of less than 3.0 g/dL (30 g/L) without the overt clinical features of anemia, hypercalcemia, renal insufficiency, lytic bony lesions, and infections and less than 10% plasma cells in the bone marrow. This patient has macroglossia, nephrotic syndrome, and acquired factor X deficiency, negating the possibility of MGUS.

Patients with multiple myeloma–associated kidney disease may have proteinuria. However, this is usually due to Bence-Jones protein rather than excessive albumin, and urinalysis would not show a 4+ protein concentration. Furthermore, patients with multiple myeloma would have a larger monoclonal protein spike (>3.0 g/dL [30 g/L]).

- AL amyloidosis should be suspected in patients with nephrotic-range proteinuria, acquired factor X deficiency, postural hypotension, and macroglossia; it is also associated with a low-grade plasma cell dyscrasia.

Bibliography

Sanchorawala V. Light-chain (AL) amyloidosis: diagnosis and treatment. Clin J Am Soc Nephrol. 2006;1(6):1331-1341. [PMID: 17699366]

Oncology Answers

Item 54 Answer: C
Educational Objective: Evaluate a patient with early-stage breast cancer.

This patient has early-stage breast cancer (stage I) based on the tumor size (<2 cm), absent lymph node involvement, and no apparent metastases based on her symptoms, physical examination findings, and routine blood tests. The step that would be most helpful in directing the approach to management of this patient is to perform an assay for expression of estrogen and progesterone receptors to determine the optimal systemic treatment, and this evaluative step should be performed in all cases of primary breast cancer. Endocrine therapy (tamoxifen, aromatase inhibitors, fulvestrant, and megestrol acetate) is beneficial only in patients with estrogen receptor (ER)–positive or progesterone receptor (PR)–positive tumors. Patients whose tumors are hormone receptor–negative are refractory to endocrine treatment and should receive chemotherapy.

In patients with early-stage breast cancer, the routine evaluation is limited to a thorough history and physical examination, diagnostic mammography, chest radiography, and routine blood tests (including liver chemistry tests). The use of additional imaging studies or blood tests such as tumor marker measurement is not warranted in the absence of specific symptoms because they may lead to the detection of abnormalities of no significance (a false-positive test result). In early-stage disease, the positive predictive value of abnormal findings of whole-body positron-emission tomography is approximately 1%; therefore, this type of imaging modality is not recommended. The absence of metastases in a sentinel axillary lymph node has a high negative predictive value, obviating the need for and avoiding the morbidity of a complete axillary lymph node dissection. Testing for the *BRCA1* or *BRCA2* gene would not be indicated without a more compelling family history of disease.

> **KEY POINT**
> - Assay for expression of estrogen and progesterone receptors is crucial in determining the optimal systemic treatment for breast cancer and should be performed in all patients with primary breast cancer.

Bibliography
Singletary SE, Connolly JL. Breast cancer staging: working with the sixth edition of the AJCC cancer staging manual. CA Cancer J Clin. 2006;56(1):37-47. [PMID: 16449185]

Item 55 Answer: A
Educational Objective: Manage a patient with a mediastinal germ cell tumor after successful therapy.

Although bleomycin may be associated with pulmonary toxicity and cisplatin has known ototoxic effects, no delayed cardiovascular effects are associated with this patient's chemotherapeutic regimen that would require surveillance beyond age- and sex-appropriate screening. Screening recommendations for survivors of germ cell cancer are no different than those for the general population, and, for this patient, includes periodic lipid screening (every 5 years), annual blood pressure measurement (or at each office visit), and counseling regarding tobacco use.

Because his risk for cardiovascular risk is not increased, an exercise stress test is not indicated in this patient.

Cisplatin therapy is related to high-tone hearing loss, but in most patients, this long-term complication presents predominantly asymptomatically. Audiometry screening in asymptomatic individuals is not recommended because it has little impact on subsequent management.

Although this patient does remain at risk for late-onset bleomycin-induced lung injury, pulmonary function tests are not advised in the absence of symptoms. Whether the patient should wear a Medic-alert bracelet warning of the dangers of high FiO_2 during subsequent surgery is debatable.

Although dose-related nephrotoxicity may occur during cisplatin therapy, there is no risk for late renal injury or renal neoplasia, and screening renal ultrasonography is not recommended.

> **KEY POINT**
> - Nothing beyond age- and gender-based screening is recommended for long-term germ cell cancer survivors who received cisplatin or bleomycin chemotherapy.

Bibliography
O'Sullivan JM, Huddart RA, Norman AR, et al. Ann Oncol. 2003;14(1):91-96. [PMID: 12488299]

Item 56 Answer: B
Educational Objective: Treat gastric cancer.

This patient requires chemotherapy, radiation, and surgical resection for treatment of gastric cancer. Chronic *Helicobacter pylori* infection is associated with the development of gastric ulceration and subsequent gastric cancer. Other medical conditions associated with an increased risk for gastric cancer include chronic atrophic gastritis, intestinal metaplasia, pernicious anemia, gastric adenomatous polyps, Ménétrier disease (also referred to as giant hypertrophic gastritis), and familial adenomatous polyposis. Patients often present with vague abdominal complaints, early satiety, and weight loss. Clinical signs and symptoms of gastric cancer at diagnosis may include anemia, fecal occult blood, hypoproteinemia, and abnormal liver chemistry studies. Rarely, an abdominal mass is discovered on examination and is often predictive of unresectable disease. Gastric cancer is relatively uncommon in the United States but has a higher prevalence in other countries. This malignancy occurs more frequently in men than in women, and blacks have a 50% increased risk for developing gastric cancer compared with whites. Surgical treatment remains the standard of care for patients with early gastric cancer and is curative in approximately 50% of patients with localized disease, who constitute only 10% to 20% of all patients with gastric cancer. Improved survival has been demonstrated in patients with early-stage gastric cancer who received adjuvant chemotherapy and radiotherapy compared with surgery alone. Other studies have shown improved results with preoperative chemotherapy or chemoradiotherapy. Although clinical studies to support postoperative versus preoperative chemotherapy or chemotherapy versus chemoradiotherapy are still lacking, oncologists have concluded that neither surgery, chemotherapy, nor radiation therapy alone is adequate for curative therapy of patients with gastric cancer.

Although proton-pump inhibitors and antibiotics may eradicate *H. pylori* infection and improve outcomes in patients with mucosa-associated lymphoid tissue (MALT) lymphoma, such therapy is not effective in patients with gastric cancer.

KEY POINT

- **Patients with locally advanced gastric cancer require combined chemotherapy, radiation therapy, and surgical resection.**

Bibliography

Macdonald JS, Smalley SR, Benedetti J, et al. Chemoradiotherapy after surgery compared with surgery alone for adenocarcinoma of the stomach or gastroesophageal junction. N Engl J Med. 2001;345(10):725-730. [PMID: 11547741]

Item 57   Answer: D

Educational Objective: Treat metastatic hepatocellular carcinoma.

This patient requires sorafenib therapy. Cirrhosis is the most important risk factor for the development of hepatocellular carcinoma, regardless of the cause of the cirrhosis. The most common causes of cirrhosis leading to hepatocellular carcinoma are chronic hepatitis B and hepatitis C viral infections and alcoholic liver disease. Patients with cirrhosis with a compatible imaging study and a serum α-fetoprotein level greater than 500 ng/mL (500 μg/L) can be diagnosed with hepatocellular carcinoma without a biopsy. Metastatic hepatocellular carcinoma, the diagnosis in this patient, is associated with poor overall survival and an average life expectancy of 6 to 8 months. The most appropriate treatment for this patient is sorafenib therapy.

A phase III randomized clinical trial recently showed improvement in time to disease progression and overall survival in patients with advanced hepatocellular carcinoma treated with sorafenib (a small-molecule-receptor tyrosine kinase inhibitor that targets differences between normal tissue and malignant cells by inhibiting vascular endothelial

growth factor receptors, platelet-derived growth factor receptors, and other oncogenic signaling pathways). Patients in the treatment arm had a median overall survival of 46.4 weeks compared with 34.3 weeks for those in the placebo arm. The progression-free rate at 4 months was 62% for patients given sorafenib compared with 42% for those receiving placebo.

Surgical resection and liver transplantation are the only curative treatments for localized hepatocellular carcinoma; however, patients with tumors greater than 5 cm in diameter are poor candidates for either procedure because of a high risk for recurrent disease within a few years after surgery. Surgical resection is safe and effective only in highly selected patients with excellent hepatic function and no evidence of portal hypertension. Because the underlying cause of hepatocellular carcinoma usually is not removed by surgical resection, recurrent disease is common, particularly in patients with cirrhosis or active hepatocellular injury. For these reasons, liver transplantation has become the primary treatment of choice for a few select patients with cirrhosis and limited hepatocellular carcinoma. Neither surgical resection nor liver transplantation is indicated in this patient with evidence of metastatic disease.

Treatment of unresectable hepatocellular carcinoma with standard chemotherapeutic agents such as doxorubicin has not been associated with significant improvement in patient survival. Percutaneous ethanol injection or radiofrequency ablation is indicated for patients who are poor candidates for surgical resection or liver transplantation because of medical, surgical, or psychosocial contraindications. However, ethanol injection is usually not effective in patients with tumors greater than 3 cm in diameter and is not indicated for patients with metastatic disease.

KEY POINT

- **Sorafenib is beneficial in treating patients with unresectable hepatocellular carcinoma.**

Bibliography

Llovet JM, Ricci S, Mazzaferro V, Hilgard P, SHARP Investigators Study Group. Sorafenib in advanced hepatocellular carcinoma. N Engl J Med. 2008;359(4):378-390. [PMID: 18650514]

Item 58   Answer: A

Educational Objective: Manage a patient with newly diagnosed ovarian cancer.

This patient requires laparotomy with surgical cytoreduction and staging. Early ovarian cancer is frequently asymptomatic, but the most common symptoms are abdominal swelling, abdominal pain, gastrointestinal symptoms, abnormal vaginal bleeding, and fatigue. Ovarian masses with irregular borders and solid or bilateral masses are more likely to represent malignant tumors. Transvaginal ultrasound has more resolution to detect minimal morphologic changes. However, no universally accepted criteria exist for the sonographic diagnosis of ovarian cancer, although scoring systems featuring explicit and reproducible criteria have been developed. An elevated CA-125 level is not diagnostic for ovarian cancer because it is frequently elevated in many benign conditions and other intra-abdominal cancers. CT scans of the abdomen and pelvis may reveal findings of extensive carcinomatosis, or liver metastases may provide staging information but will rarely change management. At this point, the patient requires surgical cytoreduction and staging of ovarian cancer. Staging is determined surgically by diffuse sampling of abdominal and pelvic structures and surfaces rather than clinically by imaging studies and measurement of serum cancer markers. Up to 30% of patients whose disease appears to be clinically limited to the ovary will be found to have metastatic disease at the time of surgery. The staging procedure consists of laparotomy with en bloc resection of the primary tumor, ovaries, and uterus; partial infracolic omentectomy; selective lymphadenectomy; bowel resection as indicated; sampling of the diaphragm; removal of all visible and resectable tumor; and appendectomy. Patients with optimally debulked cancer, meaning no visible tumor greater than 1 cm remaining after completion of the staging procedure, have better outcomes than patients with suboptimally debulked cancer. Optimal debulking occurs in more than 80% of surgical procedures when performed by a fully trained gynecologic oncologist.

Performing a left oophorectomy would be inadequate in the accurate staging of this patient's disease. Pelvic irradiation does not play a role in the treatment of suspected ovarian cancer. Decisions regarding chemotherapy should be made after full staging is completed.

KEY POINT

- The first and most important step in managing a patient with suspected ovarian cancer is maximal surgical cytoreduction and accurate staging by laparotomy.

Bibliography

Winter WE 3rd, Maxwell GL, Tian C et al. Tumor residual after surgical cytoreduction in prediction of clinical outcome in stage IV epithelial ovarian cancer: a Gynecologic Oncology Group Study. J Clin Oncol. 2008;26(1):83-89. [PMID: 18025437]

Item 59   Answer: D

Educational Objective: Manage a patient with stage IV non-small cell lung cancer metastases.

This patient likely has recurrent non-small cell lung cancer (NSCLC) with a solitary, surgically accessible metastasis to the brain, and surgical resection of the metastasis is the most appropriate next step in management. Patients with good performance status and a surgically accessible single (or few) metastatic lesion(s) to the brain and minimal or no evidence of extracranial disease are most likely to benefit from surgical intervention. Surgical resection of this patient's brain metastasis is required for quick symptomatic

relief, to control progression of brain metastases, and to provide histologic confirmation of metastasis. This approach is now appropriate for a wider range of patients with brain metastases owing to the improved safety associated with neuroanesthesia and the procedure itself. Following surgery, this patient may also receive radiation therapy to the lesion, either with external-beam radiation or stereotactic surgery. Although combined-modality treatment with radiation therapy does not prolong survival compared with surgery alone, it does reduce the incidence of recurrent disease and the need for repeated therapy. Retrospective series have suggested that some patients without evidence of other systemic disease have prolonged survival following resection of brain metastases.

Highly chemosensitive cancers, such as metastatic testicular germ cell tumors and central nervous system lymphoma, will respond to chemotherapy alone. However, NSCLC does not respond well to chemotherapy. Because this patient is symptomatic, she should not receive chemotherapy with erlotinib alone but should undergo surgical resection.

Temozolomide is an alkylating agent used in the treatment of primary and metastatic brain tumors. The combination of temozolomide followed by whole-brain radiation therapy may prove to be more effective than radiation alone in the treatment of metastatic tumors and is currently undergoing evaluation in clinical studies. However, radiation therapy is generally reserved for patients with surgically inaccessible tumors or tumors that are not otherwise appropriate for surgical resection and is not the best therapy for this patient.

Best supportive care (comfort care without chemotherapy or surgery) is not appropriate for this patient because of her previously intact performance status and evidence of a surgically accessible solitary site of recurrence, both of which make her eligible for surgical resection and its potentially positive impact on symptoms, metastatic progression, and survival.

KEY POINT

- Surgical excision of a solitary brain metastasis should be considered for patients with good performance status, minimal, or no evidence of extracranial disease, and a surgically accessible, single brain metastasis amenable to complete excision.

Bibliography

Mintz A, Perry J, Spithoff K, Chambers A, Laperriere N. Management of single brain metastasis: a practice guideline. Curr Oncol. 2007;14(4):131-143. [PMID: 17710205]

Item 60   Answer: A

Educational Objective: Manage a patient with follicular lymphoma who received no prior therapy.

Follicular lymphoma constitutes approximately 40% of cases of non-Hodgkin lymphoma in the United States.

The disease is considered incurable beyond stage I, but patients can have a relatively long survival (median survival, 8 to 12 years). Indications to begin palliative treatment include the presence of symptoms, threat to vital organ function, issues concerning appearance because of enlarged lymph nodes, and patient preference. This patient has gradually progressive lymphadenopathy after 3 years of observation. He has cosmetic concerns, some restricted activity, and discomfort from the enlarged axillary lymph nodes. Combination chemotherapy, such as cyclophosphamide, vincristine, and prednisone with rituximab, is a reasonable treatment for debulking his disease. Adding rituximab, a monoclonal antibody targeting CD20+ antigen, to the regimen is associated with an improved clinical outcome with higher response and survival rates and longer intervals until disease progression.

Radiation therapy alone may be curative in those few patients with stage I disease, but multimodality therapy has not been shown to result in cure or prolonged survival versus alternative therapeutic combinations for patients with advanced-stage disease. Therefore, there is no role for high-dose chemotherapy followed by stem cell transplantation in this patient. Studies have failed to demonstrate improved survival for patients treated with adjuvant chemotherapy with or without radiation, and this treatment is associated with an increased incidence of hematopoietic stem cell disorders. Therefore, combined-modality therapy is not used in patients with follicular lymphoma.

If biopsy were to be considered, excisional biopsy (not fine-needle aspiration biopsy) of rapidly enlarging lymph nodes would be appropriate to evaluate the presence of a second, more aggressive, type of lymphoma. However, because this patient describes a history of gradually increasing generalized lymphadenopathy for several years, there is no indication for obtaining an additional biopsy.

Observation is not appropriate because of his symptoms, examination findings, and radiographic evidence of progressive disease.

KEY POINT

- **Indications for initiation of palliative treatment of follicular lymphoma include the presence of symptoms, threat to vital organ function, issues concerning appearance because of enlarged lymph nodes, and patient preferences.**

Bibliography

Marcus R, Imrie, Belch A, et al. CVP chemotherapy plus rituximab compared with CVP as first-line treatment for advanced follicular lymphoma. Blood. 2005;105(4):1417-1423. [PMID: 15494430]

Item 61   Answer: C

Educational Objective: Manage a patient at high risk for *BRCA* mutation.

Testing for *BRCA1* and *BRCA2* gene mutations should be done if (1) the individual has personal or family history features suggestive of genetic cancer; and (2) the test results will help to establish the diagnosis or influence the management of the patient or family members at risk. This patient clearly has a history suspicious for the *BRCA* mutation as shown by her Ashkenazi Jewish heritage and the presence of breast, ovarian, and male breast cancer in the family. A family history associated with an increased risk for breast cancer in women of Ashkenazi Jewish descent includes any first-degree relative (or two second-degree relatives on the same side of the family) with breast or ovarian cancer. This patient's father should undergo genetic testing considering his history of breast cancer and her paternal grandmother's history of ovarian cancer and breast cancer at a very young age, the combination of which confers a high likelihood for the *BRCA* mutation. If the patient's father is positive for the *BRCA* gene mutation, the patient has a 50% chance of carrying this gene mutation. The patient's mother may have sporadic breast cancer but should undergo testing if the patient's father tests negative because the mother was younger than 50 years of age at diagnosis and is of Ashkenazi Jewish descent. If the mother's test results are also negative, there is no reason for this 20-year-old patient to undergo testing. If the parents were deceased, it would be appropriate to test the patient. Otherwise, genetic testing in this patient would not begin until she reaches 25 years of age.

Prophylactic mastectomy and oophorectomy may become appropriate at a later time depending on the results of genetic counseling and testing but would not be indicated prior to information gained through such counseling and testing. Several retrospective experiences and a few prospective observational studies have suggested up to a 90% or higher proportional reduction of cases of new breast cancer after prophylactic mastectomy, and patients with *BRCA1* or *BRCA2* abnormalities appear to gain substantial benefit because of their high risk for breast cancer. In those women at high risk for cancer because of *BRCA1* and/or *BRCA2* abnormalities, oophorectomy may be an acceptable risk-reduction strategy, because it not only reduces breast cancer risk by approximately 50%, but it also reduces the risk for ovarian cancer, which is also greatly increased in these patients. Early initiation of mammography and clinical screening should be especially considered in high-risk individuals, based on family history or the identification of predisposing genetic mutations, although there are limited prospective data to support this strategy. Some experts recommend the initiation of screening 5 to 10 years earlier than the age when breast cancer occurred in a first- or second-degree relative or at the age of 25 years. As such, it is probably premature to begin screening in this 20-year-old woman.

There are no randomized trials of breast MRI in patients with a genetic predisposition to breast cancer. Despite the lack of outcome data, guidelines from the American Cancer Society recommend the integration of both mammography and breast MRI for breast cancer surveillance in high-risk women. Therefore, the use of MRI and mammography may be considered in this patient if she proves to have a genetic mutation that places her at risk for breast cancer at the time when screening is appropriate.

> **KEY POINT**
>
> - Patients with a family history suggestive of genetic cancer should be advised to undergo genetic counseling and testing.

Bibliography

American Society of Clinical Oncology. American Society of Clinical Oncology Policy Statement Update: Genetic testing for cancer susceptibility. J Clin Oncol. 2003;21(12):2397-2406. [PMID: 12692171]

Item 62　　Answer:　B

Educational Objective: Treat early-stage, aggressive, B-cell non-Hodgkin lymphoma using a combined-modality approach.

This patient has early-stage, diffuse, large B-cell non-Hodgkin lymphoma, which can be aggressive and should be treated with cyclophosphamide, doxorubicin, vincristine, and prednisone with rituximab (R-CHOP) for three cycles followed by involved-field radiation therapy. Combined-modality therapy minimizes the exposure to a longer course of chemotherapy (six cycles). Although initial studies reported that this approach was superior to chemotherapy alone, follow-up studies showed that overall survival was equivalent. However, the abbreviated course of chemotherapy plus radiation therapy is associated with less long-term toxicity (for example, doxorubicin-induced cardiotoxicity) than a longer course of chemotherapy.

Radiation therapy alone is not indicated because the relapse rate is at least 50% when only irradiation is used.

Treatment of this aggressive lymphoma in a young man without comorbidities is associated with a cure rate of at least 75%. Therefore, observation is inappropriate.

The addition of the monoclonal antibody rituximab to combination chemotherapy has been the first major therapeutic advance for patients with diffuse large B-cell lymphoma in more than 20 years, improving the cure rate by 10% to 15%. Rituximab alone is associated with a 30% response rate but no chance of cure.

> **KEY POINT**
>
> - Treatment of early-stage, diffuse, large B-cell non-Hodgkin lymphoma with an abbreviated course of chemotherapy followed by involved-field radiation therapy is associated with excellent long-term survival and decreased toxicity.

Bibliography

Zelenetz AD, Advani RH, Buadi F, et al. Non-Hodgkin's lymphoma. Clinical practice guidelines in oncology. J Natl Compr Canc Netw. 2006;4(3):258-310. [PMID: 16507273]

Item 63　　Answer:　C

Educational Objective: Treat a nonseminoma.

This patient requires right radical orchiectomy followed by chemotherapy. He has a stage IIIB intermediate-risk nonseminomatous testicular germ cell tumor based on the radiographic findings and highly elevated α-fetoprotein (AFP) and β subunit of human chorionic gonadotropin (β-hCG) levels. Although β-hCG concentrations may be elevated in patients with seminomatous or nonseminomatous tumors, AFP is increased only in patients with nonseminomas. Definitive diagnosis of testicular cancer is made by radical inguinal orchiectomy. The full staging evaluation includes measurement of serum lactate dehydrogenase, AFP, and β-hCG concentrations and a CT scan of the chest, abdomen, and pelvis. The tumor-node-metastasis (TNM) staging system is widely used in the staging of testicular cancer. Stage I disease is limited to the testis and surrounding adnexa. Stage II disease involves the testis and the retroperitoneal or para-aortic lymph nodes. Stage III disease suggests spread beyond the retroperitoneal lymph nodes, such as into the mediastinal or supraclavicular lymph nodes, and extranodal metastases. Patients with metastatic disease can be further categorized into favorable, intermediate, or poor prognostic groups based on histologic type (seminoma vs. nonseminoma), level of serum tumor markers (AFP, β-hCG, lactate dehydrogenase), and site of the primary tumor (mediastinum or nonmediastinum). For this patient with stage IIIB cancer, the optimal treatment is radical orchiectomy followed by immediate postoperative chemotherapy. After completion of cisplatin-based chemotherapy, he has a 70% to 80% chance of cure despite distant metastases.

Chemotherapy alone is ineffective in patients with testicular cancer, as all patients with seminomas or nonseminomas of any stage require radical orchiectomy before adjuvant therapy is begun. Radiation therapy is not indicated because nonseminomas are generally radiation-insensitive. Seminomas, which represent approximately 50% of all germ cell tumors, are very radiosensitive. Retroperitoneal lymph node dissection is recommended for patients with early-stage disease who are unable or unwilling to adhere to a strict postoperative surveillance program.

Surgical resection of any residual masses is recommended after the planned course of chemotherapy, as these masses often include viable residual tumor or chemotherapy-resistant teratoma.

> **KEY POINT**
>
> - Treatment of intermediate-stage nonseminoma consists of radical orchiectomy followed by chemotherapy.

Bibliography

Krege S, Souchon R, Schmoll HJ; German Testicular Cancer Study Group. Eur Urol. 2001;40(4):372-391. [PMID: 11713391]

Item 64   Answer: A

Educational Objective: Diagnose superior sulcus tumor.

This patient most likely has a superior sulcus tumor, and a CT of the chest is the most appropriate next diagnostic test. Superior sulcus tumors are characterized by radiating shoulder pain, neurologic abnormalities including upper extremity weakness due to involvement of the brachial plexus, and Horner syndrome (unilateral constricted pupil, facial dryness, and ptosis) caused by damaged sympathetic nerves. Fourteen percent to 50% of patients with Horner syndrome have superior sulcus tumors. The ptosis noted in this patient's neurologic examination is suggestive of this syndrome. The initial diagnostic test for most patients is chest radiography and is likely to reveal an apical mass and bone destruction. CT of the chest will better delineate the tumor and help to establish staging of the disease by identifying the extent of parenchymal disease, pleural disease, and mediastinal lymphadenopathy.

MRI of the cervical spine would likely also identify the tumor in this patient but would not give an accurate estimation of the extent of mediastinal disease. The patient's arm and hand symptoms, which are dermatomal in distribution, with the addition of Horner syndrome, clearly localize the lesion to the cervical spine. An MRI of the brain would therefore not be indicated.

Electromyography (EMG) is the clinical study of the electrical activity of muscle fibers. EMG is used to evaluate weakness and to establish a diagnosis in patients with neurogenic disorders and inflammatory myopathies. However, although EMG will identify the nature of the patient's weakness as neuropathic, it will not diagnose the cause and is not the appropriate initial diagnostic test in patients with suspected superior sulcus tumors.

Shoulder pain occurs in up to 35% of the general population. The most common cause is irritation of the subacromial bursa or rotator cuff tendon from mechanical impingement between the humeral head and the coracoacromial arch. Stiffness or loss of motion suggests glenohumeral arthritis or adhesive capsulitis, whereas referred pain is not exacerbated by shoulder movement. The patient does not have pain with movement of the shoulder and does have pain radiating to the hand, suggesting a radiculopathy rather than instrinsic shoulder disease; therefore, an MRI of the shoulder is not indicated.

KEY POINT

- Superior sulcus tumors are characterized by neck pain radiating to the shoulder, arm, and hand, and may be associated with weakness and/or atrophy and Horner syndrome.

Bibliography

Archie VC, Thomas CR Jr. Superior sulcus tumors: a mini-review. Oncologist. 2004;9(5):550-555. [PMID: 15477640]

Item 65   Answer: E

Educational Objective: Manage a patient with an ovarian tumor of low malignant potential and no invasive implants.

Patients with completely resected ovarian cancer of low malignant potential (previously referred to as borderline tumors) without invasive implants do not require postoperative adjuvant therapy other than close observation and monitoring. Ovarian tumors with low malignant potential are well-differentiated tumors located on the serosal surface without invasion of the surrounding tissue that usually occurs in younger women and are considered a distinct entity. These tumors are not linked to hereditary syndromes; therefore, affected patients do not require genetic testing. Ovarian tumors of low malignant potential respond poorly to both intraperitoneal and intravenous chemotherapy. It is very rare for these tumors to degenerate into a more aggressive form. Radiation therapy produces a poor response in patients with tumors and is therefore not indicated. In addition, the radiation field would require whole-abdomen radiation, which would cause excessive toxicity.

KEY POINT

- Patients with completely resected ovarian cancer of low malignant potential without invasive implants do not require postoperative adjuvant therapy.

Bibliography

Morgan RJ Jr, Alvarez RD, Armstrong DK, et al. Ovarian cancer. Clinical practice guidelines in oncology. J Natl Compr Canc Netw. 2006;4(9):912-932. [PMID: 17020669]

Item 66   Answer: B

Educational Objective: Treat spinal cord compression.

This patient requires urgent anterior surgical decompression of the spinal cord. Spinal cord compression is most commonly associated with renal, prostate, breast, and lung cancer and represents a true oncologic emergency that must be diagnosed and treated promptly. This condition is characterized by severe, progressively increasing back pain. Neurologic symptoms often develop later in the presentation. The thoracic spine is the most common location of spinal cord compression. Diagnostic confirmation of this condition is done most commonly with MRI of the spine. Establishing the diagnosis before motor weakness or other neurologic deficits develop is important to avoid permanent loss of neurologic function, which occurs in a significant percentage of patients with spinal cord compression.

A multicenter study showed that patients who underwent anterior decompressive surgical resection of metastatic epidural spinal cord compression due to cancer had better ambulatory outcomes compared with patients treated with radiation therapy alone. Patients with known highly radiosensitive tumors, such as leukemia, lymphoma, myeloma, and germ-cell tumors, were excluded from this study. This patient may be eligible to receive adjuvant radiation therapy following successful surgical debulking of the tumor.

Chemotherapy seems a rational therapeutic modality for treating both the compressive lesion and tumor elsewhere in his body; however, the substitution of paclitaxel for docetaxel (two drugs from the same class) is unlikely to benefit this patient who is probably resistant to chemotherapy.

This patient's tumor is no longer responding to hormonal therapy. Although antiandrogen therapy is often continued even when patients with prostate cancer progress, the addition of a new antiandrogen agent (leuprolide) would not be likely to have much impact and is not recommended in this patient.

KEY POINT

- Anterior decompressive surgical resection of cancer-induced metastatic epidural spinal cord compression has better ambulatory outcomes compared with radiation therapy alone.

Bibliography

Witham TF, Khavkin YA, Gallia GL, Wolinsky JP, Gokaslan ZL. Surgery insight: current management of epidural spinal cord compression from metastatic spine disease. Nat Clin Pract Neurol. 2006;2(2):87-94. [PMID: 16932530]

Item 67   Answer: E
Educational Objective: Treat a hepatic tumor in a patient with previous colon cancer.

Surgical resection of this patient's solitary lesion is indicated. The primary anatomic location of metastatic colon cancer is the liver. Between 20% and 30% of patients with metastatic disease following curative surgery for colon cancer will have isolated hepatic metastases. In these patients, regional treatment of hepatic metastases may be an alternative to systemic chemotherapy and result in better survival. This patient with previous colon cancer has a solitary site of recurrent disease after a 3-year disease-free period. Surgical resection is potentially curative in approximately 25% of patients with these findings.

Contraindications to resection include tumors that are too large, unfavorable anatomic location, multiple tumors, poor hepatic function, and poor performance status. However, even in patients who are initially not candidates for surgical resection of hepatic metastases, chemotherapy may convert previously inoperable lesions into lesions amenable to surgical intervention. Other local ablative techniques include cryosurgery, chemoembolization, ethanol ablation, and radiofrequency ablation. These options may be considered for local control in a patient who is not a surgical candidate. Although these techniques are unlikely to be curative, they may prolong progression-free survival.

KEY POINT

- Surgical resection of an isolated hepatic metastasis or small number of hepatic metastases from a previous colon cancer is potentially curative in approximately 25% of patients.

Bibliography

Pfister DG, Benson AB 3rd, Somerfield MR. N Engl J Med. 2004;350(23):2375-2382. [PMID: 15175439]

Item 68   Answer: B
Educational Objective: Treat metastatic breast cancer.

This patient received the standard 5 years of adjuvant therapy with tamoxifen and had a cancer recurrence. Initial management of patients with estrogen receptor (ER)–positive tumor status and metastatic breast cancer usually consists of serial endocrine therapies, including tamoxifen, aromatase inhibitors, fulvestrant (an ER down-regulator), and megestrol acetate. In a patient with boney metastases, hormonal therapy is usually combined with bisphosphonate therapy; the combination of anastrozole and zoledronic acid is the most appropriate therapy for this patient at this time. Randomized clinical trials and evidence from a meta-analysis support the use of an aromatase inhibitor (anastrozole, letrozole, or exemestane) as first-line hormonal therapy for metastatic breast cancer in postmenopausal women because it is associated with superior response rates, time to progression, and overall survival compared with first-line tamoxifen therapy. Bisphosphonate therapy prevents skeletal complications resulting from osteolytic bone involvement in patients with breast cancer. Clinical practice guidelines from the American Society of Clinical Oncology recommend the use of intravenous bisphosphonates, such as zoledronic acid or pamidronate, for women with radiographic lytic metastatic bone disease. The evidence demonstrating benefit of oral bisphosphonate therapy such as alendronate in the treatment of bone metastases is conflicting, with some studies failing to show any effect on preventing bone-related complications. Therefore, in this patient, an intravenous bisphosphonate such as zoledronic acid is indicated to reduce the incidence of morbidity (including bone pain), analgesic use, and fracture.

Chemotherapy is not indicated in the initial treatment of ER-positive metastatic disease because hormonal therapy is better tolerated and is more effective in producing an improvement in quality of life for the longest duration. Although chemotherapy might be considered in patients with metastatic cancer with a large tumor burden in the vital organs for whom faster-acting chemotherapy might be life-saving, it is not appropriate at this time in this patient who may benefit from hormonal therapy.

- The use of an aromatase inhibitor as first-line hormonal therapy for metastatic breast cancer in postmenopausal women is associated with superior response rates, time to progression, and overall survival compared with first-line tamoxifen therapy; an intravenous bisphosphonate is indicated for treatment of lytic bone metastases.

Bibliography

Mouridsen H, Chaudri-Ross HA. Efficacy of first-line letrozole versus tamoxifen as a function of age in postmenopausal women with advanced breast cancer. Oncologist. 2004;9(5):497-506. [PMID: 15477634]

Item 69 Answer: D

Educational Objective: Diagnose superior vena cava syndrome.

Superior vena cava (SVC) syndrome is caused by gradual compression of the superior vena cava. The most common cause, accounting for approximately 70% of cases, is lung cancer, for which this patient is at significant risk due to his long smoking history. SVC syndrome typically has an insidious onset, with dyspnea as the most common presenting symptom. Other symptoms include cough, upper extremity swelling, chest pain, and dysphagia (due to esophageal compression). Common physical findings in SVC syndrome include venous distention of the neck and chest wall, facial edema, plethora, and cyanosis. Radiographic findings are characteristic for mediastinal widening, found in two thirds of patients, and pleural effusion, found in one quarter of patients.

This patient's clinical picture, including the presence of facial swelling, venous distention, and dysphagia in the setting of a long-standing smoking history, is most suggestive of SVC syndrome secondary to lung cancer. A contrast-enhanced CT scan is the most useful test to diagnose SVC syndrome and to detect the presence of a mediastinal mass; it may also provide an opportunity for CT-guided needle biopsy. CT findings indicating SVC obstruction include intraluminal filling defects of the SVC, decreased opacification of the innominate vein or SVC below the level of obstruction, and external compression of mediastinal venous channels.

Other than cough, the patient lacks supportive evidence for pneumonia such as fever, chills, sputum production, and an infiltrate on the chest radiograph.

Heart failure is unlikely in the absence of an S_3, pulmonary crackles, peripheral edema, and venous congestion on chest radiograph. Similarly, pulmonary embolism is a cause of dyspnea, but like pneumonia and heart failure, cannot explain the patient's other symptoms or clinical findings such as dysphagia, head fullness, venous distention, and mediastinal widening on chest radiograph.

- Common findings in superior vena cava syndrome include venous distention of the neck and chest wall, facial edema, plethora, cyanosis, and mediastinal widening and pleural effusion on radiography.

Bibliography

Wilson LD, Detterbeck FC, Yahalom J. Clinical practice. Superior vena cava syndrome with malignant causes [erratum in N Engl J Med. 2008 Mar 6;358(10):1083]. N Engl J Med. 2007;356(18):1862-1869. [PMID: 17476012]

Item 70 Answer: A

Educational Objective: Diagnose multiple endocrine neoplasia type 2A.

This patient should undergo genetic screening for the *RET* mutation. The *RET* proto-oncogene encodes a putative tyrosine kinase receptor.

Although greater than 80% of cases of medullary thyroid carcinoma (MTC) are sporadic, this disease may be associated with multiple endocrine neoplasia type 2A (MEN-2A), MEN-2B, or familial non-MEN. MEN-2A consists of MTC (95% to 100% penetrance), hyperparathyroidism (10% to 20% penetrance), and pheochromocytoma (40% to 50% penetrance); MEN-2B consists of MTC, pheochromocytoma, mucosal neuromas, and a marfanoid body habitus. Inherited forms of MTC are associated with germ-line mutations in the *RET* proto-oncogene, and a commercial assay allows screening for familial disease in patients presenting with a new diagnosis of MTC. Calcitonin and carcinoembryonic antigen are markers for MTC; persistent or rising levels suggest active disease.

This patient likely has the MEN-2A syndrome based on the finding of MTC on thyroid biopsy, her significant hypertension and tachycardia, and the sudden death of her mother at a young age of a hypertensive cerebral hemorrhage, suggesting the possibility of pheochromocytoma. Further clues are suggested by the multinodular nature of the patient's thyroid gland. Sporadic MTC typically presents as a single dominant thyroid mass, whereas MTC in patients with MEN-2A is typically bilateral and multicentric. Virtually all patients with MEN-2A develop MTC, and development of this disease is often the first expressed abnormality, usually occurring in the second or third decade of life. MEN-2A is inherited as an autosomal-dominant disorder. Pheochromocytomas are present in approximately half of patients with MEN-2A. Parathyroid hyperplasias are present less commonly than pheochromocytomas. Because of this patient's hypertension, she should undergo screening for pheochromocytoma, and her serum calcium level should be measured to screen for hyperparathyroidism. She should also undergo screening for the *RET* oncogene and, if positive, at-risk members of her family should also undergo screening for the *RET* oncogene because MTC is a life-threatening disease that can be cured or prevented by early thyroidectomy.

Although differentiated epithelial carcinomas of the thyroid (papillary and follicular cancers) often concentrate iodine, thus permitting treatment with radioactive iodine, medullary thyroid tumors do not concentrate radioiodine and must be treated with thyroidectomy. Patients with metastatic or recurrent disease are treated with chemotherapy or radiotherapy.

MEN-2A syndrome is not associated with an increased risk of breast cancer. Provided the patient continues to have normal clinical breast examinations, screening mammography may commence at age 40 years.

Because MTC is caused by C-cell proliferation and C cells are not thyroid-stimulating hormone–responsive, levothyroxine is not recommended at this time; thyroid hormone replacement therapy should be initiated immediately after surgery if thyroidectomy is performed, with the goal of making the patient euthyroid.

KEY POINT

- Patients with a new diagnosis of multiple endocrine neoplasia type 2A should undergo genetic screening for the *RET* mutation.

Bibliography

Kouvaraki MA, Shapiro SE, Perrier ND, et al. RET proto-oncogene: a review and update of genotype-phenotype correlations in hereditary medullary thyroid cancer and associated endocrine tumors. Thyroid. 2005;15(6):531-544. [PMID: 16029119]

Item 71   Answer: C

Educational Objective: Manage a patient with extensive-stage small cell lung cancer.

Because occult or overt metastatic disease is present in almost all patients with small cell lung cancer (SCLC), the more complicated staging system of non–small cell lung cancer does not apply. Patients with tumor beyond the confines of a radiation port are considered to have extensive-stage disease. This patient has extensive-stage SCLC, and the most appropriate next step in management is chemotherapy. SCLC is highly responsive to multiple chemotherapeutic drugs, and chemotherapy dramatically prolongs survival in affected patients compared with best supportive care. Palliative benefits from chemotherapy may occur even in patients with a poor performance status, weight loss, or severe organ dysfunction.

At diagnosis, 30% of patients with SCLC have localized disease that can be encompassed within a radiation therapy port, usually with confinement to one hemithorax lymph node, the mediastinum, and supraclavicular lymph nodes. Such patients are designated as having limited-stage disease. For patients with limited-stage SCLC, two meta-analyses showed a 5% absolute improvement in 3-year survival rates for those who underwent chemotherapy and radiation therapy compared with those who underwent chemotherapy alone. The current standard treatment modality for patients with limited-stage SCLC consists of cisplatin and etoposide with chest radiation therapy during the first two to three cycles of chemotherapy. Risks of treatment-related death are also higher with combined-modality therapy. In one meta-analysis, the risk of toxic death with combined-modality therapy as compared with chemotherapy alone was 2.54 [CI, 1.90-3.18]. Older and frail patients may not be good candidates for combined-modality therapy. This patient has extensive-stage disease, and radiation therapy, with its attendant morbidity, is not indicated.

Because this patient already has documented metastatic disease, procuring evidence of bone marrow involvement is not necessary. In fact, given the relative invasiveness of this procedure, even in patients suspected to have limited-stage disease, routine bone marrow examination is not performed unless laboratory studies indicate cytopenia or an elevated serum lactate dehydrogenase concentration.

If left untreated, patients with SCLC rarely survive more than a few months. For patients with extensive-stage disease, 60% to 80% respond to chemotherapy, and complete responses are observed in up 15% to 20%; therefore, best supportive care and early hospice referral would not be appropriate unless the patient were to refuse chemotherapy. Hospice is warranted in patients with terminal disease for whom the life expectancy is 6 months or less.

Brain metastases are a particularly common problem in patients with SCLC, and multiple reports have indicated that intracranial metastases from SCLC are responsive to chemotherapy; therefore, the appropriate strategy in this patient with asymptomatic brain metastases would be to postpone whole-brain radiation until after systemic therapy has been initiated and the response can be assessed. In the presence of symptomatic brain metastases, treatment with brain radiotherapy is indicated but not before administration of chemotherapy.

KEY POINT

- Small cell lung cancer is a chemosensitive disease, and treatment should be offered even if the patient has poor performance status or organ dysfunction secondary to disease burden.

Bibliography

Simon GR, Turrisi A; American College of Chest Physicians. Management of small cell lung cancer: ACCP evidence-based clinical practice guidelines (2nd edition). Chest. 2007;132(3 Suppl):324S-339S. [PMID: 17873178]

Item 72   Answer: D

Educational Objective: Treat a patient with early-stage breast cancer and *HER2* overexpression.

This patient has high-risk breast cancer characterized by lymph node involvement and an *HER2*-positive tumor status. Patients with estrogen receptor (ER)–positive tumors are managed with endocrine therapy, and patients whose tumors are ER-negative or are refractory to endocrine treatment should receive chemotherapy. In addition, this patient's *HER2* overexpression warrants the addition of trastuzumab to the chemotherapy. Testing breast biopsies by immunohistochemical staining for *HER2*/neu protein overexpression and/or by fluorescent in situ hybridization (FISH) for gene amplification should be done on all breast biopsies and is now as much the standard of care as is estrogen-receptor measurement. Several large, randomized trials have demonstrated that 52 weeks of adjuvant trastuzumab therapy reduces the risk for breast cancer recurrence in women with *HER2* overexpression by approximately 50% and may even reduce mortality by as much as 30%. Trastuzumab is life-saving therapy but is expensive and occasionally toxic and must be administered only to the 30% of women whose tumors have the appropriate target. Patients should undergo monitoring of left ventricular function before trastuzumab treatment, and frequently during and after treatment, because of its association with serious cardiac toxicities, including reduced left ventricular ejection fraction and severe heart failure.

Endocrine therapy such as tamoxifen or anastrozole is beneficial only in patients with ER-positive and progesterone receptor–positive tumors and would therefore not be appropriate in this patient.

Bevacizumab is indicated only in patients with *HER2*-negative metastatic breast cancer and would not benefit this patient with *HER2* overexpression. In addition, bevacizumab has not been studied in the adjuvant setting. In this patient with a positive *HER2* tumor status, providing chemotherapy only without the addition of an agent targeted against *HER2* overexpression is inadequate therapy.

KEY POINT

- Treatment with adjuvant chemotherapy plus trastuzumab reduces the risk of recurrence and mortality in patients with early-stage, *HER2*-positive breast cancer.

Bibliography

Romond EH, Perez EA, Bryant J, et al. Trastuzumab plus adjuvant chemotherapy for operable HER2-positive breast cancer. N Engl J Med. 2005;353(16):1673-1684. [PMID: 16236738]

Item 73   Answer: A
Educational Objective: Provide postoperative management for a patient with stage III colon cancer.

This patient with stage III colon cancer is at high risk for disease recurrence because of the large number of involved lymph nodes. He is likely to benefit from systemic chemotherapy using an oxaliplatin-based regimen, because this treatment has been shown to improve disease-free survival in patients with lymph node–positive colon cancer.

There is no role for adjuvant radiation therapy in patients with colon cancer. Adjuvant radiotherapy is useful in patients with rectal cancer in whom the risk for local recurrence is greater. Observation alone is warranted only in patients with stage I or good-risk stage II cancer. Patients with lymph node–positive colon cancer have a high recurrence risk, and adjuvant chemotherapy will reduce this risk significantly.

KEY POINT

- Adjuvant chemotherapy with an oxaliplatin-based regimen has been shown to improve disease-free survival in patients with lymph node–positive colon cancer.

Bibliography

André T, Boni C, Mounedji-Boudiaf L, et al; Multicenter International Study of Oxaliplatin/5-Fluorouracil/Leucovorin in the Adjuvant Treatment of Colon Cancer (MOSAIC) Investigators. N Engl J Med. 2004;350(23):2343-2351. [PMID: 15175436]

Item 74   Answer: E
Educational Objective: Treat papillary thyroid cancer.

The four main types of thyroid cancer are papillary (75%), follicular (15% to 20%), medullary (less than 5%), and anaplastic (less than 5%). Papillary thyroid cancer and follicular thyroid cancer are treated with total thyroidectomy followed generally by therapy with radioiodine-131 (^{131}I). Radioiodine ablation serves the dual purpose of destroying normal thyroid tissue remnants, which would otherwise produce thyroglobulin and therefore be mistaken for persistent cancer, and of eradicating any microscopic foci of residual tumor.

There is no evidence that external-beam radiotherapy prolongs life, although it can relieve symptoms. There is a high incidence of esophageal and tracheal side effects after external beam radiation to the neck. Because these complications may be lifelong, external beam-radiation is not considered as first-line therapy for thyroid cancer, particularly differentiated thyroid cancer. It may be considered in patients who are not surgical candidates or when there is a high likelihood of residual cancer or relapse.

There is no role for the routine adjunctive use of chemotherapy in patients with differentiated thyroid cancer. Differentiated thyroid cancer cells have a slow doubling-time; most chemotherapeutic agents have little effect on growth or apoptosis. Trials of doxorubicin, cyclophosphamide, cisplatin, and etoposide in poorly differentiated or anaplastic thyroid carcinoma have not shown clear or durable responses.

KEY POINT

- Papillary thyroid cancer and follicular thyroid cancer are treated with total thyroidectomy followed generally by therapy with iodine-131.

Bibliography

Sherman SI, Angelos P, Ball DW, et al; National Comprehensive Cancer Network Thyroid Carcinoma Panel. Thyroid carcinoma. J Natl Compr Canc Netw. 2007;5(6):568-621. [PMID: 17623612]

Item 75   Answer: D

Educational Objective: Manage an elderly patient with prostate cancer and medical comorbidities.

Although screening by prostate-specific antigen (PSA) measurement does result in detection of some cases of cancer, no definitive benefits resulting from such detection have been reported. In this older patient, observation or watchful waiting is the most appropriate management.

According to the U.S. Preventive Services Task Force (USPSTF), there is inadequate evidence to suggest that treatment of patients younger than 75 years with screening-detected prostate cancer results in improved outcomes compared with treatment of patients with clinically detected prostate cancer. Adequate evidence indicates that the incremental benefits of treatment of patients 75 years of age or older with screening-detected prostate cancer are small to none. Moderate-to-substantial harms, including erectile dysfunction, urinary incontinence, bowel dysfunction, and death, in addition to small harms, including prostate biopsy-induced pain and discomfort and psychological effects of false-positive test results, are associated with prostate cancer screening. Because prostate cancer symptoms may not develop in many patients who receive treatment for screening-detected prostate cancer during their lifetime, consideration of these harms is important.

In view of the recommendations from the USPSTF and the evidence supporting those recommendations, repeating the PSA, bone scan, and transrectal prostate biopsy are all inappropriate choices for this 80-year-old man.

KEY POINT

- In men age 75 years or older, the U.S. Preventive Services Task Force found adequate evidence that the incremental benefits of treatment for prostate cancer detected by screening are small to none.

Bibliography

U.S. Preventive Services Task Force. Screening for prostate cancer: U.S. Preventive Services Task Force recommendation statement. Ann Intern Med. 2008;149(3):I85-I91. [PMID: 18678845]

Item 76   Answer: D

Educational Objective: Manage a patient with stage IA non–small cell lung cancer.

This patient has pathologic stage IA non–small cell lung cancer (NSCLC). It is designated "A" because the tumor is less than 3 cm. She should receive periodic physical examination and surveillance imaging. Lobectomy, the surgical removal of a single lobe, is the optimal procedure for patients with early-stage NSCLC. The 5-year survival in patients with pathologic stage I disease after a complete surgical resection is 55% to 70%. The rationale for surveillance following the initial treatment of NSCLC is to detect recurrent disease or a second primary lung tumor early enough to allow for an intervention to result in an improved long-term outcome, such as increased survival or heightened quality of life. Although there are no randomized trials of surveillance strategies in patients with NSCLC, intermittent radiographic follow-up is recommended.

Combined-modality treatment with chemotherapy and surgery or radiation therapy is recommended for patients with stage III disease. Although controversial, many experts recommend systemic chemotherapy and local radiation therapy, usually to the tumor, hilum, and ipsilateral mediastinal lymph nodes, for stage III disease to prevent local recurrence and improve survival. However, radiation therapy is not indicated for patients with stage I and II NSCLC but rather has resulted in a detrimental effect on survival in these patients; therefore, radiation therapy is not appropriate for this patient.

Multiple clinical trials of chemotherapy using contemporary platinum-based doublets and a meta-analysis have demonstrated a significant survival advantage for patients with stage II lung cancer and have noted a survival benefit for a subset of patients with stage IB NSCLC; however, the data from these studies do not support the use of adjuvant chemotherapy in patients with stage IA disease outside of a clinical trial. In fact, adjuvant cisplatin-based chemotherapy has been suggested to have a deleterious effect in patients with stage IA NSCLC.

The small-molecule epidermal growth factor receptor inhibitor erlotinib was initially developed for use as second-line therapy in patients with advanced disease who do not respond to a cytotoxic chemotherapy regimen. In this setting, erlotinib was shown to increase survival, with the magnitude of benefit similar to that of second-line chemotherapy. Although studies are underway, there are no data to support use of erlotinib in the adjuvant setting in the absence of a clinical trial, and it is not indicated in a patient with stage IA disease.

KEY POINT

- Resection alone, with periodic physical examination and surveillance imaging, is appropriate therapy for patients with stage IA non–small cell lung cancer.

Bibliography

Pisters KM, Evans WK, Azzoli CG, et al; Cancer Care Ontario; American Society of Clinical Oncology Adjuvant Chemotherapy and Adjuvant Radiation Therapy for Stages I-IIIA Resectable Non Small cell Lung Cancer Guideline. J Clin Oncol. 2007;25(34):5506-5518. [PMID: 17954710]

Item 77   Answer: A

Educational Objective: Treat stage II rectal cancer.

This patient has T3N0M0 stage II rectal cancer and is likely to benefit from a combined-modality approach. Stage II rectal cancer is treated with surgery and adjuvant chemoradiation therapy. Recurrence and death in stage II and III rectal cancer are decreased when radiation therapy is added to the recommended surgical and chemotherapy approaches. Preoperative chemoradiation with low anterior resection is becoming the treatment of choice to reduce the need for permanent colostomy, local recurrences, and long-term toxicity. However, in a randomized study comparing preoperative to postoperative chemoradiation, disease-free survival and overall survival were similar. Possible complications of radiation therapy include proctitis, intestinal obstruction, stricture, and fistula, often occurring long after treatment.

Radiation therapy as an adjunct to surgery for rectal cancer has been shown to reduce local recurrence but has not improved survival. Radiation therapy alone or chemotherapy alone is inadequate treatment of stage 2 rectal carcinoma.

KEY POINT

- **Surgery and adjuvant combined chemotherapy and radiation therapy is the standard treatment for patients with stage II and III rectal cancer.**

Bibliography

Bosset JF, Collette L, Calais G, et al; EORTC Radiotherapy Group Trial 22921. Chemotherapy with preoperative radiotherapy in rectal cancer [erratum in N Engl J Med. 2007;357(7):728]. N Engl J Med. 2006;355(11):1114-1123. [PMID: 16971718]

Item 78   Answer: D

Educational Objective: Diagnose Epstein-Barr virus–related nasopharyngeal cancer.

Nasopharyngeal cancer is squamous cell carcinoma (SCC) that occurs in the epithelial lining of the nasopharynx. Nasopharyngeal carcinoma occurs relatively rarely in most populations. However, it is one of the most common cancers in southern China, with age-adjusted incidence rates of up to 55 per 100,000. The most common clinical manifestations are headache and a neck mass. Because of the asymptomatic nature of the disease and the prolonged period between occurrence of initial symptoms and diagnosis, most patients present with advanced disease, including bone metastases with the potential for skull-base invasion and possible cranial nerve involvement. If the patient is found to have early-stage disease, she should be treated with radiotherapy. Surgery is generally not recommended owing to the technical difficulty of removing the tumor in this anatomic location. Whether radiotherapy combined with chemotherapy results in better patient outcomes remains under investigation.

Epstein-Barr virus (EBV) has been shown to be the primary pathologic cause of nasopharyngeal carcinoma. EBV is a transforming virus and has been causally linked to various malignancies, including Burkitt lymphoma, tumors in HIV-infected patients, Hodgkin lymphoma, nasopharyngeal and other head and neck carcinomas, and T-cell lymphoma.

The classic clinical presentation of Burkitt lymphoma includes a rapidly growing tumor mass and very high serum lactate dehydrogenase (LDH) and uric acid levels. Three different types of Burkitt lymphoma are usually described, including the endemic (African) form that typically presents with jaw or facial tumors; the sporadic type that usually presents in the abdomen; and immunodeficiency types that often involve the lymph nodes. The patient's ethnicity, normal LDH and uric acid concentration, and lack of history or evidence of immunosuppression make Burkitt lymphoma unlikely.

Hodgkin lymphoma can first develop in young adulthood and in patients middle-aged and older. The classic presentation is asymptomatic lymphadenopathy or a mediastinal mass on chest radiograph. Lymphadenopathy is most commonly found in the neck, followed by the axilla, and then the inguinal lymph nodes. Other clinical findings may include hepatomegaly (rare) and splenomegaly. This patient's ethnicity and tumor location make Hodgkin lymphoma an unlikely diagnosis.

Multiple myeloma is characterized by the neoplastic proliferation of a single clone of plasma cells producing a monoclonal immunoglobulin. In this disease, large masses composed of malignant plasma cells called *plasmacytomas* can grow in bones and soft tissues, but a diagnosis of multiple myeloma is unlikely in a patient with a normal blood count, calcium concentration, lactate dehydrogenase level, kidney function, and urinalysis.

KEY POINT

- **Epstein-Barr virus is believed to be the primary etiologic agent in the pathogenesis of nasopharyngeal carcinoma.**

Bibliography

Chien YC, Chen JY, Liu MY. Serologic markers of Epstein-Barr virus infection and nasopharyngeal carcinoma in Taiwanese men. N Engl J Med. 2001;345(26):1877-1882. [PMID: 11756578]

Item 79   Answer: D

Educational Objective: Treat a patient with ductal carcinoma in situ of the breast.

The incidence of pure ductal carcinoma in situ (DCIS) has been increasing, most certainly as a result of widespread screening interventions. Local therapy is appropriate for patients with DCIS, consisting of mastectomy, or, preferably, wide-excision resection and radiation therapy, but not chemotherapy. Patients with DCIS are at increased risk for new or locally recurrent breast cancer in the contralateral or ipsilateral breast. In patients with estrogen receptor–positive tumors, tamoxifen, in addition to lumpectomy, seems to decrease the risk of a new breast cancer event. In the National Surgical Adjuvant Breast and Bowel Project (NSABP) B-24 trial, 1804 women with DCIS were randomized to take tamoxifen or placebo for 5 years after a lumpectomy and radiation therapy. Women in the tamoxifen group had fewer breast cancer events at 5 years than those taking placebo (8.2% vs. 13.4%).

Adjuvant chemotherapy offers no proven benefit in patients with DCIS. Raloxifene is appropriate only for primary prevention of breast cancer in postmenopausal women and, furthermore, is not used to treat DCIS. Megestrol acetate would be appropriate as a second- or third-line hormonal therapy for DCIS but is not used as preventive therapy.

KEY POINT

- **Tamoxifen is indicated for patients with ductal carcinoma in situ after lumpectomy and radiation therapy to reduce the risk for local recurrences and second primary breast cancer.**

Bibliography

Burstein HJ, Polyak K, Wong JS, Lester SC, Kaelin CM. Ductal carcinoma in situ of the breast. N Engl J Med. 2004;350(14):1430-1441. [PMID: 15070793]

Item 80   Answer: B
Educational Objective: Diagnose nonseminoma.

This patient's ultrasound is suggestive of a neoplasm (nonseminomatous testicular germ cell tumor) based on the elevated serum α-fetoprotein (AFP) level. When the consideration of cancer first arises, serum tumor markers including AFP and the β subunit of human chorionic gonadotropin (β-hCG) should be measured. Although β-hCG concentrations may be elevated in patients with seminomatous or nonseminomatous tumors, AFP is increased only in patients with nonseminomatous tumors. Scrotal ultrasound can distinguish intrinsic from extrinsic testicular lesions and solid from cystic lesions. Although this patient's surgical biopsy specimens may show seminomatous components, patients with a pure seminoma do not have an elevated serum AFP level. Germ cell malignancies (seminomas and nonseminomas) are the most common solid tumors in young men between the ages of 15 and 34 years and are highly curable. Radical orchiectomy is required for definitive histologic staging and treatment, followed by additional staging studies such as a CT scan of the abdomen and pelvis and radiograph of the chest.

Neisseria gonorrhoeae epididymitis most often is accompanied by pain and penile discharge, which this patient does not have, and would not cause the elevated serum tumor markers or ultrasonographic findings noted in this patient. Testicular torsion presents with acute, severe pain and occasionally nausea and vomiting, and the affected testicle is often elevated and horizontally oriented. Testicular torsion would also not cause the laboratory and ultrasonographic abnormalities noted in this patient.

KEY POINT

- **An elevated serum α-fetoprotein level is indicative of a nonseminoma; seminomas are associated with a normal α-fetoprotein level.**

Bibliography

Kuczyk M, Bokemeyer C, Hartmann JT. Advances in our understanding of the biology, new diagnostic approaches and recent treatment strategies for testicular germ cell cancer. World J Urol. 2004;22(1):1. [PMID: 15057561]

Item 81   Answer: B
Educational Objective: Manage a patient with limited-stage, small cell lung cancer.

This patient should undergo prophylactic cranial irradiation. Brain metastases are diagnosed in 10% to 14% of patients with small cell lung cancer (SCLC) at presentation and more than 50% of SCLC patients during the course of their illness. The brain is a frequent site of first relapse in patients after complete therapeutic response. Prophylactic cranial irradiation should therefore be considered for patients with SCLC who have a response to initial chemotherapy. A meta-analysis of the use of prophylactic cranial irradiation based on randomized clinical trials largely applied to patients with limited-stage SCLC has demonstrated not only a reduction in central nervous system relapse but also an improvement in long-term survival by approximately 5%. Therefore, prophylactic cranial radiation in this patient is preferred to expectant observation.

Studies of maintenance therapy with topotecan or oral etoposide for patients who responded to first-line chemotherapy showed an improvement in progression-free survival but not in overall survival, apparently due to the emergence of chemotherapy resistance. By prolonging the duration of treatment, cumulative toxicities occur. Therefore, this patient should not be treated with maintenance chemotherapy with topotecan.

SCLC vaccination is not an effective therapy for SCLC. This was demonstrated in preliminary studies of BEC2, an anti-idiotypic antibody that mimics gangliosides expressed on SCLC tumors but not on normal cells. In these studies, the combination of BEC2 plus Bacillus Calmette-Guérin was able to induce anti-BEC2 and anti-GD3 antibodies and cause the death of SCLC cells; however, a phase III study in patients who received the vaccine after induction chemotherapy did not result in prolonged survival.

SCLC is considered a systemic disease; patients who present with seemingly localized disease almost always have concurrent micrometastases, and surgical therapy for cure is not an option. Surgery will not benefit this patient but only add increased morbidity.

- Prophylactic cranial irradiation reduces central nervous system relapse and improves survival in patients with limited-stage, small cell lung cancer.

Bibliography

Prophylactic Cranial Irradiation Overview Collaborative Group. Cranial irradiation for preventing brain metastases of small cell lung cancer in patients in complete remission. Cochrane Database Syst Rev. 2000;(4):CD002805. [PMID: 11034766]

Item 82   Answer: B

Educational Objective: Diagnose anthracycline-induced cardiomyopathy.

Anthracycline therapy with agents such as doxorubicin can cause progressive cardiomyopathy, which can occur acutely during treatment, within weeks to months following treatment, or years after treatment. This patient's physical examination findings indicating left ventricular failure demonstrated by a dilated left ventricle with a poor ejection fraction are most compatible with dilated cardiomyopathy. Several chemotherapeutic agents are known to cause myocardial necrosis and subsequent cardiomyopathy, including the anthracyclines (doxorubicin, daunorubicin, idarubicin, and epirubicin) and mitoxantrone. In the case of the anthracyclines, the toxicity is related to the cumulative dose.

Tamoxifen therapy is associated with thromboembolic complications, but only while the patient is receiving the therapy rather than 2 years following therapy, as in this patient. In addition, the patient's findings of dilated cardiomyopathy are not compatible with acute pulmonary embolism that may present with dyspnea but no specific findings or evidence of acute right-sided heart failure.

Radiation therapy can cause cardiac side effects; the most common manifestations are pericardial disease, coronary artery disease, cardiomyopathy, valvular dysfunction, and conduction abnormalities. Most cases of radiation-induced cardiac disease occur late in the course of the patient's disease, often 10 years or more following treatment, and occur more frequently with left-sided breast cancers than right, particularly if the internal mammary lymph nodes were not included in the radiation field. Therefore, radiation therapy to the right breast 2 years ago is less likely than doxorubicin to be the primary cause of this patient's dilated cardiomyopathy.

Cyclophosphamide has been associated with acute severe cardiotoxicity that appears to be dose-related and occurs most often as part of infusion therapy related to bone marrow transplantation preparative regimens. Pathologic findings in cyclophosphamide-induced cardiotoxicity include transmural hemorrhage and pericardial effusion and, occasionally, pericarditis. Late cardiac effects of cyclophosphamide are unknown.

- Anthracycline therapy is associated with an increased risk for cardiomyopathy.

Bibliography

Doyle JJ, Neugut AI, Jacobson JS, Grann VR, Hershman DL, et al. Chemotherapy and cardiotoxicity in older breast cancer patients: a population-based study. J Clin Oncol. 23(34):8597-8605. [PMID: 16314622]

Item 83   Answer: C

Educational Objective: Treat a patient with early-stage laryngeal cancer.

External-beam radiation is the most appropriate treatment for this patient who has stage II (T2) laryngeal cancer. Laryngeal cancer is often discovered at an earlier stage than other types of head and neck cancer, because hoarseness tends to occur relatively early in the course of the disease. Given the fundamental role that the larynx plays in human speech and communication, taking into consideration both survival and functional consequences of the treatment approach is crucial. The American Society of Clinical Oncology guideline recommends that all patients with T1 or T2 laryngeal cancer, with rare exception, should be treated initially with intent to preserve the larynx. One larynx-preservation option is external-beam radiation therapy, which provides good local control and survival rates in patients with small tumors. Voice-sparing surgery has a role in patients with small, T1 lesions.

The initiation of chemotherapy is not necessary in this patient because he has local, and potentially curable, disease. Initial therapy for such patients is radiation therapy or surgery. In contrast to the setting of lymph node–positive or locally advanced disease, the benefit of concurrent chemoradiotherapy or induction chemotherapy in patients with early-stage disease is not well-studied and not recommended.

The American Society of Clinical Oncology recommends that to ensure an optimum outcome with a laryngeal-sparing approach, a multidisciplinary team is necessary, and the patient should be fully informed about the advantages and disadvantages of larynx-preservation options compared with total laryngectomy. With the patient clearly indicating a preference for sparing his voice, proceeding with a laryngeal-sparing approach seems most appropriate after fully informing the patient of all the options.

Cetuximab is a monoclonal antibody that is directed against the epidermal growth factor receptor, which is over-expressed in most head and neck tumors. Cetuximab has been investigated in patients with advanced head and neck squamous cell carcinoma, and, when combined with radiation, it has been found to improve local control and overall survival rates. However, this patient has early-stage disease and could receive curative therapy with surgery or radiation alone.

- Larynx-preservation therapy such as external-beam radiation or voice-sparing surgery is curative and preferred over laryngectomy in patients with early-stage cancer of the larynx.

Bibliography

Pfister, DG, Laurie, SA, Weinstein, GS, et al; American Society of Clinical Oncology. American Society of Clinical Oncology clinical practice guideline for the use of larynx-preservation strategies in the treatment of laryngeal cancer. J Clin Oncol. 2006;24(22):3693-3704. [PMID: 16832122]

Item 84 Answer: B

Educational Objective: Treat recurrent large B-cell non-Hodgkin lymphoma.

Diffuse large B-cell lymphoma is the most common of the non-Hodgkin lymphomas, constituting 30% of newly diagnosed cases. Most patients with localized disease are curable with R-CHOP (rituximab plus CHOP [cyclophosphamide, doxorubicin, vincristine, and prednisone]) chemotherapy, with or without radiotherapy. R-CHOP is curative in more than half of patients with advanced-stage disease. Patients who have a relapse may still be cured by stem-cell transplantation consolidation after they respond to re-induction therapy with an aggressive combination-chemotherapy regimen. Because this patient is young and has no comorbidities, treatment should be of curative intent. His best chance for cure or long-term remission is ifosfamide, carboplatin, and etoposide with rituximab followed by high-dose chemotherapy with autologous hematopoietic stem cell rescue. The patient completed his first chemotherapy treatment 2 years ago and is likely to still have chemosensitive disease. The presence of chemosensitivity is important in predicting the efficacy of stem cell transplantation because patients with chemoresistant disease do not have good outcomes even with high-dose chemotherapy.

Doxorubicin can cause an irreversible, and sometimes fatal, cardiomyopathy, and the risk is directly related to the cumulative dose. This patient is close to exceeding his lifetime limit for doxorubicin. Only three or four more doses of this agent can be given before the risk of chronic heart failure becomes clinically significant. Therefore, re-treatment with cyclophosphamide, doxorubicin, vincristine, and prednisone with rituximab is not indicated.

Single-agent rituximab can induce a 30% to 40% response rate in patients with relapsed, diffuse, large B-cell lymphoma but is not curative.

Whole-body radiation therapy followed by stem cell transplantation would increase the risk for a secondary myelodysplastic syndrome and secondary acute myeloid leukemia and is therefore rarely used in this setting.

- Patients with recurrent, large B-cell non-Hodgkin lymphoma may be cured with aggressive combination chemotherapy followed by high-dose chemotherapy with autologous hematopoietic stem cell rescue.

Bibliography

Zelenetz AD, Advani RH, Buadi F, et al; National Comprehensive Cancer Network. Non-Hodgkin's lymphoma. Clinical practice guidelines in oncology. J Natl Compr Canc Netw. 2006;4(3):258-310. [PMID: 16507273]

Item 85 Answer: B

Educational Objective: Treat a patient with breast cancer and a small, focal tumor.

This patient should undergo breast-conserving therapy plus sentinel lymph node biopsy. Breast conserving-therapy consists of excision of the primary tumor followed by radiation to the remaining ipsilateral breast tissue. Breast-conserving therapy is generally indicated for patients with focal disease and small tumors for which conservation will offer a good cosmetic result. However, patient preferences must be considered in the surgical decision-making process. Randomized clinical trials have shown that the survival rate for women undergoing breast-conserving therapy is equivalent to that of those who undergo mastectomy, with breast-conserving therapy resulting in improved cosmetic outcomes and less morbidity than mastectomy. Most patients treated with lumpectomy without radiation therapy have a high risk for local recurrence. In addition, sentinel lymph node biopsy is a safe and accurate method for screening the axillary lymph nodes for metastases in women with small breast tumors.

Mastectomy would be indicated in patients who are not eligible for breast-conserving therapy because complete excision cannot be achieved unless mastectomy is performed, the tumor cannot be accessed by radiation, or radiation is contraindicated.

The two most highly effective breast cancer risk-reduction strategies have been prophylactic mastectomy and endocrinologic manipulation, but these interventions are not indicated for most women who do not have a high risk for breast cancer, such as those with BRCA1 or BRCA2 genetic abnormalities. There is no such indication for a prophylactic mastectomy of the right breast in this patient.

- Lumpectomy with sentinel lymph node biopsy followed by breast irradiation is the appropriate management of women with small, focal breast cancer.

Bibliography

Veronesi U, Paganelli G, Viale G, et al. A randomized comparison of sentinel-node biopsy with routine axillary dissection in breast cancer. N Engl J Med. 2003;349(6):546-553. [PMID: 12904519]

Item 86   Answer: C

Educational Objective: Diagnose spinal cord compression due to bone metastases.

This patient most likely has spinal cord compression due to bone metastases from recurrent prostate cancer. The three most common malignancies responsible for spinal cord compression are prostate, breast, and lung cancer. His history of prostate cancer with a Gleason score of 8 places him at high risk for recurrence. His signs and symptoms are consistent with spinal cord compression, and the elevated serum alkaline phosphatase level suggests bone metastases. The initial symptom in patients with epidural spinal cord compression due to tumor usually is spinal or radicular pain that may precede the onset of neurologic symptoms, which may include weakness, numbness, or sphincter disturbances. Spinal cord compression is an oncologic emergency, and MRI of the thoracolumbar spine is needed to confirm the diagnosis and assist in treatment planning. Clinicians should have a low threshold of suspicion for spinal cord compression in a patient with known cancer or a risk for recurrent cancer. The absence of neurologic findings should not alter that strategy. Patients whose cord compression is discovered after developing neurologic deficits are more likely to remain functionally impaired after intervention.

Radionuclide bone scanning is very sensitive for detecting bone metastases and has the advantage of visualizing the entire skeleton, but it has a high false-positive rate and provides no information about thecal sac compression. Because a bone scan cannot confirm a diagnosis of spinal cord compression, it is an inappropriate diagnostic test in this emergent setting.

The clinical feature of bilateral lower extremity weakness accompanied by hyperreflexia localizes the process to the spinal cord. An MRI of the brain would therefore be an inappropriate diagnostic test.

Plain radiographs are used to diagnose compression fractures of the thoracic spine. In a patient such as the one presented, major vertebral body collapse or pedicle erosion is approximately 80% predictive of spinal cord compression, but a false-negative result occurs in nearly 20% of patients with spinal cord compression. Therefore, plain radiography is not the best diagnostic test for this patient.

KEY POINT

- The triad of back pain, muscle weakness, and loss of bowel or bladder control is suggestive of spinal cord compression.

Bibliography

Loblaw DA, Perry J, Chambers A, Laperriere NJ. Systematic review of the diagnosis and management of malignant extradural spinal cord compression. J Clin Oncol. 2005;23(9):2028-2037. [PMID: 15774794]

Item 87   Answer: C

Educational Objective: Manage a patient with asymptomatic metastatic prostate cancer.

This patient has metastatic prostate cancer involving the bones. Because his initial Gleason score was 8 and serum prostate-specific antigen level was 20 ng/mL, he had a high risk for prostate cancer recurrence despite definitive treatment. However, his disease is most likely hormone sensitive at this time. Because he is asymptomatic, hormonal therapy with surgical castration or gonadotropin hormone–releasing hormone (GnRH) agonists such as leuprolide is the treatment of choice. GnRH therapy causes impotence, hot flushes, gynecomastia, and loss of libido, as does orchiectomy. Patients may experience tumor-flare reactions with the use of GnRH agonists, which initially cause an increase in luteinizing and follicle-stimulating hormones. These hormones lead to a transient increase in testosterone, which can exacerbate prostate cancer symptoms. The risk for tumor flare is diminished in patients with a lower volume of disease. This reaction can be prevented by a brief course of concomitant antiandrogen therapy with agents such as bicalutamide, nilutamide, or flutamide.

Although docetaxel-based chemotherapy has been shown to improve survival, this agent is generally indicated only for patients with hormone-refractory cancer. Several studies have demonstrated an improvement in overall survival with docetaxel-based chemotherapy in this setting. Median overall survival of patients with metastatic hormone-refractory prostate cancer is about 19 months. Hospice care is premature, as multiple sequential medical interventions are likely to improve this patient's overall and progression-free survival. Observation is inappropriate, because his disease is likely to progress without any intervention.

Samarium-153 is a radionuclide that is taken up by bone. It may be useful in treating prostate cancer with painful bone metastases but may cause bone marrow suppression and should be used only in patients whose cancer is no longer responsive to other therapies.

KEY POINT

- Surgical castration or gonadotropin hormone–releasing hormone (GnRH) agonists are first-line therapies for an asymptomatic patient with metastatic prostate cancer.

Bibliography

Ramirez ML, Keane TE, Evans CP. Managing prostate cancer: the role of hormone therapy. Can J Urol. 2007;14 Suppl 1:10-8. [PMID: 18163939]

Item 88 Answer: E

Educational Objective: Manage a patient concerned about her risk for ovarian cancer.

There is no evidence that any screening tests, including physical examination, CT imaging, transvaginal ultrasonography, or CA-125 measurement, are beneficial in women of average risk for ovarian cancer. Ovarian cancer screening is not recommended for patients at average risk because tests lack sensitivity and specificity, and no survival benefit from earlier diagnosis and therapy has been shown.

An increased risk of ovarian cancer is noted in women with a family history of multiple affected family members over several generations or a family history of ovarian cancer at an early age as well as in women with *BRCA1/BRCA2* genetic risk or the hereditary nonpolyposis colorectal cancer syndrome. Although data demonstrating survival benefit are lacking, the NIH consensus conference has recommended performing screening in those high-risk women with serum CA-125 measurement and transvaginal ultrasonography every 6 to 12 months, beginning at age 35 years or at least 10 years earlier than the age at which the youngest family member was diagnosed with ovarian cancer. Some oncologists would recommend bilateral oophorectomy in these women after child-bearing is completed.

Abdominal and pelvic CT imaging is not recommended for use in ovarian cancer screening, even in high-risk patients, because of the low yield and risk of additional radiation exposure.

KEY POINT

- Ovarian cancer screening is not recommended for patients at average risk because tests lack sensitivity and specificity, and no survival benefit from earlier diagnosis and therapy has been shown.

Bibliography

Walsh CS, Karlan BY. Contemporary progress in ovarian cancer screening. Curr Oncol Rep. 2007;9(6):485-493. [PMID: 17991357]

Item 89 Answer: C

Educational Objective: Treat metastatic renal cell carcinoma.

This patient has metastatic renal cell carcinoma, which is incurable. However, two new oral agents that delay disease progression (sunitinib and sorafenib) have recently been approved by the U.S. Food and Drug Administration. These drugs are small-molecule-receptor tyrosine kinase inhibitors that target differences between normal tissue and malignant cells by inhibiting vascular endothelial growth factor receptors, the most important growth factors involved in tumor angiogenesis, as well as other oncogenic signaling pathways. Sunitinib is one option for first-line therapy in patients with advanced metastatic renal cell

carcinoma. This agent has been shown to improve progression-free survival and is associated with a response rate of 31% compared with 5% for interferon alfa.

Another new intravenous agent, temsirolimus, has been approved for use in patients with metastatic renal cell carcinoma. This agent inhibits the mammalian target of rapamycin (mTOR).

Hospice care is indicated for patients with a terminal illness, poor performance status, and a prognosis of 6 months or less. Hospice care is not indicated in this patient because of his good performance status and reasonable expectation for survival of greater than 6 months with treatment despite his metastatic disease.

Until recently, biologic agents such as interferon alfa and interleukin-2 were the treatment of choice for renal cell carcinoma, but these drugs have many toxic effects and provide only minimal benefit. Interleukin-2 may result in a small complete remission rate in young patients but is associated with significant toxicity and lengthy hospitalization.

Trastuzumab is a monoclonal antibody directed at *HER2* and is used to treat patients with *HER2*-positive breast cancer.

Vinblastine chemotherapy has little activity in renal cell carcinoma, and there are far more effective therapies available.

KEY POINT

- Sunitinib and sorafenib are small-molecule tyrosine kinase inhibitors that improve progression-free survival in patients with metastatic renal cell carcinoma.

Bibliography

Motzer RJ, Basch E. Targeted drugs for metastatic renal cell carcinoma. Lancet. 2008;370(9605):2071-2073. [PMID: 18156012]

Item 90 Answer: C

Educational Objective: Manage cancer of the tongue.

Oral-cavity cancer is characterized by nonhealing, persistent ulcers, plaques, papules, or erosions. Because most cases of head and neck squamous cell carcinoma (approximately 80%) are attributed to alcohol and tobacco use, patients with a history of nonhealing, persistent ulcers and risk factors for oral cavity cancer should undergo fine-needle aspiration of suspicious lesions and endoscopic evaluation to rule out signs of metastatic disease. This patient's current symptoms combined with his oral ulcer history and alcohol and tobacco use are suspicious for oral cancer. For patients in whom malignancy is confirmed, appropriate imaging, including CT scan, should be performed. If there is no evidence of metastatic disease, then surgery is recommended for small, anterior, and well-lateralized lesions. Radiation therapy is preferred for large T1 lesions and for T2 tumors for which resection would result in impairment of normal speech and/or swallowing.

Treatment with clotrimazole is appropriate for patients with candidiasis. Candidiasis is a local infection of moist skin folds and mucosal surfaces (mouth and vagina) caused by *Candida* species. In adults, it is most often diagnosed in patients with diabetes or in those who have otherwise altered their skin and mucous membrane ecology with antibiotics or have been immunosuppressed with chemotherapy or radiation therapy. It also occurs in patients with diseases such as AIDS. Oral candidiasis is characterized by white or yellow patches on an erythematous base that bleeds if the patch is scraped off. This patient's presentation is not consistent with oral candidiasis, and therapy with clotrimazole is therefore not indicated.

Treatment with topical triamcinolone is appropriate for patients with aphthous ulcers. Aphthous ulcers are small, painful, shallow ulcers that are most commonly located on the buccal and labial mucous membranes and less commonly on the tongue and floor of the mouth. The onset of single or multiple ulcers can occur at anytime from childhood to maturity but is less common with aging. Most heal spontaneously within 1 to 2 weeks. The occurrence of a nonhealing ulcer of 4 weeks' duration in a older individual with risk factors for oral cancer should not be treated with triamcinolone or carefully observed; instead, it is imperative that immediate evaluation be done to rule out cancer of the tongue.

KEY POINT

• Persistent or nonhealing oral ulcers, particularly in the setting of smoking and/or alcohol use, may be suggestive of squamous cell carcinoma and require prompt biopsy.

Bibliography
Kademani D. Oral cancer [erratum in Mayo Clin Proc. 2007;82(8):1017]. Mayo Clin Proc. 2007;82(7):878-887. [PMID: 17605971]

Item 91   Answer: A

Educational Objective: Manage hypogammaglobulinemia in a patient with chronic lymphocytic leukemia.

Chronic lymphocytic leukemia (CLL) is the most common adult leukemia of the western world and is characterized by abnormal accumulation of morphologically mature–appearing lymphocytes with a characteristic immunophenotype (CD5+, CD20+, and CD23+ B cells) in the blood, bone marrow, or lymphatic tissues. Complications of pancytopenia, such as hemorrhage or infection, are a major cause of death. Immunologic aberrations peculiar to CLL include autoimmune hemolytic anemia, immune thrombocytopenia, and depressed immunoglobulin levels. Most of these patients (up to 70%) experience infectious complications, with up to 55% dying from infection.

Hypogammaglobulinemia is a treatable cause of immunodeficiency in patients with CLL, and treatment with intravenous immune globulin is indicated in this patient who has had two episodes of pulmonary infection requiring hospitalization during the previous 18 months. In patients with hypogammaglobulinemia, immunoglobulin is the treatment of choice to reduce both frequency and severity of bacterial infections. Treatment with high-dose intravenous immune globulin is associated with a decrease in the incidence of major bacterial infections. The impact on mortality is unproven.

Splenectomy may be considered in selected patients with CLL and persistent cytopenia due to hypersplenism or symptoms related to splenomegaly refractory to chemotherapy. However, there is no role for surgery in this patient with recurrent infection.

There is no clinical trial that demonstrates the efficacy of prophylactic antibiotics to prevent recurrent infection in patients with CLL. Because this patient's absolute neutrophil count is greater than 4000/µL (4×10^9/L) and the major immune deficiency appears to be hypogammaglobulinemia, treatment with intravenous immune globulin is more likely to reduce the incidence of recurrent infection than prophylactic antibiotics.

Given this patient's history of recurrent serious infection, immediate measures should be taken to address the CLL-associated hypogammaglobulinemia rather than to observe and perform repeat monitoring of the complete blood count.

KEY POINT

• Hypogammaglobulinemia is a treatable cause of recurrent, serious infection in patients with chronic lymphocytic leukemia, requiring treatment with intravenous immune globulin.

Bibliography
Zelenetz AD, Advani RH, Buadi F, et al; National Comprehensive Cancer Network. Non-Hodgkin's lymphoma. Clinical practice guidelines in oncology. J Natl Compr Canc Netw. 2006;4(3):258-310. [PMID: 16507273]

Item 92   Answer: D

Educational Objective: Treat early-stage, well-differentiated ovarian cancer.

Patients diagnosed with low-risk, early-stage ovarian cancer (stage I, grade 1 disease confined to one or both ovaries with an intact capsule and no ascites) after thorough surgical staging have a greater than 90% survival rate without postoperative chemotherapy. Randomized trials have not shown any benefit to using postoperative adjuvant chemotherapy in these patients, who should be followed with close observation and monitoring. Platinum-based therapy, such as intravenous carboplatin and paclitaxel, is therefore inappropriate for this patient but is the preferred platinum-containing doublet for patients with high-risk, early-stage ovarian cancer (stage IC or II, grade 3 tumor or clear cell histology). Intraperitoneal chemotherapy is associated with excellent survival results in patients with optimally debulked stage III disease, which this patient does not have. The use of platinum and paclitaxel has been shown to improve survival compared with other chemotherapy regimens. Non–platinum-based chemotherapy is inappropriate because all patients with ovarian cancer who require post-operative chemotherapy need a platinum-based regimen.

KEY POINT

- Patients diagnosed with stage I, grade 1 ovarian cancer after thorough staging have a greater than 90% survival rate without receiving postoperative chemotherapy.

Bibliography

Morgan RJ, Alvarez RD, Armstrong DK, et al; National Comprehensive Cancer Network. Ovarian Cancer. Clinical practice guidelines in oncology. J Natl Compr Canc Netw. 2006;4(9):912-939. [PMID: 17020669]

Item 93   Answer: C

Educational Objective: Manage axillary lymph node metastasis in a patient with occult primary breast cancer.

Although most cases of unilateral axillary lymphadenopathy in women are benign, when a malignancy does occur, it is most commonly breast cancer. Other tumors manifested by axillary lymph node metastasis include those of the lung, thyroid, head and neck, skin, and gastrointestinal tract. The primary site remains unknown in about 30% of patients. Patients with axillary lymphadenopathy, negative imaging studies, and positive findings on immunohistochemical analysis supportive of a diagnosis of occult breast cancer should receive treatment according to established guidelines for stage II breast cancer. Immunohistochemical staining results positive for carcinoembryonic antigen, CK-7, estrogen receptor (ER)/progesterone receptor (PR), mammaglobin, CA-125, and BRST2, and negative for CK-20 and TTF-1 may be suggestive of occult breast cancer. Although this patient's immunohistochemical staining results are ER/PR negative, this does not rule out breast cancer because ER/PR expression is negative in up to 30% of patients with breast cancer. In addition, less than 30% of breast adenocarcinomas are TTF-1 negative. Therefore, this patient should undergo axillary lymph node dissection and concurrent modified radical mastectomy.

Chest CT scan would be an appropriate diagnostic step if lung cancer remained high on the list of diagnostic possibilities following a negative chest radiograph and would also be useful in the staging of confirmed lung cancer. However, this patient has no risk factors for lung cancer, and the tumor's immunohistochemical staining results make lung cancer an unlikely possibility.

A thyroid ultrasonographic examination is useful in patients with suspicious thyroid nodules. An ultrasound showing a solid or mixed solid and cystic nodule is 95% sensitive for thyroid cancer, although the specificity is quite low (18%). Solid or mixed nodules would be further evaluated with fine-needle aspiration. Because this patient does not have any thyroid nodules on palpation and the immunohistochemical stain of the tumor is most supportive of breast cancer, a thyroid ultrasound examination is not indicated.

Aerodigestive panendoscopy, which consists of laryngoscopy, bronchoscopy, and esophagoscopy, as well as dedicated CT of the head and neck, should be performed as part of the diagnostic evaluation for patients with metastatic cancer to the cervical lymph nodes. Unilateral axillary lymphadenopathy would be an unusual location for metastatic cancer from the aerodigestive tract, but not impossible. However, the patient is at low risk for aerodigestive tract cancer, and the immunohistochemical stain supports the diagnosis of breast cancer.

KEY POINT

- Patients with axillary lymph node metastasis and no detectable primary tumor should be treated for stage II breast cancer.

Bibliography

Varadarajan R, Edge SB, Yu J, Watroba N, Janarthanan BR. Prognosis of occult breast carcinoma presenting as isolated axillary nodal metastasis. Oncology. 2006;71(5-6):456-459. [PMID: 17690561]

Item 94   Answer: B

Educational Objective: Understand the association between autoimmune diseases and non-Hodgkin lymphoma.

This patient has most likely has a lymphoma associated with Sjögren syndrome. The life-time risk of lymphoma in patients with Sjögren syndrome is approximately 5%, which is 40 to 44 times higher than that in the general population. The diagnosis of lymphoma occurs at a mean of approximately 7 years after the diagnosis of Sjögren syndrome. The patient's increasing lymphadenopathy suggests non-Hodgkin lymphoma, which is most often mucosa-associated lymphoid tissue (MALT) lymphoma and is generally low grade.

When patients present with a neck mass, excisional biopsy should be performed to determine histologic cell type. Diagnosis generally falls into one of three categories: 1) epithelial tumors, such as squamous cell carcinoma, adenocarcinoma, or anaplastic tumors; 2) lymphoma; or 3) melanoma. Because this patient has no risk factors for head and neck cancer and she has a long history of Sjögren syndrome, lymphoma is much more likely than squamous cell carcinoma.

This patient's Sjögren syndrome does not place her at increased risk for thyroid cancer, metastatic spread to preauricular lymph nodes would be distinctly unusual, and her thyroid examination is normal, making metastatic thyroid cancer much less likely than lymphoma.

Plasmacytomas are tumors composed of plasma cells identical to those seen in multiple myeloma. Plasmacytomas can occur in bone and soft tissue. Soft-tissue plasmacytomas are most often located in the head and neck region, including the parotid gland and lymph nodes. Plasmacytomas are relatively rare manifestations of multiple myeloma (3%) and are a less likely cause of this patient's lymphadenopathy than lymphoma.

Lymphadenitis would be unlikely in a patient without fever or tender lymph nodes.

KEY POINT

- Lymphoma is a well-known manifestation of Sjögren syndrome that usually presents later in the course of the disease.

Bibliography

Mellemkjaer L, Pfeiffer RM, Engels EA, et al. Autoimmune disease in individuals and close family members and susceptibility to non-Hodgkin's lymphoma. Arthritis Rheum. 2008;58(3):657-666. [PMID: 18311836]

Item 95   Answer: C

Educational Objective: Prevent tumor lysis syndrome.

Prior to the initiation of induction chemotherapy, this patient should receive vigorous intravenous hydration and allopurinol to prevent the tumor lysis syndrome. Tumor lysis syndrome is an oncologic emergency resulting from spontaneous or treatment-induced lysis of malignant cells. Tumor lysis syndrome is characterized by hyperkalemia, hyperuricemia, hyperphosphatemia, hypocalcemia, and acute renal failure. The onset of tumor lysis syndrome is within 1 to 5 days of induction chemotherapy. Patients at the highest risk are those with acute leukemia and high-grade lymphoma; the syndrome is less commonly associated with solid tumors. Risk factors for tumor lysis syndrome include a high leukocyte count, high pretreatment levels of lactate dehydrogenase or uric acid, compromised renal function, and the concomitant use of nephrotoxic agents.

The role of urinary alkalinization with sodium bicarbonate is controversial. There are no randomized clinical trials that support the use of sodium bicarbonate for prevention of tumor lysis syndrome. In addition, in patients with hyperphosphatemia, urine alkalinization has the potential to promote tissue deposition of calcium phosphate at the time of rapid cell death during chemotherapy. In 2008, an international expert panel recommended against the use of sodium bicarbonate in the prevention of tumor lysis syndrome except in patients who are acidemic. The panel could not reach consensus regarding the use of sodium bicarbonate in patients receiving allopurinol but concluded that alkalinization should be avoided in patients with hyperphosphatemia. This patient has mild hyperphosphatemia, and the best approach is to avoid urinary alkalinization.

The routine use of myeloid growth factors during induction chemotherapy for acute myeloid leukemia is not generally recommended. Growth factors are associated with a shortened duration of neutropenia, but clinical studies have documented variable effects on the incidence of severe infection, antibiotic use, and duration of hospitalization.

The Infectious Diseases Society of America does not recommend routine antibiotic prophylaxis for neutropenic patients based on evidence that it does not clearly confer a survival advantage; antibiotic side effects; and the potential for development of antibiotic resistance. Although certain circumstances may warrant antibiotic prophylaxis, the appropriate antibiotic in such cases should have broad activity against enteric bacteria. Because vancomycin does not provide protection against a broad array of enteric organisms, its use in this patient is inappropriate.

KEY POINT

- Vigorous intravenous hydration and allopurinol are indicated to prevent the tumor lysis syndrome in high-risk patients (those with acute leukemia and high-grade lymphoma).

Bibliography

Coiffier B, Altman A, Pui CH, Younes A, Cairo MS. Guidelines for the management of pediatric and adult tumor lysis syndrome: an evidence-based review. J Clin Oncol. 2008;26(16):2767-2778. [PMID: 18509186]

Item 96   Answer: C

Educational Objective: Evaluate the risk for endometrial cancer as a complication of adjuvant tamoxifen therapy.

Tamoxifen therapy is associated with an increased relative risk for endometrial cancer of 2.5, with risk increasing with longer periods of treatment. The risk extends beyond the time when tamoxifen is discontinued. A retrospective review of women taking tamoxifen therapy found that endometrial cancer was only present in women with symptoms such as vaginal bleeding or discharge. Ninety percent of patients with endometrial cancer will have an abnormal pink or brown vaginal discharge, and 80% of these patients will have abnormal bleeding, most often postmenopausal. The diagnosis is established with an endometrial biopsy. A low threshold for performing an endometrial biopsy should be used in patients with irregular vaginal bleeding who are over age 40, have postmenopausal bleeding or vaginal discharge, or are at high risk for endometrial cancer, including patients taking tamoxifen therapy. Patients in the perimenopausal stage of life should have periods that become lighter and spaced further apart. Any other perimenopausal pattern of bleeding should be evaluated. In the absence of clinical symptoms suggesting endometrial cancer, routine sampling of endometrial tissues has not been shown to be cost-effective.

Tamoxifen therapy is not associated with an increased risk for acute myeloid leukemia, ovarian cancer, or colon cancer.

KEY POINT

- **Tamoxifen use is associated with an increased risk for endometrial cancer.**

Bibliography

Swerdlow AJ, Jones ME; British Tamoxifen Second Cancer Study Group. Tamoxifen treatment for breast cancer and risk of endometrial cancer: A case-control study. J Natl Cancer Inst. 2005;97(5):375-384. [PMID: 15741574]

Item 97   Answer: E

Educational Objective: Diagnose tamoxifen-induced pulmonary embolism.

This patient's vital signs and shortness of breath, chest pain, and hypoxemia after a long flight are suggestive of a pulmonary embolism. Furthermore, patients who take tamoxifen, especially those who are also receiving chemotherapy, have an increased risk for thromboembolic disease. This risk is two to three times higher in older women who take tamoxifen.

An uncommon side effect of cyclophosphamide is interstitial pneumonitis, which can be fatal. This reaction is most commonly reported in patients receiving low doses of cyclophosphamide for prolonged durations, and the onset is usually insidious. Interstitial pulmonary fibrosis has been reported in patients receiving high-dose cyclophosphamide over a prolonged period. Alkylating metabolites and acrolein may be responsible for cyclophosphamide pulmonary toxicity. The patient's short course of cyclophosphamide, abrupt onset of symptoms, and normal pulmonary examination and chest radiograph make this reaction unlikely. Cyclophosphamide has been associated with severe cardiotoxicity characterized by acute heart failure, which can be intractable and fatal within a few days' time. Acute cardiac toxicity has been restricted to patients receiving large doses over relatively short durations as part of preparative regimens for bone marrow transplantation.

Cardiomyopathy is a well-recognized acute and chronic side-effect of doxorubicin, but this would not explain the patient's pleuritic chest pain, clear lungs, abnormal alveolar-arterial oxygen gradient, and normal chest radiograph.

The use of radiation therapy has improved the survival of patients with early-stage breast cancer. Modern radiotherapy techniques have reduced, but not eliminated, the risk for thoracic radiation–related complications, which may include pericarditis, coronary artery disease, and valvular heart disease. However, most complications are delayed, usually occurring 10 years or more after therapy.

Therefore, a radiation-related complication seems unlikely in this patient.

Surgery within 3 months of the index event is a well-recognized risk factor for venous thromboembolic disease, but breast-conserving surgery 1 year ago is unlikely to be related to this current episode of probable pulmonary embolism.

KEY POINT

- **The risk for thromboembolic disease is increased in patients taking tamoxifen, particularly in the setting of chemotherapy.**

Bibliography

Duggan C, Marriott K, Edwards R, Cuzick J. Inherited and acquired risk factors for venous thromboembolic disease among women taking tamoxifen to prevent breast cancer. J Clin Oncol. 2003;21(19): 3588-3593. [PMID: 14512389]

Item 98   Answer: B

Educational Objective: Diagnose bladder cancer.

This patient most likely has bladder cancer, which is associated with smoking and advancing age. The diagnosis is often delayed because symptoms may occur intermittently and are similar to those caused by less serious disorders such as urinary tract infections, prostatitis, and renal calculi. Cystoscopy and biopsy are required for diagnosis.

Isolated genitourinary bleeding would be unusual in a patient with a primary hemostasis disorder. Therefore, coagulation studies are not needed. Even if a bleeding disposition were discovered, the patient would still require cystoscopic evaluation to rule out bladder neoplasia.

The absence of pyuria and the negative leukocyte esterase make a urinary tract infection unlikely. Urine culture results are likely to be negative, and therapy with an alternative antibiotic would not be helpful. Because ciprofloxacin has antimicrobial activity against most urinary tract pathogens, failure of this patient's symptoms to resolve after an initial course indicates that he is unlikely to have an infection. A second course of a different antibiotic is therefore not indicated. A urine culture is inappropriate because an infection is unlikely in this patient. In addition, this patient has already received an antibiotic, which will interfere with culture results. Finally, it is important to recall that infections can occur in the presence of bladder cancer, and the presence of a urinary tract infection in an adult at risk for bladder cancer does not rule out the diagnosis of bladder cancer; such patients require careful follow-up monitoring.

KEY POINT

- **Symptoms of bladder cancer may mimic those of more benign disorders, such as urinary tract infection; diagnosis is established by cystoscopy and biopsy.**

Bibliography

Barocas DA, Clark PE. Bladder cancer. Curr Opin Oncol. 2008;20(3): 307-314. [PMID: 18391631]

Item 99   Answer: C
Educational Objective: Diagnose bisphosphonate-induced osteonecrosis of the jaw in a patient with breast cancer.

The figure shows exposure of a portion of the bone of the left mandible near a tooth extraction socket. Osteonecrosis of the jaw is an increasingly reported complication occurring most commonly in cancer patients taking bisphosphonates, particularly intravenous ones such as zoledronic acid. The use of corticosteroids such as dexamethasone increases this risk. This complication is most commonly reported following a dental procedure. Other risk factors are older age and longer follow-up time to presentation.

Preventive measures include informing patients about avoidance of dental procedures during administration of bisphosphonate therapy in addition to educating them about the risks for this side-effect. Eradicating dental problems prior to bisphosphonate administration and careful monitoring of patients for this condition during bisphosphonate therapy are important. Treatment of osteonecrosis of the jaw should be preceded by a discussion of the benefits versus harms of discontinuing bisphosphonates. Therapeutic options include limited débridement, antibiotic therapy, topical mouth rinses, hyperbaric oxygen therapy, and, for refractory cases, surgical resection of necrotic bone.

This patient has had no recent trauma to suggest temporomandibular joint dislocation. In addition, patients with dislocated jaws are unable to close the mouth and present with excess saliva, neither of which is present in this patient. Patients who take letrozole do report musculoskeletal symptoms; however, letrozole-induced bone pain is usually characterized as joint pain or stiffness and cannot explain the oral findings in this patient.

Breast cancer metastatic to the jaw occurs rarely, and this patient's recent bone scan revealed stable metastatic disease without changes over the past 6 months, which would make such a diagnosis unlikely.

KEY POINT

- Osteonecrosis of the jaw is an increasingly reported complication in cancer patients who take bisphosphonates, particularly with intravenous agents such as zoledronic acid.

Bibliography

Woo SB, Hellstein JW, Kalmar JR. Systematic review: bisphosphonates and osteonecrosis of the jaws [erratum in Ann Intern Med. 2006;145(3):235]. Ann Intern Med. 2006;144(10):753-761. [PMID 16702591]

Item 100   Answer: B
Educational Objective: Manage recurrent ovarian cancer.

Patients who were treated for ovarian cancer with a platinum-based regimen and who maintain a platinum-free interval (the time from the completion of primary platinum-based treatment to the time of recurrence) of more than 6 months are considered to have platinum-sensitive disease. Platinum-resistant patients who are re-challenged with platinum have a response rate of less than 20%, whereas the response rate for platinum-sensitive patients is 25% to 69%. Response rates to repeat administration of platinum increase with increasing platinum-free intervals. Administering a second course of chemotherapy with a platinum-based regimen is therefore preferable for this patient in the absence of contraindications. Although she has residual neuropathy, many platinum-containing doublets are available that have tolerable degrees of neurotoxicity.

Non–platinum-containing regimens are not indicated for a patient with known platinum-sensitive disease because they will be less effective. In a randomized study of paclitaxel against cyclophosphamide, doxorubicin, and cisplatin in patients with platinum-sensitive ovarian cancer, a significant improvement in disease-free and overall survival was observed in the cisplatin arm.

Radiation therapy to the pelvis and abdomen would cause excessive toxicity.

Tumor debulking surgery may be appropriate for patients with an isolated site of disease and a long disease-free interval. Patients who appear to benefit the most have undergone optimal cytoreduction at primary surgery, achieved a complete response to front-line chemotherapy, have a prolonged disease-free interval (>12 months), and have an isolated site of recurrence; however, this patient has diffuse studding of recurrent cancer rather than large masses and is therefore less likely to benefit from attempted resection.

KEY POINT

- Platinum-based chemotherapy is the treatment of choice for patients with recurrence of platinum-sensitive ovarian cancer and who relapse more than 6 months after completion of initial therapy.

Bibliography

Bukowski RM, Ozols RF, Markman M. The management of recurrent ovarian cancer. Semin Oncol. 2007;34(2 Suppl 2):S1-15. [PMID: 17512352]

Index

Target cells, in thalassemia, 26, 27f
T-cell lymphoma, 95f, 96. *See also* Lymphoma
Temsirolimus, in renal cancer, 94
Testicular cancer, 90–92, Q63, Q80
  lymphadenopathy in, 105
Testis, undescended, cancer and, 91
Thalassemia, 26–27, Q24
  hemolytic anemia in, 23–24
Thalidomide, for multiple myeloma, 14
Therapeutic apheresis, 35
  platelet, for essential thrombocythemia, 4
Thrombin, 36–37, 36f, 37f
Thrombocythemia, essential, 4–5, Q21
Thrombocytopenia, 39t, 40–42, 41t, 42f
  causes of, 45
  heparin-induced, 41t, 43–44, Q42
  immune, in chronic lymphocytic leukemia, 102
  in pregnancy, 57
  in thrombotic thrombocytopenic purpura, 44–45
Thrombocytopenic purpura, thrombotic, 24, 44–45
  in pregnancy, 58
Thrombolytics, 50
Thrombophilia, 47–53
  congenital, 47–49
  diagnosis of, 49–50
  in pregnancy, 58–60, 58t
Thrombopoietin, 9, 10
  recombinant, for immune thrombocytopenic purpura, 43
Thrombopoietin receptor agonists, 10
Thrombosis/thromboembolism, 47–55
  acute chest syndrome and, 28t
  in antiphospholipid syndrome, 49–50, 49t
  in antithrombin deficiency, 48, 50
  in cancer, 54
  deep venous, 53–54, Q9, Q47
  in disseminated intravascular coagulation, 38–40
  in essential thrombocythemia, 4–5
  Factor V Leiden and, 47
  genetic factors in, 47
  in heparin-induced thrombocytopenia, 44
  management of, 53–54, 55t, Q9, Q22, Q26, Q47
  pathophysiology of, 47–49. *See also* Thrombophilia
  in polycythemia vera, 5
  postphlebitic syndrome and, 54
  in pregnancy, 58–60, 58t, 59f
  prevention of, 50–53, Q14, Q20
  in protein C deficiency, 49–50
  in protein S deficiency, 49–50
  pulmonary embolism and, 53–54
  risk factors for, 48t
  venous, 53–54
Thrombotic microangiopathies, 44–45
Thrombotic thrombocytopenic purpura, 24, 44–45, Q23
  in pregnancy, 58
Thyroid cancer, 86–88, 87t, Q74
Total iron-binding capacity, in iron-deficiency anemia, 18
Total joint arthroplasty, anticoagulation for, 52
Transfusion(s), 32–35
  acute lung injury and, 33–34, Q7
  allergic reactions to, 34
  alloimmunization in, 32, 35
  alternatives to, 35
  blood group compatibility in, 32

blood products for, 33
circulatory overload and, 34
complications of, 33–34
cryoprecipitate, 33
for disseminated intravascular coagulation, 40
erythrocyte, 32, 33
  alloimmunization in, 32, 35
  iron overload from, 29, 30
  for myelofibrosis, 6
  for sickle cell disease, 29, 56
fever and, 34
graft-versus-host disease and, 34
hemolytic reactions in, 32, 33, Q39
indications for, 33
iron overload from, 29, 30
leukoreduction in, 33
in liver disease, 38
massive, 34
for myelodysplastic syndromes, 3
plasma, 33
platelet, 32, 33, Q31
posttransplant, Q51
safety precautions for, 32
sepsis and, 34
for sickle cell disease, 29
  in pregnancy, 56
for thalassemia, 27
for thrombotic thrombocytopenic purpura, 45
for warm antibody hemolytic anemia, 32
Transplantation
  bone marrow, 10–11
  renal, erythrocytosis after, 31
  stem cell. *See* Stem cell transplant
Trastuzumab, for breast cancer, 66
Tumor lysis syndrome, 107, Q95
Tyrosine kinase inhibitors, for chronic myeloid leukemia, 6

Ultrasonography, in venous thromboembolism, 54
Uremia. *See also* Renal disease
  peripheral blood smear in, 23, 23f
  platelet dysfunction in, 46

Vascular endothelial growth factor, in renal cancer, 94
Vasoocclusive crisis, in sickle cell disease, 27
Venous thrombosis. *See* Thrombosis/thromboembolism
Viral infections, cancer and, 61
Vitamin B$_{12}$ deficiency, 19–21, 20, 21f, Q38
Vitamin K deficiency, coagulopathy and, 38, 39t, Q37
von Hippel-Lindau disease, cancer in, 94
von Willebrand disease, 38, 39t, 46, Q5
Vorinostat, for mycosis fungoides, 101

Waldenström macroglobulinemia, 16
Warfarin, 51–53. *See also* Anticoagulants
  dosage of, 51–52
  indications for, 51–52
  INR for, 52
  perioperative management of, 52–53
  in pregnancy, 59
  for venous thromboembolism, 54, 55t
Warm antibody hemolytic anemia, 24, 25f, 25t
  transfusion for, 32
Wells criteria, for venous thrombosis, 54